the Unofficial Guide™ to Dieting Safely

Janis Jibrin, M.S., R.D.

Macmillan • USA

Macmillan General Reference
A Simon & Schuster Macmillan Company
1633 Broadway
New York, New York 10019-6785

ISBN: 0-02-862521-8

Manufactured in the United States of America

10 9 8 7 6 5 4 3 2 1

First edition

For my father, a natural cook who can cut back on fat and still make it taste good. And for my grandmother, Elaine Richmond, who practiced "all things in moderation" for 98 years.

Acknowledgments

Thanks to my editor, Nancy Gratton, for her skill and encouragement; to Adrian Brown, MD, for her insights that went into the eating disorders chapter; and to Kelly Brownell, Ph.D., for his generous loan of the Weight Loss Readiness Test.

Contents

The *Unofficial Guide* Reader's Bill of Rights..............xiii

The *Unofficial Guide* Panel of Experts xvii

Introduction..xix

I Getting Started.....................................1

1 Healthy Weight, Unhealthy Approaches.......3
Weight Debate...4
What's Too Fat? 5
  Body Mass Index *5*
  Percent Body Fat....................................*9*
Healthy Weight 12
  Apple-Shaped and Pear-Shaped *13*
  Shed Pounds, Drop Risk..........................*14*
Is Diet Just a Four-Letter Word? 20
Dieting's Legacy: Weight Loss Myths............22
  Deprivation Myth *22*
  The Thin Myth.......................................*23*
  Repeated Diet Failure Myth......................*24*
  The Genes Myth *24*
  The Gluttony Myth *24*
The Dirty Side of Dieting 25
Do You Need to Lose Weight?......................28
Just the Facts..30

2 Getting Organized...................................31
Ready . . . or Not?......................................32
Ready? . . . Set . . . Test! 35
Why Change? 44
Timing..45

Setting Goals...............................46
Analyze......................................47
Pick an Area to Work On 48
Set Non-Weight Goals 49
How to Set a Realistic Weight Goal.............51
Evaluating Your Options 52
Psychological Support........................56
Rallying the Troops..........................57
Just the Facts..............................60

II Nutrition You Should Know.............61

3 How Do You Get Fat? 63
The Calorie Curse...........................64
What the Heck Is a Calorie?..............64
Storing Calories 65
Burn, Baby, Burn 66
Lean Body Mass............................68
Did Your Genes Make You Do It? 69
How Big a Role Do Genes Play?..............69
A Peek into the Fat Factory 71
Can You Fight Your Set Point? 75
What Big Macs and Sitting on
Your Bum Gotta Do with It 76
Pima Predicament...........................77
Devious Diet Culprits 78
The Slide into Sedentary 79
Booze and Cigarettes.......................80
Outwitting Your Genes 82
Just the Facts..............................83

4 Nutrition Basics to Keep You
Basically Healthy.........................85
What's in that Pizza? 85
Carbohydrate Complex.......................86
Protein Overload...........................88
Fat Flap 89
Food Labels Cut Through the Hype.............92

The Pyramid: Substance versus
Sensationalism..96
   The USDA's Pyramid.................................97
   Keeping the Pyramid Low Cal...................99
The "Other" Pyramids 101
   A Pyramid Vegetarians Can Call Their Own 101
   Mediterranean Eating............................104
Just the Facts 106

5 Vital Nutrients 107
Why Supplement? 108
Buying a Decent Supplement......................109
Getting the Most from Your Multi...............115
   Housebreaking Your Supplement 115
   Special Cases.......................................116
Phyto-What? 118
Vitamins and Minerals at a Glance..............119
Just the Facts 120

III Weighing the Options......................127

6 Getting Good Help...............................129
Consulting a Nutritionist...........................130
   Who's Legit?..131
   What to Expect from a Good Nutritionist ..133
"Chain" Weight Loss Programs 134
Shopper's Guide to Weight Loss Programs 135
The Three Biggies 137
   Weight Watchers 141
   Jenny Craig...143
   Nutri/System® and L.A.
     Weight Loss Centers...........................145
Four Stellar Programs 147
   The LEARN® Program for Weight Control ..148
   The Solution..150
   Choose to Lose Weight Loss/
     Healthy Eating Program.....................151
   The Program for Reversing Heart Disease ..152

Medically Supervised Very
Low-Calorie Programs 155

Non-Profit Support Groups 157
   TOPS (Take Off Pounds Sensibly)..............*158*
   Overeaters Anonymous (OA)...................*158*

Residential Weight Loss Programs..............159
   Duke Diet and Fitness Center,
      Durham, North Carolina....................*159*
   Structure House, Durham, North Carolina..*160*
   Green Mountain at Fox Chase *161*
   Spas *162*

Surgery 163
   Gastric Surgery....................................*163*
   Liposuction *168*

Just the Facts 169

7 Diets that Deliver, Diets that Deceive......171

Evaluating Diets 173

What's Out There 176
   Healthy Diets *176*
   Meals Out of the Blender......................*181*
   Out of the Scientific Mainstream.............*183*

Some Useful "Not-Entirely-Diet" Books........194

Why Do We Believe the Bad Ones? 197

Just the Facts 199

8 Diet Drugs, Weight Loss Supplements,
and Scams...201

Diet Drugs 201
   The Caveats.......................................*204*
   Here's What's Up, Doc *206*
   What We're Taking...............................*207*
   Over-the-Counter Diet Drugs *208*
   Future Drugs *209*

Fringe Fat Fighters...................................213

Ergogenic Aids 223

Outrageous Scams....................................226

Exercise Equipment..................................228

Quack Watch 232

Just the Facts 235

IV Eating Habits Rx 237

9 The Weight Loss Head Trip 239

Watch Your Attitude 240
  Take Care of Yourself 241
  Take Responsibility 242
  Do It for Yourself 242
  Be Realistic 243
  See Failures as Learning Experiences 244
  Rethink Deprivation 244
  See Shades of Gray 245
  Accept Less-than-Skinny 246
  Enjoy Yourself 248

Habits of Highly Effective Weight Losers 249
  Graze Responsibly or Don't Graze at All 249
  Eat Aware 251
  Curb Cravings 255
  Diffuse Emotional Eating 258
  Slow It Down 260
  Home in on Hunger 261
  Derail Deprivation 264

Eating Out 264
  Civilized Social Eating 264
  Assert Your Restaurant Rights 266

Support System 268

Just the Facts 272

10 What to Eat 273

Pinpointing the Problem 275
  The Food Record 275
  Do It Slowly and Permanently 280

Eating More of the Good Stuff 282
  Turn Up the Vegetable Volume 282
  Figuring in Fruit 284
  Gaining Grains 286
  Controlling "Healthy" Carbs 287
  How Much Water Should You Drink? 288

Eating Less of the Bad Stuff 290
  Putting the Microscope on Fat 290
  Slimmer Snacks 292
  How Sweet It Still Can Be 293
  Is Sugar Bad for You? 293
  Greaseball Cures 295

How Critical Are Calories? 299

Cooking Light..303
   Get It Right from the Start *304*
   Give Your Cooking a Makeover.................*305*

Fat and Sugar Substitutes 307
   Fat Replacers......................................*307*
   Sugar Substitutes................................*310*
   Are Sugar and Fat Substitutes Worth It? ..*312*

Just the Facts 315

11 Staying Psyched.................................317

The Exercise Advantage 318

How Much Do You Need?............................319

Best Maintenance Diet...............................320

What Helps You Stay the Course? 324

Diet Drugs 333

Outmaneuvering Saboteurs........................333
   Stress and Negative Emotions..................*334*
   Sabotaging Spouses..............................*334*

Just the Facts 337

**12 Eating Disorders Aren't Just for
Skinny People 339**

When Do Your Food Habits
Become a "Disorder"?...............................340

That Binge High 344

Binge-Eating Disorder................................345
   Official Definition.................................*345*
   What It Does to You *348*

Bulimia Nervosa (Bulimia)..........................348
   Official Definition.................................*348*
   What It Does to You *350*

Anorexia Nervosa (Anorexia)......................351
   Official Definition.................................*352*
   What It Does to You *353*

Getting Help 354
   The Basics *355*
   Finding Treatment................................*359*
   *Binge-Eating Disorder
      Treatment Specifics*...........................*361*
   Bulimia Treatment Specifics *362*

Anorexia Treatment Specifics 363
Hospitalization for Anorexia 365
Medication 365

What Causes Eating Disorders? 366
The Impossible Ideal 366
Psychological Links 368
Who Gets Eating Disorders? 370
Did Your Diet Make You Do It? 371

Just the Facts 374

V Get Moving 375

13 You've Got to Keep Moving 377

Outside Beauty 378
Exercise and Weight Loss 379
Exercise and Weight Maintenance 382
Exercise Combats Age-Related Muscle Loss 383

Inner Beauty 385

Improved Mood 393

Eating for Exercise 395
Nutritional Nuances for the Exerciser 395
Vitamin Requirements that
    Increase with Exercise 400

Where to Begin 401
Meet Your Exercise Match 403
Incidental Exercise 405
Safety Screening 405

Just the Facts 408

14 Getting Physical 409

Getting Started 410
How Much Is Enough? 411
Mapping Out Your Strategy 412
Staying Motivated 413

Aerobic Exercise 416
Walking Works 420
Happy Hiking 422
Running/Jogging 422
Swimming 423
Classes 424
Aerobic Exercise Machines 430

Strength Training 432

Your Body "Weight"...............................*433*
Stretching and Flexibility.......................*436*

Exercise Safety..*436*
Stay Hydrated......................................*436*
Warm-Up *437*
Cool-Down..*437*

Exercising Good Sense with Your Dollars......*438*
Evaluating Instructors............................*438*
Hiring a Personal Trainer *439*
Don't Get Gypped by a Gym....................*440*
Before You Sign Up...............................*441*
Do Your Homework on Home
Exercise Equipment...........................*443*

Just the Facts *444*

A Recommended Reading List.......................**445**

B Resources..**451**

C Menus for You..**463**

D Fast-Food Fat and Calorie Counts **473**

E Brand Name Calorie, Fat, and Fiber Counts......**483**

F Blank Food Records for You to Use **499**

Index **509**

The *Unofficial Guide* Reader's Bill of Rights

We Give You More Than the Official Line

Welcome to the *Unofficial Guide* series of Lifestyles titles—books that deliver critical, unbiased information that other books can't or won't reveal—*the inside scoop*. Our goal is to provide you with the *most accessible, useful* information and advice possible. The recommendations we offer in these pages are not influenced by the corporate line of any organization or industry; we give you the hard facts, whether those institutions like them or not. If something is ill-advised or will cause a loss of time and/or money, we'll give you ample warning. And if it is a worthwhile option, we'll let you know that, too.

Armed and Ready

Our hand-picked authors confidently and critically report on a wide range of topics that matter to smart readers like you. Our authors are passionate about their subjects, but have distanced themselves enough from them to help you be armed and protected and help you make educated decisions as you go through your process. It is our intent that, from having read this book, you will avoid the pitfalls everyone else falls into and get it right the first time.

Don't be fooled by cheap imitations; this is the genuine article *Unofficial Guide* series from Macmillan Publishing. You may be familiar with our proven track record of the travel *Unofficial Guides,* which have more than three million copies in print. Each year thousands of travelers—new and old—are armed with a brand new, fully updated edition of the flagship *Unofficial Guide to Walt Disney World,* by Bob Sehlinger. It is our intention here to provide you with the same level of objective authority that Mr. Sehlinger does in his brainchild.

The Unofficial Panel of Experts

Every work in the Lifestyle *Unofficial Guides* is intensively inspected by a team of three top professionals in their fields. These experts review the manuscript for factual accuracy, comprehensiveness, and an insider's determination as to whether the manuscript fulfills the credo in this Reader's Bill of Rights. In other words, our Panel ensures that you are, in fact, getting "the inside scoop."

Our Pledge

The authors, the editorial staff, and the Unofficial Panel of Experts assembled for *Unofficial Guides* are determined to lay out the most valuable alternatives available for our readers. This dictum means that our writers must be explicit, prescriptive, and, above all, direct. We strive to be thorough and complete, but our goal is not necessarily to have the "most" or "all" of the information on a topic; this is not, after all, an encyclopedia. Our objective is to help you narrow down your options to the best of what is available, unbiased by affiliation with any industry or organization.

In each *Unofficial Guide* we give you:

- Comprehensive coverage of necessary and vital information
- Authoritative, rigidly fact-checked data
- The most up-to-date insights into trends
- Savvy, sophisticated writing that's also readable
- Sensible, applicable facts and secrets that only an insider knows

Special Features

Every book in our series offers the following six special sidebars in the margins that were devised to help you get things done cheaply, efficiently, and smartly.

1. "Timesaver"—tips and shortcuts that save you time.
2. "Moneysaver"—tips and shortcuts that save you money.
3. "Watch Out!"—more serious cautions and warnings.
4. "Bright Idea"—general tips and shortcuts to help you find an easier or smarter way to do something.
5. "Quote"—statements from real people that are intended to be prescriptive and valuable to you.
6. "Unofficially . . ."—an insider's fact or anecdote.

We also recognize your need to have quick information at your fingertips and have thus provided the following comprehensive sections at the back of the book:

1. **Glossary:** Definitions of complicated terminology and jargon.

2. **Resource Guide:** Lists of relevant agencies, associations, institutions, web sites, etc.

3. **Recommended Reading List:** Suggested titles that can help you get more in-depth information on related topics.

4. **Important Documents:** "Official" pieces of information you need to refer to, such as government forms.

5. **Important Statistics:** Facts and numbers presented at-a-glance for easy reference.

6. **Index.**

Letters, Comments, and Questions from Readers

We strive to continually improve the *Unofficial* series, and input from our readers is a valuable way for us to do that.

Many of those who have used the *Unofficial Guide* travel books write to the authors to ask questions, make comments, or share their own discoveries and lessons. For lifestyle *Unofficial Guides,* we would also appreciate all such correspondence, both positive and critical, and we will make best efforts to incorporate appropriate readers' feedback and comments in revised editions of this work.

How to write to us:
Unofficial Guides
Macmillan Lifestyle Guides
Macmillan Publishing
1633 Broadway
New York, NY 10019
Attention: Reader's Comments

The *Unofficial Guide* Panel of Experts

The *Unofficial* editorial team recognizes that you've purchased this book with the expectation of getting the most authoritative, carefully inspected information currently available. Toward that end, on each and every title in this series, we have selected a minimum of three "official" experts comprising the "Unofficial Panel" who painstakingly review the manuscripts to ensure factual accuracy of all data; inclusion of the most up-to-date and relevant information; and that, from an insider's perspective, the authors have armed you with all the necessary facts you need—but the institutions don't want you to know.

For *The Unofficial Guide to Dieting Safely,* we are proud to introduce the following panel of experts

Joy Bauer, MS, RD Ms. Bauer maintains a thriving private practice in New York City with reviewer Lisa Mandelbaum. In her practice, she provides counseling on a wide number of nutritional issues, including weight management, eating disorders, cardiac rehabilitation, sports nutrition, food allergies, and pregnancy. In addition, Joy is affiliated with Columbia Presbyterian Medical Center, where she oversees ongoing research on eating disorders. Joy regularly lectures and conducts workshops on nutrition and fitness for schools and businesses; she recently completed a five-year post as the director of nutrition and fitness for the "Heart Smart Kids" program that she designed for the Mount Sinai Medical Center Department of Pediatric Cardiology. Joy is also author of *The Complete Idiot's Guide to Eating Smart.*

Lisa Mandelbaum, MS, RD Ms. Mandelbaum maintains a nutritional counseling practice with reviewer Joy Bauer. In addition, she is the nutritional specialist and coordinator of patient care and counseling at Peak Wellness, a medical center in Greenwich, Connecticut. At the center, Lisa provides nutritional counseling and leads community outreach programs at local schools and businesses.

Ann Marie Miller Ms. Miller is the Fitness Training Manager for New York Sports Clubs, a network of more than 35 clubs in the metropolitan New York area. Ann has presented numerous fitness workshops and fitness instructor training courses. As a Reebok Master Trainer, she has led fitness classes across America and Europe. Ann is also an avid runner and competitive cyclist who completed the 1997 London Marathon. She has appeared as a fitness expert on FOX-TV, Lifetime, and the *Today Show,* and has been featured in such publications as *Glamour, Mademoiselle, Good Housekeeping, New York Magazine,* and the *New York Times.*

Introduction

Being overweight in a country that worships skeletal supermodels can make you a little desperate and a little susceptible to unproven, ineffective, and risky weight loss diets, pills, and supplements. This guidebook will help you keep your head while you lose weight. I'll show you what's out there, pointing out what works, what doesn't, what's safe, and what's not. I'll steer you toward the worthwhile books, programs, and techniques. Anyone can lose weight on any diet that reduces calories. But no one's found a guaranteed way of maintaining that weight loss. However, some recent encouraging research describes techniques that give you a real shot at keeping it off. I'll tell you about it.

Before going any further, I've got to come clean. I have used one gimmick in this book: I put "dieting" in the title, but the book doesn't advocate dieting at all. In fact, I do my best to convince you *not* to diet, at least not in the traditional, severely calorie restrictive fashion. The book is about the best (and worst) approaches to losing weight. If dieting kept your weight off over the long haul, I'd promote it. But it doesn't.

So why put "dieting" in the title? Because, frankly, it's what makes people buy this book. "Dieting," for most people, is synonymous with weight loss. And rightly so—you go on a diet, you cut calories, and you lose weight. But then you get sick of the diet, the foods are too restrictive, the calories too low, the hunger too unbearable, so you go off the diet and gain the weight right back again.

How about the "safely" part of this title? Now that's something I will deliver on. One thing you get from years of nutrition graduate school and years of counseling people is a sixth sense for unhealthy fad diets and weight loss supplements. Not only do these diets rip you off nutritionally, but they also take a toll on your self-esteem when you "fail" yet again. ("Failure" is actually sanity; you'd have to be out of your mind to swear off carbohydrates, or eat cabbage soup all day!) Happily, the same diet that's safe and healthy, is also the most effective at getting you down to a healthy weight.

The definition of "healthy weight" is still a raging nutrition controversy. I've tried not be schizoid about it, but the book does reflect the split in the obesity field over this question. On the one hand they (obesity researchers, doctors, nutritionists) want us to drop down to a healthy weight to lower our risk of disease. But other nutrition experts argue that fat can be fit, and that the link between obesity and disease risk hasn't been solidly nailed down yet. And, they argue, much of obesity is genetic; that number on your scale is the result of physiology beyond your control, and the price of lowering that number is too high to pay in terms of pain and suffering. The "lose weight" advocates counter that even if it's genetic, it's still worth fighting the genes and getting down to a less risky, if not slender, weight. And, they point out, being overweight also has to do with how many double cheeseburgers you're eating. Genetics take at least 50,000 years to change; in just 20 years the level of obesity has jumped from a quarter to a third of the population. That's overeating and underexercising, not genes.

So the line I try to walk in this book is: There's no need to whittle yourself down to "thin" or to even lose weight at all if your body weight isn't harming you physically or emotionally. But if your weight is putting you at medical or psychological risk and you want to drop some pounds, this book will steer you to the safest, most effective ways, and away from the fraudulent or dangerous. And, as those of you who've tried lots of diets and programs know, weight loss is chancy business: even the "best," most reputable programs are no guarantee of permanent weight loss.

Also, while I recognize the mental and physical damage wrought by restrictive dieting, by the futility of trying to turn a pear-shape into a willow, I gotta say that there are lots of positives to weight loss. In the largest study of people who've lost weight and kept it off, most reported that weight loss "greatly improved their quality of life, health and well-being, mood, mobility, and level of energy." (From the National Weight Control Registry research, more on this throughout the book.)

On average, it's guesstimated that a third of the obesity in this country can be blamed on genetics. That's on average. For some of you genetics is just a little bit to blame, for others it could be driving 90 percent of your weight problem. If it's just a little to blame and the rest is bad diet and exercise habits, then it's a matter of gathering the drive to make some big changes. If you do, you'll lose weight and keep it off without your body fighting you all the way. But if your body fat is largely genetic and if you're genetically large, then don't kill yourself trying to get skinny. But it's worth a shot at "healthy weight"—something in between overweight and Cindy Crawford.

In the meantime, of course, society's party line is: Be thin. You get this message from your doctor, from Calvin Klein billboards, from countless weight loss books, and it's implicit in the looks that pass between the fat-free romantic leads on the big and small screens. It's a message that fuels the millions of cases of eating disorders in this country. But this is an *Unofficial Guide,* so I don't have to go by the party line. So thin is not the message or goal of this book; healthy weight is. If that's "thin" for your body, great. If it's a little more meaty, but healthy, that's great too. Anyway, thin, skinny, wall-of-muscle, waif, bony, social X-ray—these physical types just aren't in the genetic cards for most people. And, as I said, the party line that advocates them isn't holding up so well. Many of the leading experts in the field of weight loss are urging us to reconsider thin. To reconsider losing weight at all, in some cases. Chapters 9 and 12 will help you combat that impossible thin ideal and cope with disordered eating.

Then there's the other party line running through in the weight loss literature: that you can lose the weight, but you might as well forget about keeping it off because only 5 percent ever do. The studies "proving" this used subjects that weren't typical of the general overweight population. New research is finally starting to look into the millions of success stories out there and it indicates that a realistic, reasonable goal weight is certainly within your grasp. So, chalk up two more goals for this *Unofficial Guide:* instilling the belief that it is possible to maintain your weight loss and giving you the tools to do so.

What if you've been on countless diets and are still overweight? I can't guarantee that this book will solve your weight problems for good; no one can make that promise (although so many do). But since I'm not pushing any one program or strategy (in fact, I'm presenting most everything out there), you're bound to find something in this book that works for you.

Many of you already know what to do, how to eat and exercise, but just haven't been able to stick with it. For some reason, you just weren't ready yet. But most weight loss books and commercial diet programs expect you to be ready to plunge into a whole new way of living. Maybe you are ready to make less drastic changes. That's what you'll find out from the readiness quiz generously loaned to us by weight loss expert Kelly Brownell. The quiz, the sections on readiness and stages of change, and the food/mood diary offered here all offer powerful insight into what's been holding you back. Armed with that information, you can adopt some of the strategies that, based on the limited but encouraging research, work the best. For instance, if you're problem is emotional, stress-related eating, you can turn to Chapter 9 to find out how various experts suggest handling it. Also, you can try one of the programs or books that have successfully treated the problem.

Be careful out there. The field of nutrition, and especially weight loss, is rife with quackery. Some are psychopaths, who prey on your desperation without regard to your health; others are well-meaning but misguided. They are the scariest ones because they really believe what they're selling. Some of the nicest people I've interviewed for magazine stories are quacks. Some are MDs. They came up with a theory 20 years ago—say, that combining certain foods and avoiding others will keep you thin. They milk their theories for all they're worth in book after book, often attracting quite a following. In Chapters 6, 7, and 8 you'll find out which books, techniques, programs, and pills are unsubstantiated and which you can rely on.

The thing is, you'll lose weight on even the quackiest books, as long as they keep calories low. The thing that's still confounding quacks and professionals alike is how to help you *keep* your weight off. Though the weight maintenance field is still pretty barren, there's some promising stuff out there. Some programs are showing long-term results, and researchers are turning to those who've kept their weight off to try to bottle what they have. I've included war stories from the research, from quasi-research, and from the anecdotes related to me from formerly overweight people I interviewed.

One strategy that consistently pops up in studies of successful weight maintainers is exercise. The great thing about exercise is that you not only lose weight, but you lose lots more body fat than you would through dieting alone. In this guide, you'll find out how much and what type of exercise will help you lose weight and keep it off. If you hate to exercise, you'll be relieved to read that simple *walking* works, and that splitting your exercise time in four 15-minute segments a day also works. And you'll get a sense of how to get started. But to really fine-tune your exercise regimen, I've suggested some good books, and you can get more information about specific types of exercise in the resource list in the Appendix.

A final reminder: I'm not selling you "my" diet. Nor do I have a stake in promoting anyone else's theory. What I've done is combed the scientific literature, talked to the head honchos in academic and clinical circles, talked to counselors on the front lines, and culled insights from my own counseling experience to put forward the strategies that give you the best chance at succeeding. I wish you success.

Getting Started

GET THE SCOOP ON...
The doablity of weight loss ▪ Measuring fatness
▪ Why fat is risky ▪ Dieting's new reputation ▪
Why lose weight?

PART I

Healthy Weight, Unhealthy Approaches

Alright, I tricked you. This book really isn't about dieting, it's about *losing weight safely*. It's about the state-of-the-art approaches to getting your weight down and keeping it that way. "Dieting" is in the title because people still equate it with weight loss, but as you'll find out in this chapter, dieting and permanent weight loss don't mix. And I'm only interested in helping you lose weight safely, and safely maintain that weight loss.

How much you should weigh, and how to lose it, are among the most controversial, explosive topics in the health field today. Two opposing camps are battling it out: the fat acceptance movement spreading the anti-dieting gospel, and the medical community, alarmed at the epidemic of diabetes and other obesity-related diseases. There may be a compromise position, called "healthy weight." This is a relatively new concept that has emerged from large-scale research studies linking body weight to disease risk. Turns out that you don't have to be skinny to be

3

healthy—great news for many overweight people, for whom "skinny" means fighting an unwinnable battle against powerful genetic forces.

You'll get a pretty good idea of what's a healthy weight for you by the time you finish this chapter. In Chapter 3, you can zero in on it more specifically, if you want (there's a strong case to be made for *not* setting a specific goal weight). Also, I'll tell you what the anti-dieting flap is all about and run through the misconceptions that are the legacy of decades of dieting.

Weight debate

Since you may have heard otherwise, let's get something straight: You *can* lose weight, and you *can* keep it off. That grim statistic that floats around—that only 5 percent of people ever keep the weight off—appears to be the scientific equivalent of an urban myth: No one knows where it came from. While it's true that studies of very obese people coming out of hospital-based weight loss programs show that most regain the weight, there are no good statistics on what happens to everyone else.

The truth is, no one knows what percent of people who lose weight keep it off over the long haul. But new research, including the Weight Registry Study of 2,000 successful "losers" shows that many people do keep the weight off—tremendous amounts of weight—for 5, 10, 40 years or more. It's certainly not a one-size-fits-all experience. The "success stories" sprinkled throughout this book— people I've interviewed who've kept off 15 to 70 pounds for 1 to 20 years—testify to the many different legitimate approaches. However, as you'll see, there are some basics that most adhere to. You just have to find a way that's right for you.

Unofficially . . .
At any given time, 15 to 35 percent of Americans are on a diet. We spend $30 to $50 billion a year on weight loss programs, pills, exercise programs, special diet foods, and other diet-related paraphernalia.

And for many of you, especially if you've got uncooperative genes, keeping your weight off isn't going to be easy. Sorry, I'm not going to push a fantasy of easy, painless weight loss—you can go to a zillion hokey diet books for that. But I will tell you about the light at the end of the weight loss tunnel: The longer you manage to keep it off, the easier it gets, according to the people I've spoken to who've done it and the nutrition experts who study it.

What's too fat?

Don't get too hung up on definitions of overweight and obesity, since the nutrition community itself hasn't come to a consensus on these terms. What's really important are the body weights and measurements which are related to health and disease. "Overweight" sounds less scary than "obese," but I'll use obese a lot in this chapter because it relates to body fat, while overweight does not, necessarily.

For instance, a muscle-bound body builder might be overweight, but certainly not overfat. We'll use measurements, recognized by much of the scientific community, that rely on percent body fat and the body mass index (BMI), a calculation made from your weight and height measurements.

Body mass index

Until recently, the standard for ideal body weights were the height/weight charts put out in 1959 by the Metropolitan Life Insurance Company (revised in 1983). Twenty percent over the ideal was considered obese. These weights were based on a company study looking at the heights and weights associated with the lowest mortality. Critics of the charts pointed out that the sample population was not representative of society and that the charts

Unofficially . . .
While the cutoff points for these terms are still controversial, the scientific community is starting to line up behind the following definitions: *Overweight* means a high weight for height, and that weight comes from all tissues—muscle, bone, and fat as well as water. *Obesity* specifically means "overfat."

were confusing because they were based on frame size, which is hard to measure ("big-boned," "medium-boned," or "small-boned"). Table 1.1 shows what was considered ideal if you're 5'5" or 5'10", according to the 1983 charts:

TABLE 1.1   THE OLD WAY

For 5'5"	Women (lbs.)	Men (lbs.)
Small Frame	117–130	134–140
Medium Frame	127–141	137–148
Large Frame	137–155	144–160
For 5'10"		
Small Frame	132–145	144–154
Medium Frame	142–156	151–163
Large Frame	152–173	158–180

Compared to the BMI charts (see Table 1.2), the Metropolitan table's high end for the 5'5" male (160 pounds) would be considered a slightly risky BMI of 26 or 27. And the high of 180 pounds for the 5'10" male is also a little over the healthy BMI cutoff of 25.

The BMI chart is rapidly replacing the old ideal weight-for-height charts because it better indicates obesity, not just excess weight. On both the BMI chart and the old ideal height/weight charts, a muscular, heavy (since muscle weighs more than fat) football player could be mistakenly classified as obese. But the BMI chart better adjusts for this.

The real value of the BMI chart is that it relates certain weights-for-heights with disease risk. Basically, after a BMI of 25, the higher your BMI, the greater your risk for heart disease, cancer, and other obesity-related illnesses described later on in this chapter. The risk is just a little higher between 25 and 27 than it is under 25. After a BMI of 27 the risk steadily increases.

Exactly where "overweight" and "obese" fall on the BMI chart is still controversial. A government-sponsored expert panel on obesity recently took a crack at it, defining overweight as a BMI of 25 to 29.9 and obese as a BMI of 30 or above. (A BMI of 25 is about 20 percent over ideal weight by the old height/weight standards.) By these measures, 97 million American adults—55 percent of the population—are considered overweight or obese. Many obesity experts, including Surgeon General C. Everett Koop, who now heads Shape Up America!, criticized the new guidelines, saying that they are unnecessarily stringent and may discourage those who have a hard time making it down to a BMI of under 25. Previous definitions were more generous; the National Center for Health Statistics defined overweight as a BMI of 28 for men and 27 for women. Interviews with the experts I consulted for this book indicate that a BMI of 27 or under is usually a healthy weight; anything over 27 starts getting risky.

Remember, the BMI chart is not infallible. Even with a BMI of 25, 26, or 27 you may not be overfat if you've been working out and much of your weight comes from muscle. Standing naked in front of the mirror still can't be beat for determining whether too much of that weight comes from those rolls of fat padding that bod.

Researchers have linked certain BMIs with increased risk for various diseases. Although BMI gets closer to measuring "overfat" and healthy weight than the old height/weight charts, it's still a

TABLE 1.2 BODY MASS INDEX (BMI)

	Good Weights						Borderline			Increasing Risk												
									BMI													
Height	19	20	21	22	23	24	25	26	27	28	29	30	31	32	33	34	35	36	37	38	39	40
4'10"	91	96	100	105	110	115	119	124	129	134	138	143	148	153	158	162	167	172	177	181	186	191
4'11"	94	99	104	109	114	119	124	128	133	138	143	148	153	158	163	168	173	178	183	188	193	198
5'	100	106	111	116	122	127	132	137	143	148	153	158	164	169	174	180	185	190	195	201	206	211
5'1"	100	106	111	116	122	127	132	137	143	148	153	158	164	169	174	180	185	190	195	201	206	211
5'2"	104	109	115	120	126	131	136	142	147	153	158	164	169	175	180	186	191	196	202	207	213	218
5'3"	107	113	118	124	130	135	141	146	152	158	163	169	175	180	186	191	197	203	208	214	220	225
5'4"	110	116	122	128	134	140	145	151	157	163	169	174	180	186	192	197	204	209	215	221	227	232
5'5"	114	120	126	132	138	144	150	156	162	168	174	180	186	192	198	204	210	216	222	228	234	240
5'6"	118	124	130	136	142	148	155	161	167	173	179	186	192	198	204	210	216	223	229	235	241	247
5'7"	121	127	134	140	146	153	159	166	172	178	185	191	198	204	211	217	223	230	236	242	249	255
5'8"	125	131	138	144	151	158	164	171	177	184	190	197	203	210	216	223	230	236	242	249	256	262
5'9"	128	135	142	149	155	162	169	176	182	189	196	203	209	216	223	230	236	243	250	257	263	270
5'10"	132	139	146	153	160	167	174	181	188	195	202	209	216	222	229	236	243	250	257	264	271	278
5'11"	136	143	150	157	165	172	179	186	193	200	208	215	222	229	236	243	250	257	265	272	279	286
6'	140	147	154	162	169	177	184	191	199	206	213	221	228	235	242	250	257	265	272	279	287	294
6'1"	144	151	159	166	174	182	189	197	204	212	219	227	235	242	250	257	265	272	280	288	295	302
6'2"	148	155	163	171	179	186	194	202	210	218	225	233	241	249	256	264	272	280	287	295	303	311
6'3"	152	160	168	176	184	192	200	208	216	224	232	240	248	256	264	272	279	287	295	303	311	319
6'4"	156	164	172	180	189	197	205	213	221	230	238	246	254	263	271	279	287	295	304	312	320	328

To use this chart, find your height on the left column and move your finger over to the weight that's closest to yours. For instance, if you're 5'5" tall and weigh 156 pounds, you've got a body mass index (BMI) of 26. (*Chart source: W/H—George A. Bray, MD, copyright, 1988.*)

fairly crude estimator, and one that is insensitive to individual differences in body fat and muscle. So don't panic if your BMI is in the risky zone, especially if it's around 27 or 28, and especially if the mirror tells you that you've got lots of muscle and little body fat.

Percent body fat

Another way of measuring overweight is to calculate the percentage of body fat. Over 27 percent body fat is considered overweight for a woman, while 32 percent is considered obese. Since men naturally carry less body fat than women, their cutoff point is lower: 23 percent body fat is overweight, and 28 percent indicates obesity. Getting an accurate body fat measure is not that easy; and some of the tools used at health clubs can be pretty useless. Here's what's out there:

■ **Underwater (also called hydrostatic) weighing.** Although it's a more accurate measure than some, this procedure probably isn't worth the hassle. And if you're claustrophobic, forget it, unless you need a desensitization shocker! Underwater weighing is just what is sounds like: Clothed only in a thin bathing suit, you get into a little capsule, exhale, and hold your breath for five to 10 seconds while you're completely dunked under water. Those with lots of body fat must be strapped in with heavy, weighted belts to prevent floating. Based on the amount of water that's displaced, and your body weight in water compared to your body weight on land, scientists have come up with a formula that is a good estimator of your body fat percentage. However, as you can imagine, this is a

Bright Idea
Although they shouldn't, people often cut dairy products when they cut calories. Cutting back on our number one calcium source increases the risk for osteoporosis—a devastating bone disease—later in life. Keep using nonfat milk and other low- or no-fat dairy and buy calcium-fortified orange juice. But to keep calories in check, limit fruit juice to no more than a cup a day.

Watch Out!
With all the sedentary distractions enticing kids, like TV and computers, it's more important than ever to get them out of the house and moving their bodies. Since 1980 childhood obesity rates have increased by 42 percent. One in five teenagers is now considered significantly overweight. This jump in childhood obesity is especially worrisome because being overweight in childhood is related to cardiovascular disease later in life.

time-consuming and expensive procedure. Not many health clubs or weight loss program offices just happen to have an enormous underwater weighing machine lying around.

- **Caliper measurement.** Don't worry, these plier-like instruments don't hurt. What you should worry about is whether the person doing the measuring is well trained; otherwise your results could be meaningless. Calipers are used to measure the amount of "subcutaneous" fat, the fat right under your skin. Using calipers, the person taking your measurements grabs a fold of skin with the fat underneath and gently pulls it away from the muscle. Still holding the skin, the calipers measure the fold. Typically, this is done on your upper arm (triceps), under the shoulder blade (subscapular), just above the hip bone (suprailiac), at the waist (abdominal), and on the thighs. These numbers are plugged into a formula appropriate for your age and sex category, and body fat is estimated. This method can be very accurate if two situations coexist: The person doing the measuring is well trained (otherwise the measurements can be *way* off) and if you are under 55 years of age with a regular distribution of body fat. As we age, our subcutaneous body fat thins, and the internal or "visceral" body fat stores grow—and those fat deposits can't be measured by calipers.

- **Girth measurements.** By plugging measurements of the upper arm, abdomen, buttocks, thigh, and calf into a formula, body fat can be estimated. Although this requires just one simple tool—a tape measure—the calculations are pretty involved, differing according to age and gender.

- **Bioelectrical or electrical impedance.** In this method, electrodes are placed on your hands and feet and an electric current is shot through your body. It sounds dreadful, but it's actually painless. Unfortunately, it's also unreliable. The principal behind it is that electric current passes more easily through lean tissue but slows down or is impeded by fat tissue. By measuring the impedance to the flow of an electric current throughout the body this instrument indirectly measures the percentage of body fat. "Problem is, you get different readings depending on which manufacturer made the instrument," according to Ken Ellis, Ph.D., Director of the Body Composition Laboratory at the USDA Children's Nutrition Research Center at Baylor College of Medicine in Houston. Also, says Ellis, the chance for error is high if the person administering the test isn't well trained. "Electrodes placed just half an inch off on the hands or legs can throw the body fat readings off by 10 percent." This test is free at some health clubs and diet programs.

- **DEXA (Dual Energy X-ray Absorptiometer).** This is just the technical name for a bone scan, and it's Ellis's top pick for measuring body fat. As the machine measures bone density it automatically determines the percent of body fat. "You get two tests in one," Ellis points out. Unfortunately, while this procedure is widely used to check out the thickness of your spine or wrist bones, the Food and Drug Administration

Moneysaver
A recent study by Kaiser Permanente found that health care costs were 25 percent greater for those with BMIs of 30 to 34.9 and 44 percent greater for BMIs of 35 or higher, when compared to costs for people in the healthy BMI range of 20 to 24.9.

(FDA) hasn't yet approved it for scanning the whole body. But if you live near a teaching hospital or major weight loss clinic, they may be running a study using the DEXA. Experimental use is kosher with the FDA.

Healthy weight

What is a "healthy weight"? "Healthy weight" is the new buzzword, the new goal promoted by nutrition experts. It's the weight range considered to pose the fewest health risks—19 to 25 on the BMI chart. Besides helping you to look and feel better generally, getting down to a healthy weight can greatly reduce your risk of developing big-time killers later on, like heart disease and diabetes. That's because the more body fat you have, the more likely you are to develop health problems. Being slightly overweight may not raise your risk for any disease, but being obese for 10 to 30 years doubles the likelihood of dying prematurely. While there's no clear cutoff point along the BMI chart at which your weight changes from healthy to unhealthy, risk seems to increase gradually after a BMI of 25. A BMI of 28 or greater is linked to a three to four-fold increase in developing stroke, heart disease, or diabetes compared to the general population.

As you can see from the BMI chart, "healthy weight" does not necessarily mean "thin." It's amazing how relatively small weight losses—5 to 10 percent of body weight—can make such huge differences in disease risk. If you're a 5'9" male weighing 189 pounds (and the mirror tells you that way too much of your poundage is body fat), your BMI is an unhealthy 28. Lose 10 percent of your body weight—19 pounds—and you've gone down to a much healthier BMI of 25. Losing 10 percent of your body weight is often enough to bring blood sugar, blood pressure, and blood cholesterol down to normal levels.

What if you fall in between the weights and heights listed in the BMI chart? Plug your measurements into this equation:

$$\frac{704 \times (\text{your weight in pounds})}{(\text{your height in inches})^2}$$

Figure 1.1   Calculating your BMI

If you weigh 155 pounds and are 65.5 inches tall, you get the following:

$$\frac{704 \times 155}{65.5^2} = \frac{109,120}{4,290} = 25.4$$
$$(\text{round to } 25)$$

Figure 1.2   A BMI sample calculation

By this calculation, your BMI is 25, which is in the healthy, low-risk zone—so, as you can see, a healthy BMI isn't necessarily skinny.

Apple-shaped and pear-shaped

Your "love handles" are another way to get a handle on disease risk. You may have heard it before: "apple-shaped" people—those with big bellies—are at higher risk for heart disease, high blood pressure, and diabetes than "pear-shaped" people, who carry more weight in their hips and thighs. You can't control where your body chooses to deposit fat—you're genetically programmed to be more apple-like or pear-like. But you can control how *much* fat is parked on those hips or that belly. By losing weight you can become a "safe apple," no longer at increased risk for disease.

Unofficially . . .
We're raising a sluggish generation: Daily enrollment in high school physical education classes has fallen from 42 percent in 1991 to 25 percent in 1995 and the trend continues downward.

Bright Idea
Eating more vegetables may stave off that middle-age spread. American Cancer Society scientists tracked 80,000 middle-age people for 10 years and found that those who ate the most vegetables (19 servings per week) had the flattest bellies.

An unsafe apple is a woman with a waist-to-hip ratio greater than .85 or a man with a waist-to-hip ratio greater than .95. Here's how to calculate your waist-to-hip ratio:

1. With a tape measure, circle your waist—that's the smallest part of your torso between your rib cage and belly button. Write that number down. For this example, let's say you're a man and the number is 41.

2. Now measure your hips, the largest measurement around the widest part of your buttocks. Write it down. For example: 46.

3. Divide your waist measurement by your hip measurement. $41 \div 46 = .89$, which is in the safe zone.

Shed pounds, drop risk

Why bother losing weight? Perhaps you shouldn't, if your weight isn't affecting your mental or physical well-being (that is, if you have no weight-related medical conditions such as diabetes or high blood pressure). If your BMI is under 27, you may not be at any increased risk. But if your body weight has moved beyond a medically healthy point, losing just 10 percent of your current weight can make an enormous difference in how you feel, and perhaps, enough of a difference in how you look to satisfy you. Also, a 10 percent loss may be one you can actually sustain.

Successful "losers" in the ongoing National Weight Control Registry overwhelmingly reported that keeping their weight down greatly improved their quality of life, health and well-being, mood, mobility, and energy level. Interestingly, few of these people are thin, but they are maintaining their weight in the healthy range. But if your BMI is past the 27 mark and you're feeling it, getting down to the healthy weight zone will decrease your risk for the following conditions:

▪ **Heart disease.** Heart disease is the leading cause of death in the U.S. for both women and men, causing 32 percent of men's deaths and 42 percent of women's deaths. The type of heart disease most affected by obesity is "coronary heart disease," in which the coronary arteries, those leading to the heart, start getting clogged up with cholesterol and other gunk. As the arteries narrow, the heart muscle itself can't get enough nutrients and oxygen and starts to falter. A heart attack happens when the arteries are so clogged they finally close off, or a clot that would normally pass through now obstructs the artery. Being overweight increases your chances of developing heart disease because it triggers high blood cholesterol, diabetes, and high blood pressure—all causes of heart disease.

▪ **Diabetes.** There's an epidemic of Type II diabetes in this country, the type you develop as an adult. Being overweight and sedentary has a lot to do with it. Diabetics have faulty insulin, a hormone responsible for regulating blood sugar and for storing fat. A healthy person's insulin efficiently clears the blood sugar and fat byproducts from the last meal, but diabetics must spew out a large amount of their "inefficient" insulin to clear the blood. Eventually, even high levels of insulin don't work and the resulting high blood sugar wreaks havoc on the organs, causing blindness, foot disease, and

Watch Out!
Hispanics
and African
Americans have
obesity rates
that are 10 to 20
percent higher
than whites,
while Native
Americans and
Hawaiians have a
10 to 40 percent
greater preva-
lence of
unhealthy
weight.

other problems. The high volume of circulating fats finds its way to the arteries, clogging them up and causing heart disease and stroke. Plus, all that insulin sends a message to store fat, rather than to burn it. Gaining weight can cause Type II diabetes, especially if it runs in your family. Losing weight can usually get rid of this type of diabetes, especially when exercise is part of the weight loss regimen.

▪ **Cancer.** If we ate a balanced diet, got regular exercise, and stuck to a healthy body weight, about 30 to 40 percent of all cancer cases would be eliminated. Whereas some cancers are caused by unbalanced diets (too much meat and fat, few fruits, vegetables, and whole grains), other cancers—of the colon, rectum, prostate, gallbladder, breast, uterus, cervix, and ovaries—are also related to being overweight. To reduce cancer risk, experts recommend keeping your body mass index between 18.5 and 25.

▪ **Gallstones.** The gallbladder, a three-inch long organ that lies beneath the liver, helps us digest fat by releasing bile, a detergent-like liquid that breaks up the fat particles in that doughnut, salad dressing, or another fatty food you just swallowed. Being overweight ups your chances of developing gallstones, hard clumps made of cholesterol and other material. Gallstones usually don't bother you, but for the minority of people who have symptoms, the attacks are painful, leading to 500,000 operations yearly. But quick weight loss isn't the answer, in fact, it can bring on gallstones. If you're overweight and have gallstones, the gradual weight loss promoted in this book is your best course of action.

■ **Gout.** Gout is a type of arthritis in which painful, needle-like crystals accumulate in the joint spaces, causing inflammation, swelling, and pain, most commonly in the big toe. The crystals are made of uric acid, a naturally occurring substance in the body that rises to too-high levels in people with gout. Uric acid forms from the breakdown of protein, alcohol, and another compound in food called purine. Organ meats, lima beans, certain varieties of seafood, and a few other foods are high in purines. Overeating protein-rich and purine-rich foods contributes to gout in susceptible people. Therefore, the overeating that goes on in obesity is a setup for gout. Also, obesity makes it harder for the body to excrete uric acid. Weight loss, especially on a diet that keeps a lid on protein, alcohol, and purines, helps treat gout.

■ **Osteoarthritis of the spine, hip, or knee.** As you get heavier, you place undue stress on these joints and this wears away cartilage, the bone-like substance that makes up joints. This worn-down cartilage is osteoarthritis, which ranges in severity from mild stiffness and aching joints to severe pain and disability. Lose weight through diet and exercise and do your joints a big favor.

Even if your knees are the problem, walking a treadmill seems to be a good thing: In one study, 48 overweight women with osteoarthritis of the knees walked a treadmill three times a week, for up to 45 minutes per session. They also met weekly with a nutritionist who helped them follow a reduced-calorie diet that set a 30 percent limit on fat. The

Bright Idea
If your degree of overweight is not placing you at medical risk and you are fed up with dieting, go to the following sources for inspiration on accepting your body:

■ Healthy Weight website: www. healthyweight-network.com

■ Size Acceptance website: www. bayarea.net/ ~stef/Fatfaqs/ size.html

payoff: After six months, the women lost an average of 15.5 pounds, and most had a lot less knee pain. Using something called the Womach pain score, 40 percent of the women reported only half as much pain as they had known before the exercise and diet regimen. A third of the women experienced a 50 percent improvement in functions such as walking up stairs. And compared to when they began the study, on average, the women walked 15 percent farther on a six-minute walking test.

If you're obese, dropping 10 to 15 pounds cuts the risk of getting osteoarthritis by half, according to the research of David Felson, MD, professor of medicine and public health at Boston University School of Medicine, Department of Arthritis. "Besides extra pressure on the joints, obesity may also exert some metabolic influences that affect bone and cartilage," says Felson. Otherwise, why would obese women get more osteoarthritis of the hand, an area that wouldn't be stressed from being overweight?

Additional health problems associated with obesity include:

- **Breathing problems such as snoring and sleep apnea** (brief periods where breathing stops). Excess fat tissue around the neck closes off the airways, causing breathing disorders. Weight loss is by far the most effective treatment for snoring, as shown in a University of Florida study. Nineteen overweight male snorers who went on a weight loss program for six months reduced the number of times they snored per hour. Men who lost over 13 pounds cut snores back to just 12 per hour. Weight loss is explicitly used as part of the treatment for sleep apnea.

- **Psychological trauma.** Since thinness is next to godliness in this culture (especially for women), overweight people often feel unattractive, ashamed, and depressed. It takes a tremendous amount of confidence to feel good about your body when you're overweight. But, as you'll see in Chapter 9, with some help you can feel very differently about your body.

The point is that you don't have to strive for an unrealistic, too-thin weight goal—just losing enough weight to put you in the healthy range can make a tremendous difference in how you feel. For most overweight people, losing 10 percent of their body weight is often enough to normalize the following factors:

- Blood cholesterol, reducing risk for heart disease
- Blood pressure, reducing risk for heart disease
- Blood glucose levels, reducing risk for diabetes
- The stress on knees and ankles, reducing the risk and symptoms of osteoarthritis

If exercise is part of your weight loss strategy, you'll really notice a difference in how you feel. Here's what you can look forward to:

- Increased energy
- Diminished hunger
- Better sleep
- Better mood
- Greater body tone (even if you still have more body fat than you'd like)
- Greater endurance

- Stronger bones, thereby decreasing the risk for osteoporosis, a bone-thinning disease

- Quicker recovery from illness, and less risk if you have to have an operation

- Savings in medical bills and insurance premiums

Is diet just a four-letter word?

Do you have to diet to keep off the weight? Recently, "diet" has become a dirty word in some nutrition circles. We're in the midst of an anti-diet—or "undieting"—movement, a backlash against all the low-calorie, structured diets ubiquitous in magazines and best-selling diet books over the past 30 years. The year 1998 began with an editorial in the prestigious *New England Journal of Medicine* that railed against dieting, suggesting that it isn't always medically necessary. The article ended on this dramatic note: "Countless numbers of our daughters and increasingly many of our sons are suffering immeasurable torment in fruitless weight loss schemes and scams, and some are losing their lives." While *The 5 Day Miracle Diet* is still on the shelves, more and more diet books have anti-dieting titles such as *Living Without Dieting* or *Never Diet Again*.

Some of the beliefs of the undieting movement are valid: Dieting *can* be physically harmful and gaining back the weight *does* erode self-esteem; overweight people *are* unfairly discriminated against; and there really *is* no proof that dieting results in sustained weight loss. But another key premise— that obesity may not be so bad for your health— flies in the face of an impressive collection of solid scientific research. In fact, former Surgeon General

Timesaver
Feel guilty about going out to exercise when you don't spend enough time with the kids? If they're still infants, invest in a jogging carriage. If they're old enough, take them walking with you. You'll set a good exercise example they may keep for life.

C. Everett Koop, who is leading a national campaign (called Shape Up America!) to reduce obesity, was so infuriated by the *New England Journal* article that he sent out a press release attacking its weak scientific premise and irresponsible message.

So are diets dead? The restrictive low-calorie ones that have you walking around in a hungry daze dreaming about jelly doughnuts are pretty much passé. But some version of a "diet" has its place, especially for the initial weight loss. About half the successful "losers" in the National Weight Registry used some sort of formal diet program to lose the weight—Weight Watchers, liquid meal replacements, or sessions with a dietitian. Some people do better with structure, and a diet plan that tells them what they should eat for breakfast, lunch, and dinner for the next month may really help them take the weight off. For others, this approach doesn't work: They either exercise more; eat less of what they normally eat; eat lower-fat, lower-calorie foods; or use some combination of the three. And face it, whenever you cut back on calories to lose weight, you're doing some type of dieting.

The difference is that there are healthy diets and unhealthy diets—approaches to losing weight that help you maintain your new weight and super-restrictive diets limited to a few foods that practically guarantee a relapse to your old ways and old weight.

What seems to be more important than the terminology—"dieting" vs. "lifestyle eating changes"—is your attitude about eating. The "success stories" I interviewed for this book don't perceive themselves as being "on a diet." They honestly

Watch Out!
Make a mental
note *not* to let
those fast-food
commercials on
TV pull you into
a fast-food
restaurant.
Researchers from
Johns Hopkins
University
tracked 1,059
men and women
for a year and
found that
women, but not
men, who
watched more
television also
ate more fast
food and were
more obese.

don't feel deprived, at least not enough to be unhappy about it. Ditto for the successful "losers" tracked by other researchers working in this field.

Dieting's legacy: weight loss myths

If you've been through a number of "miracle" diets over the years, you may have gotten some wrong-headed messages. Throw them out along with that stack of old diet books.

Deprivation myth

Many people think that you have to cut way back on calories, avoid certain foods, and/or feel hungry and deprived to lose weight. But while deprivational techniques may work to take the weight off, even if you can stand it for more than a few weeks or months, they won't help you to keep it off over the long haul. In the 1980s, when Oprah Winfrey lost about 80 pounds on a liquid diet, she gained it all back within a few months. Deprivation dooms dieters to this horrible cycle:

Figure 1.3 The devastating deprivation cycle

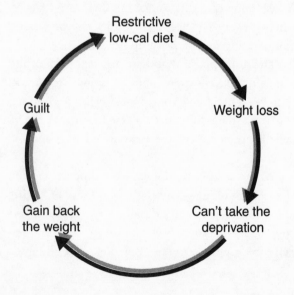

This approach simply doesn't work: While up to 35 percent of Americans say they're on a diet, about half are overweight and a third qualify as obese. Diets in the traditional sense of the word don't work in the long term. Plus, to add insult to injury, they wear down your self-esteem, making you feel like a failure. To break the cycle, you have knock out the restrictive diet part and replace it with a healthy, not-too-low-calorie approach to eating. You won't lose weight as quickly, but you'll have a heck of a better chance at keeping it off.

If you throw in exercise along with the healthy diet, you've just raised your odds of success another few notches. Even if the new way of eating still leaves you feeling a bit deprived, a little fiddling with the diet to include foods you love and a little psychological work can put an end to those feelings. Successful "losers" say that they switched from thinking "Poor me, I can't eat the way I used to" to "I feel in control because I'm choosing to eat well now." And most people who've kept weight off for years say that just changing the way they eat hasn't been enough—some sort of regular exercise was also critical.

The thin myth
This one says that you can, and should, look like a fashion model. The truth is, some of us won't be skinny for life. However, *all* of you can get down to a healthy weight and, with the right combination of diet, exercise, and attitude, stay there. You see, most bodies just weren't designed to be skinny, and trying to get there and stay there involves such an overwhelming effort (like near starvation) that very few people can achieve it. Because of nature or nurture, or some combination of the two, becoming

and staying skinny is just too difficult. However, a healthy weight is much more doable, and that weight will be different for each individual.

Repeated diet failure myth

"You're likely to remain fat if you've lost and gained weight a number of times." Or so goes this fallacy. But who hasn't lost and gained? There's no evidence that a history of yo-yo dieting—cycles of weight loss and gain—necessarily dooms you to remain overweight. In fact, most of the successful "losers" in the National Weight Registry and most of the success stories interviewed for this book had long histories of yo-yoing. The average person totaled a combined loss of 220 pounds over several attempts. The last attempt "took," partly because people made use of strategies they'd learned during previous weight loss efforts.

The genes myth

This myth says that you're doomed to be fat because you have "fat genes." But as you'll find out in Chapter 3, being overweight is usually the result of a complex interaction between genetics and environment. Only a few very rare genetic disorders (and you'd know it if you had one) make excess body fat virtually inevitable.

The gluttony myth

"You're fat because you're a glutton." But it's not clear that overweight people eat more than normal weight people. Instead, it's probable that their bodies just hang on to calories more tightly. Meanwhile everything in our society works against sticking to lower levels of caloric intake. Just look around you: 7-Elevens open all night, McDonald's stands in Wal-Mart, pizza ads on TV just when you thought you

> 66
> Trying not to eat is like trying not to breathe. Sooner or later, your body will take over and you will gasp for breath. If dieting is too restrictive, your body will take over and demand a binge.
> —John Foreyt, Ph.D., Director of the Nutrition Research Clinic at Baylor College of Medicine in Houston, and co-author of *Living Without Dieting* (Warner Books, 1994).
> 99

were full . . . An overabundance of food, food used as stress relief, lack of exercise, and those so-called "fat genes" make gaining weight almost inevitable and keeping it off very tricky.

But keep in mind that lots of people *do* keep it off. Throughout this book you'll hear their stories, and while you'll see that there's no single "right" way to do it, you will discover that it usually involves some sort of commitment to physical activity (even walking) and a gradual change in dietary habits. Dietary *habits*, mind you, not *diet*.

The dirty side of dieting

Although getting down to a healthy weight improves your health in the long run, a quack fad diet can make the weight loss process a risky one. The more drastic the diet, the worse the side effects. Here's a list of dieting's "dirty side" compiled by Frances M. Berg in her book *Afraid To Eat* (Healthy Weight Publishing Network, 1997). (These things shouldn't happen when you keep calories at a level that prevents hunger and induces a weight loss of no more than one to two pounds a week.)

The first four points under "Mental and Emotional Risks" are mainly due to imbalances of nutrients and hormones in the brain. For instance, after following a very low-fat diet that contains few essential fatty acids, brain cells just don't work as well. Brain cells, or neurons, are made up of fat. Deprived of it, they don't receive signals as well from each other—and sometimes they die. On very high-protein/low-carbohydrate diets, like the Atkins' diet described in Chapter 7, the body becomes glucose-deprived. Given that glucose is the cells' preferred fuel, the body has to scramble to make an alternate type of fuel out of fat, called

Unofficially . . .
Non-dieting approaches can be very effective, as shown in a University of California at San Francisco study of 22 people with an average weight of 205 pounds. For 18 weeks, they received training in strong nurturing, effective limits, body pride, good health, balanced eating, and "mastery living" (becoming physically active and feeling fulfilled). Three months into the program they lost an average of nine pounds, and they kept losing after the program ended.

Unofficially . . .
A 1998 study by the Calorie Control Council (CCC), an association of low-cal/low-fat food manufacturers, found that two out of three Americans are trying to control their weight, but that the majority said that they are NOT "on a diet." CCC's interpretation: this indicates "a growing realization among Americans that diets don't work."

RISKS OF DIETING AND WEIGHT LOSS

Mental and Emotional Risks
Apathy
Depression, anxiety
Irritability, intolerance, moodiness
Decrease in mental alertness, comprehension, and concentration
Thoughts focused on eating, weight, and hunger
Self-absorbed, self-focused, decrease in wider interests
Preoccupation with own body, judgmental of others' size
Lowered self-esteem, feels self-worth depends on being thin
Physical Risks
Weakness, fainting, fatigue
Cold intolerance
Gouty arthritis
Elevated cholesterol
Anemia
Headache
Hair loss, thinning hair
Hypotension
Abdominal pain
Muscle cramps
Aching muscles
Both slowed and increased heart rate
Heart abnormalities, arrhythmia
Death

(List reprinted with permission from *Afraid To Eat,* Frances M. Berg, Healthy Weight Publishing Network, 1997.)

ketones. Running on ketones can make you feel dizzy and "out of it." The other mental and emotional effects come from a preoccupation with food, a sense of deprivation, and the feelings of failure that arise if you go off the diet.

The physical effects of fad diets have various causes. If you don't eat enough you don't have enough fuel to run on and you're going to feel weak and tired. Diets that cut out whole food groups, like all-fruit diets (talk about diarrhea!) can lead to vitamin and mineral deficiencies, which can cause some of the symptoms listed in this section. For instance, heart problems, muscle cramps, and aching muscles are a response to low or imbalanced levels of sodium and potassium. These "electrolytes," along with calcium and magnesium, are responsible for muscle contraction, including your heartbeat. Low-calorie diets that are also low on protein sap your lean body tissue because your body starts cannibalizing its own muscle mass for fuel. Low protein also causes hair thinning, hair loss, and heart problems. Low-carbohydrate diets can also be low in fiber, causing constipation.

Most diets won't kill you. In the 1970s there were a few deaths from heart muscle shrinkage caused by liquid protein diets—those diets are now banned. However, some diets can turn into life-threatening eating disorders like anorexia or bulimia—which can eventually kill.

Another indirect side effect not on this list is that very low-calorie diets prevent you from exercising. You're just too weak and tired. That means you're not only losing muscle as your body breaks it down for fuel, but you're not building any either.

Okay, now that I've scared you to death, do you still have any doubts that very restrictive or fad dieting can be bad for you? None of the approaches recommended in this book will put you in jeopardy, at least not for the physical or physiologically induced mental risks. But any time you lose weight you are at risk for becoming food and weight preoccupied. Check out Chapters 9 and 11 for ways of

Watch Out!
Medical researchers calculate that 88 to 97 percent of all cases of Type II diabetes, 57 to 70 percent of coronary heart disease cases, 11 percent of breast cancers, and 10 percent of colon cancers that are diagnosed in overweight Americans are attributable to obesity.

overcoming those feelings. And even balanced diets can become risky if you drop the calories down too low. Here's where your judgment is critical. If you follow a diet plan on your own, or pay for a program or counselor, you've got to make sure that the diet isn't so low in calories that you start feeling the ill effects listed earlier.

Do you need to lose weight?

You may not need the BMI chart in this chapter to answer that question—the mirror is brutal enough, thank you very much. If rolls of fat stare back at you, your BMI is probably above 26, and you need to lose weight. Or you may be at a medically benign weight but you still feel uncomfortably heavy and want to get down to a weight you've been before that feels better. If being a little round doesn't bother you, and your BMI is 26 or below, and you have no risk factors for disease that your doctor thinks could be cured by losing weight (like high blood pressure), then relax. You may not need to lose weight. But we could all benefit from staying active and following a pyramid-style diet outlined in Chapter 4. That alone will automatically knock off a few pounds.

You probably shouldn't try to lose if you've gotten down to a healthy (but not skinny) weight and dropping any lower means you have to exercise like a maniac and half starve yourself. That's not worth it. And, of course, you shouldn't be losing weight if you're already thin but have a distorted body image. Find out if that's you by checking out Chapters 9 and 12.

Your weight loss experience will depend on how much weight you want to lose and on how you go about it. Do you want to fit into that wedding dress in two months or do you want to lose 60 pounds over the next few years? Can you afford a private nutritionist or a commercial weight loss program, or is this book—and maybe one or two others—going to be the extent of your investment? How you go about losing weight depends somewhat on how much you want to lose, your fears, and what motivates you

---

Success Story: Richard Drezen

Maybe it's because I met Richard in my workout class that I have a hard time picturing him 30 pounds heavier (it's also hard to believe he's 47; he looks late-30s, no problem). He's among the fittest people in the class, but he's gained and lost 30 pounds twice in the last eight years. Both times he lost it with the help of worksite Weight Watchers and gyms. "I lost it the first time in New York City, but the stress of moving to Washington, D.C., brought back old habits and I gained it all back. But I got back into Weight Watchers and took a year to slowly lose it again. I'm on lifetime Weight Watchers; I weigh in once a month, and if the weight starts coming back I won't hesitate to get back into weekly sessions." Since Richard's a "snacker" he makes sure that he's nibbling on fruits and vegetables. Another strategy that's been effective: taking lunch to work. "That way, I know I'm getting something low-fat and fairly low-calorie. So if something comes up, like an office birthday party, I still have calories to spare for a little piece of cake." He says he truly doesn't feel deprived, "Unless I have to miss a workout, then I feel bad."

---

best. By the time you finish this book, you'll have a clearer idea of the best approach for you.

Just the facts

- Don't listen to the nay-sayers; you can lose weight, especially if you set realistic goals.
- BMI and percent body fat are the ways of measuring body fat, replacing the old height/weight tables.
- Losing as little as 10 percent of your body weight makes a big difference in your health.
- Dieting is getting slammed, and justifiably. But it doesn't have to be dangerous if done right.
- Old ways of dieting are now being replaced by a focus on "healthy weight" and a combination of nutrition and exercise.
- Only you can judge whether you need to lose weight and why.

Chapter 2

GET THE SCOOP ON...
Readiness ▪ Timing ▪
Setting reachable goals ▪ Finding the right
program ▪ Support—Who needs it?

Getting Organized

This is honesty time, baby. Here's where you decide how far you're in the mood to go. Don't worry if you're not ready to go all the way just yet, there's time for that later. Sounds like a date? Well maybe it is—a date with eating and exercise changes that you may someday be married to. But before taking the big step (diet and exercise changes, that is), make sure you're ready.

Pushing ahead too quickly with major life changes (and, as you know, changing the way you eat and exercise is M-A-J-O-R) is usually the kiss of death to success. But working at your own pace prepares you for each subsequent step. Look, if this takes months or years, fine. Those "quick-loss" 1,000-calorie diets obviously haven't done the trick, plus they've saddled you with all sorts of unwarranted guilt and bad feelings.

To heck with all that! This time, take it slow, set reasonable goals and fight the urge to lose tons of weight quickly. By doing the stuff you need to do, even if it seems unrelated to dieting, you pave your way to a healthier weight. And, as touched upon in

31

"
You can't scare
someone into
treatment. When
a person is tired
of dealing with
the disorder,
they'll want help.
Sometimes loving
insistence from
an important
person can
encourage earlier
treatment.
—Vivian Hanson
Meehan,
President, ANAD
(National
Association of
Anorexia Nervosa
and Associated
Disorders)
"

Moneysaver
Most YMCAs offer
sliding-scale
membership
dues. Depending
on your local
YMCA's policy,
you can save big.
For instance, in
the Washington,
D.C., area, a
yearly health
club membership
runs about $800;
lower-income
residents can get
a membership for
$200.

Chapter 1, for many of you that weight isn't "thin." But it'll be thinner than where you are now.

Perhaps that's the hardest part—letting go of that dream of being skinny. That's the dream that sells $30 to $50 billion in weight loss aids every year and sets millions of people up for certain failure. Chapter 9 gives you suggestions from experts in the field on how to revise this dream. Some of you can be skinny without too high a cost, but for most overweight people, trying to become skinny sets them up for a losing battle against their genetics. Ironically, successful dieters say that only after they let go of the "skinny" goal were they finally able to get their weight down and keep it down. This chapter will help you figure out where to begin, help you set achievable goals, and steer you to the weight loss program that's right for you.

Ready . . . or not?

The first step in the goal-setting process is checking your readiness. You want to lose weight, to look thinner, to feel better. But how ready are you to make the changes that will get you there? Compared to your earlier efforts to lose weight, how motivated are you this time? Do you feel up to sticking it out until you lose the weight? Changing the way we eat and exercise is a big deal, and we all come at it from different stages of readiness.

You can really get tripped up if you take on more than you're ready to handle. But once you meet the process on your own level you can make real progress. You may not be losing lots of weight right away, but you'll be on the right track. You'll be succeeding, and that success will help take you to the next level.

TABLE 2.1   STAGES OF CHANGE

Stage of Change	If You're Here
1. Precontemplation. You're not even considering taking any actions to change the way you eat or exercise, or to reduce stress and other triggers to overeating.	You're already past this because you're reading this book.
2. Contemplation. You're thinking about it seriously, but still haven't done anything, like step up exercise, or make diet changes.	Keep reading. Don't dive into a drastically different lifestyle unless that approach generally works for you. If you want, try something small: Take a short walk every day, or switch from whole milk to 2% or from 2% to 1%.
3. Preparation. You're intent on changing, and you've begun to make a few inroads, such as switching to lower-fat foods.	Keep reading. Also, explore the options mentioned in this chapter and detailed in Chapters 6 and 14. Get recommendations on a nutritionist or weight loss program, or visit a few health clubs. Also, you may be ready to start using the diet diary in the Appendix. Do-it-yourselfers, start thinking about how you can change your diet to move closer to the pyramids in Chapter 4.
4. Action. You've gotten the ball rolling by making some changes in the way you eat, exercise, or relate to food.	Keep reading; this book may show more areas of change that are appropriate for you and will help with what you're currently working on.
5. Maintenance. You've really incorporated that new way of eating and exercising into your lifestyle, and you're comfortable with it.	Congrats, and be vigilant. Don't worry if you find your self backsliding, just pick up where you left off. Chapter 11 offers you guidance.

One of the main problems with many weight loss programs is that they don't meet people at their individual stages of readiness, laments obesity expert Kelly Brownell, Ph.D., in *Eating Disorders and Obesity*, by Brownell and Fairburn (Guilford Press,

1995). Most programs expect people to be ready to jump right in and cut calories drastically, join a gym, and magically erase lots of bad habits. These weight loss programs assume you are in the "action" stage in the "stages of change" chart that follows. "Thus," says Brownell, "programs are 'mismatched' to individuals who are in earlier stages."

See if you can place yourself in one of these "stages of change," adapted from a much-referenced model by University of Rhode Island psychologist James Prochaska.

Sometimes you go through all these stages, get blown off course, and go through them once again. That's okay; sometimes it takes several cycles to "set." Remember Richard Drezen, the "Success Story" profiled in Chapter 1? He lost 30 pounds on Weight Watchers, kept it off for a year, then gained it back when he moved to a new city. He didn't panic, because he knew he had it in him to do it again. And he did—this time the weight's been off for over a year.

Don't be discouraged if you're not yet at the action stage. There's still lots to do in the meantime, like figuring out what to work on when you do feel up to it, or making a few small changes just to see how it feels (Chapters 9 and 10 give you lots of ideas). Change of any kind isn't an all-or-nothing proposition. People who've lost weight and kept it off will tell you that the last time—the time that worked—they were finally "really ready." They say that they were only "kinda ready" during all the previous attempts, when they lost weight but gained it back. Those earlier experiences taught them things that worked, and these they plugged into their lifestyles when they finally did get the proper motivation. But beware: too many dieting failures

Unofficially . . .
Lose just 8 to 10 pounds and cut back sodium to 1800 mg daily and you may be able to throw that blood pressure medicine away. That's what happened to 30 percent of the 975 overweight people with high blood pressure in the National Institute of Health's TONE (Trial of Nonpharmacologic Interventions in the Elderly) study.

can be destructive, wearing down your self-esteem and self-confidence.

Ready? . . . set . . . test!

To test your readiness, take these mini-quizzes, developed by top-dog weight loss expert Kelly Brownell, Ph.D., of Yale University for his LEARN® Program for Weight Control (described in Chapter 6). These tests should not be used as the only basis for deciding when to begin a program. Use them to ask yourself questions about your readiness, not to make a final decision. And keep in mind that "overall readiness" may be a less helpful notion than thinking of readiness in different areas. For instance, most people entering a weight loss program expect to change their diet, so the majority would be in a high state of nutrition readiness. People vary more widely in their readiness to be physically active. Low scores in one area may be a signal to take action to improve readiness in that specific area before going further into your weight loss program. Remember, low readiness is not necessarily permanent; you may be more ready later on. The tests simply provide a snapshot in time to show whether the conditions are right at this moment.

THE WEIGHT LOSS READINESS TEST

Answer the questions below to see how well your attitudes equip you for a weight loss program. For each question, circle the answer that best describes your attitude. As you complete each of the six sections, add the numbers of your answers and compare them with the scoring guide at the end of each section. (For example, in Section 1, if you answered "1" on questions 1 and 2, and "5" on questions 3 to 6, your score would be $1 + 1 + 5 + 5 + 5 + 5 = 22$.)

Section 1: Goals and Attitudes

1. *Compared to previous attempts, how motivated to lose weight are you this time?*

   1. Not at all motivated
   2. Slightly motivated
   3. Somewhat motivated
   4. Quite motivated
   5. Extremely motivated

2. *How certain are you that you will stay committed to a weight loss program for the time it will take you to reach your goal?*

   1. Not at all certain
   2. Slightly certain
   3. Somewhat certain
   4. Quite certain
   5. Extremely certain

3. *Consider all outside factors at this time in your life (the stress you're feeling at work, your family obligations, and so on). To what extent can you tolerate the effort required to stick to a program?*

   1. Cannot tolerate
   2. Can tolerate
   3. Uncertain
   4. Can tolerate well
   5. Can tolerate easily

4. *Think honestly about how much weight you hope to lose and how quickly you hope to lose it. Figuring a weight loss of one to two pounds per week, how realistic is your expectation?*

1. Very unrealistic
2. Somewhat unrealistic
3. Moderately unrealistic
4. Somewhat realistic
5. Very realistic

5. *While dieting, do you fantasize about eating a lot of your favorite foods?*

   1. Always
   2. Frequently
   3. Occasionally
   4. Rarely
   5. Never

6. *While losing weight, do you feel deprived, angry, and/or upset?*

   1. Always
   2. Frequently
   3. Occasionally
   4. Rarely
   5. Never

Section 1—TOTAL Score ___

If you scored:

6 to 16: This may not be a good time for you to start a weight loss program. Inadequate motivation and commitment together with unrealistic goals could block your progress. Think about the things that contribute to this situation and consider changing them before undertaking a program.

17 to 23: You may be close to being ready to begin a program, but you should think about ways to boost your readiness before you begin.

24 to 30: The path is clear with respect to goals and attitudes.

Section 2: Hunger and Eating Cues

7. *When food comes up in conversation or in something you read, do you want to eat even if you are not hungry?*

   1. Never

   2. Rarely

   3. Occasionally

   4. Frequently

   5. Always

8. *How often do you eat because of* physical hunger?

   1. Always

   2. Frequently

   3. Occasionally

   4. Rarely

   5. Never

9. *Do you have trouble controlling your eating when your favorite foods are around the house?*

   1. Never

   2. Rarely

   3. Occasionally

   4. Frequently

   5. Always

Section 2—TOTAL Score ____

If you scored:

3 to 6: You might occasionally eat more than you would like, but it does not appear to be a result of high responsiveness to external cues. Controlling the attitudes that make you eat may be especially helpful.

7 to 9: You may have a moderate tendency to eat just because food is available. Weight loss may be easier for you if you try to resist external cues and eat only when you are physically hungry.

10 to 15: Some or most of your eating may be in response to thinking about food or exposing yourself to temptations to eat. Think of ways to minimize your exposure to temptations, so that you eat only in response to physical hunger.

Section 3: Control Over Eating

If the following situations occurred while you were on a diet, would you be likely to eat *more* or *less* immediately afterward and for the rest of the day?

10. *Although you planned on skipping lunch, a friend talks you into going out for a midday meal.*

    1. Would eat much less

    2. Would eat somewhat less

    3. Would make no difference

    4. Would eat somewhat more

    5. Would eat much more

11. *You break your diet by eating a fattening, "forbidden" food.*

    1. Would eat much less

    2. Would eat somewhat less

    3. Would make no difference

    4. Would eat somewhat more

    5. Would eat much more

12. *You have been following your diet faithfully and decide to test yourself by eating something you consider a treat.*

1. Would eat much less

2. Would eat somewhat less

3. Would make no difference

4. Would eat somewhat more

5. Would eat much more

Section 3—TOTAL Score ___

If you scored:

3 to 7: You recover rapidly from mistakes. However, if you frequently alternate between eating out of control and dieting very strictly, you may have a serious eating problem and should get professional help.

8 to 11: You do not seem to let unplanned eating disrupt your program. This is a flexible, balanced approach.

12 to 15: You may be prone to overeat after an event breaks your control or throws you off the track. Your reaction to these eating events can be improved.

Section 4: Binge Eating and Purging

13. *Aside from holiday feasts, have you ever eaten a large amount of food rapidly and felt afterward that this eating incident was excessive and out of control?*

    1. Yes

    0. No

14. *If you answered yes to question 13, how often have you engaged in this behavior during the last year?*

    1. Less than once a month

    2. About once a month

    3. A few times a month

    4. About once a week

    5. About three times a week

    6. Daily

15. *Have you ever purged (used laxatives, diuretics, or induced vomiting) to control your weight?*

   5. Yes

   0. No

16. *If you answered yes to question 15 above, how often have you engaged in this behavior during the last year?*

   1. Less than once a month

   2. About once a month

   3. A few times a month

   4. About once a week

   5. About three times a week

   6. Daily

Section 4—TOTAL Score ___

If you scored:

0 to 1: It appears that binge eating and purging is not a problem for you.

2 to 11: Pay attention to these eating patterns. Should they arise more frequently, get professional help.

12 to 19: You show signs of having a potentially serious eating problem. See a counselor experienced in evaluating eating disorders right away.

Section 5: Emotional Eating

17. *Do you eat more than you would like to when you have negative feelings such as anxiety, depression, anger, or loneliness?*

   1. Never

   2. Rarely

   3. Occasionally

   4. Frequently

   5. Always

18. *Do you have trouble controlling your eating when you have positive feelings—do you celebrate feeling good by eating?*

    1. Never
    2. Rarely
    3. Occasionally
    4. Frequently
    5. Always

19. *When you have unpleasant interactions with others in your life, or after a difficult day at work, do you eat more than you would like?*

    1. Never
    2. Rarely
    3. Occasionally
    4. Frequently
    5. Always

Section 5—TOTAL Score ___

If you scored:

3 to 8: You do not appear to let your emotions affect your eating.

9 to 11: You sometimes eat in response to emotional highs and lows. Monitor this behavior to learn when and why it occurs, and be prepared to find alternative activities.

12 to 15: Emotional ups and downs can stimulate your eating. Try to deal with the feelings that trigger the eating and find other ways to express them.

Section 6: Exercise Patterns and Attitudes

20. *How often do you exercise?*

    1. Never
    2. Rarely

3. Occasionally

4. Frequently

5. Always

21. *How confident are you that you can exercise regularly?*

    1. Not at all confident

    2. Slightly confident

    3. Somewhat confident

    4. Quite confident

    5. Extremely confident

22. *When you think about exercise, do you develop a positive or negative picture in your mind?*

    1. Completely negative

    2. Somewhat negative

    3. Neutral

    4. Somewhat positive

    5. Completely positive

23. *How certain are you that you can work regular exercise into your daily schedule?*

    1. Not at all certain

    2. Slightly certain

    3. Somewhat certain

    4. Quite certain

    5. Extremely certain

Section 6—TOTAL Score ___

If you scored:

4 to 10: You're probably not exercising as regularly as you should. Determine whether your attitudes about exercise are blocking your way, then change what you must and put on those walking shoes.

11 to 16: You need to feel more positive about exercise so you can do it more often. Think of ways to be more active that are fun and fit your lifestyle.

17 to 20: It looks like the path is clear for you to be active. Now think of ways to get motivated.

(Source: LEARN® Program for Weight Control, 7th ed., 1997 American Health Publishing. Reprinted with permission.)

After scoring yourself in each section of this questionnaire, you should be able to better judge your dieting strengths and weaknesses. Remember that the first step in changing eating behavior is to understand the conditions that influence your eating habits.

Why change?

It sounds obvious, but your answer may have a lot to do with your success. It's a well-known fact that your chances of long-term weight maintenance go way up if you're doing it to please yourself, rather than in response to pressure from your spouse, from your doctor, from images in *Vogue*, or other external forces. But even if it is your doctor that initially scared you into dieting, it can be you that emerges at the other end of the experience, ready and willing to lose weight.

See how two "Success Stories," profiled in this book, put it:

- "I was tired of feeling tired and dragged out. I remembered how much more energy I had and how much more I got accomplished when I exercised." Tom Kiley, head of the religion department in a Catholic high school, husband, and father of two.

- "Losing weight was part of my healing, learning to respect myself, to love myself. I wanted to get healthy, no matter what it meant weight-wise." Peggy Newman, singer/songwriter, wife, and mother.

For Tom and Peggy, and for success stories everywhere, the cost of being overweight had become higher than the cost of changing their habits. Is this true for you? To get an idea, write up a list of advantages to changing. Here are some to consider:

- I'll have more energy.

- I'll enjoy better health.

- I'll look better.

- I'll have more endurance, so it will be easier to do the things I enjoy, such as taking walks, playing with my kids, and dancing.

- I'll be happier. (Being thinner doesn't necessarily make you happier. But if your weight problem is due to depression, bingeing, or other emotional reasons, then resolving those issues may make you happier.)

Now weigh those reasons against disadvantages to change; for example:

- It takes a lot of time and effort

- It's too overwhelming (but if you make changes at your own pace it shouldn't be overwhelming).

- I'm afraid I'll fail and that will be depressing (but setting the right goals minimizes failure).

Timing

There are no hard and fast rules about the best time to lose weight. It's just common sense that an exceptionally hectic period is probably not the best moment to embark on something that demands focus, resolve, and top priority. Losing weight, and

Bright Idea
Interview your prospective nutritionist, therapist, or commercial weight loss counselor, as if you were interviewing a job candidate. A few sample questions to ask are:

1. What approach or philosophy do you use?

2. How long have you been doing this?

3. What are your credentials?

4. How much will it cost, including hidden costs?

especially the first few months of weight loss maintenance, definitely require all three. Okay, there's never a good time, but if you've got the following factors conspiring against you, you might be better off waiting:

- You just went away to college.
- A parent or other close person died very recently.
- You just got married.
- You just had a baby.
- You just moved to a new city.
- There are major upheavals at work.
- You just got divorced.
- You just retired from your job.
- You're working on a project that demands all your time.

But don't use circumstances as an excuse; the key issue is how the circumstance makes you feel. For instance, a job that keeps you on the road a lot does make it harder to eat well and get more exercise. But if you are basically happy with your job—not feeling too stressed out about it or other things—then this may be a fine time to start working on your weight problem. In this case, you could use help setting up ways to eat well and exercise while on the road.

Setting goals

This will make or break you. Just think of all the smaller goals NASA scientists set before putting a man on the moon—they broke the big job into manageable chunks. People who try to lose weight are notorious for their all-or-nothing mentality: If I don't get down to a size 6 or look like the cover of

Men's Health or *Vogue,* then why bother? If I slip up and binge, then I might as well give up; I'll never stick with it. Setting unrealistic goals sets you up to fail. Period. But if you can accept that this time you might not lose the weight quickly, then you're ready to set realistic, achievable goals. Here's how:

Analyze

Why do you think you're overweight? While heredity no doubt plays a role, what are the contributing lifestyle factors? You'll get a clearer sense of this when you start keeping a food diary (described in Chapter 10). Meanwhile, see if anything on this list rings a bell:

- I don't exercise enough—or at all.

- I spend lots of time on the computer or watching television.

- I eat too much at—or between—meals.

- I graze all day, without realizing the total amount I wind up eating.

- I skip a meal, then get very hungry and overeat later on, often on junk foods.

- I have more than one alcoholic drink per day.

- I don't seem to eat a *lot,* but the foods I do eat are very high in fat and calories (like french fries, burgers, and ice cream).

- I'm "good" for a few days, then I overeat for a few days, then try to be "good" again, and the cycle keeps repeating itself.

- Social eating and drinking (in restaurants, at friends' homes) is doing me in.

- I use food to cope with both good and bad stress.

- I go on very high calorie binges that feel out of control.

- I'm fine when I'm at home, but I overeat and stop exercising when I travel. And I travel a lot.

- I'm better when I travel; I go to the hotel gym and pool and order reasonable food from restaurants. But at home I'm stressed, and my eating and exercise habits go down the tubes.

- I'm depressed, which makes me feel tired, lethargic, and unmotivated.

- I feel overwhelmed by the prospect of losing weight—because I've failed when I tried before, or because I have so much to lose, or because I just don't know where to begin.

Notice how many of these issues aren't directly related to how much you eat or how little exercise you get. Many are related to other things going on in your life. Stress, or emotional eating, occurs when you eat in response to anxiety, boredom, anger, depression, loneliness, and other emotions. (More on this and other eating disorders in Chapter 12.)

Pick an area to work on

After honestly appraising your habits, decide which one to tackle. The Dieting Readiness Tests you took earlier should have helped clarify which areas need the most work. Depending on how motivated you are, you can take on your "problem area" whole hog, or start out with a few baby steps. For example, perhaps your diet isn't bad, but your problem is not getting enough exercise. Based on your level of readiness you might choose to do one of the following:

- You're highly motivated, at the "action" stage of change. In this case, you might buy a book on exercise and start following it (see the Appendix for suggestions). Or you might buy a stationary bike or join a gym and start using the equipment and exercise classes there. You might even hire a personal trainer.

- You hate to exercise and you're not very motivated. You need baby steps: one or two ten-minute walks every day, maybe with a friend to encourage you. If walking is tolerable, then increase the length of the walks gradually. If walking isn't burning enough calories and isn't enough to give you that heightened feeling of well-being, then explore other options. But test things out before you put your money into a gym or an expensive piece of equipment. Maybe you'll never like exercise much, but you can work yourself up to the minimum level that makes a difference in your life.

Set non-weight goals

If the scale depresses and terrorizes you, don't set a body weight goal. Instead, try setting other goals that will help you eat better and get more exercise. Believe me, you won't need a scale to let you know you're getting thinner. Remember, set the goal based on the "analyze" exercise you just went through. Find a problem area that you're ready to tackle and go for it. Here are some alternative goals:

- **Specific exercise goal.** For instance: I plan to walk three to seven (depending on where you are now) hours a week. If I miss a day, I'll make up for it later on in the week.

Timesaver
Before hunting through the phone book for a registered dietician, call the American Dietetic Association (ADA) at (800) 366-1655 weekdays for reliable referrals, or check "Find a Dietitian" on the ADA website, www.eatright.org. Get at least three referrals and call all three; that increases your chances of getting someone you like and that you can afford.

- **Attitude goal.** There are all sorts of attitudes that get in the way of making changes of any kind, including diet and exercise changes. One big attitude problem is not taking responsibility for your weight gain and weight loss. In a survey of 541 Weight Watcher's group leaders who'd kept their weight off for about six years, 77 percent named "taking responsibility for one's own behavior" as one of the top three factors in maintaining their weight loss. Chapter 9 runs through this and other attitudes that can help you.

- **Healthy-eating goal.** For instance: add one or two fruits and vegetables daily and curb one or two high fat foods that regularly make it to your plate. Curb, don't eliminate. For more ideas, check out Chapter 10.

- **Changed eating-habits goal.** Say you skip breakfast most days. Set a goal to eat breakfast two days a week. Even if it's not a conventional breakfast, try to get something into your stomach within two hours of waking. Next week move it to three breakfasts. You get the picture. For more on changing eating habits, consult Chapters 9 and 10.

- **Mental health goal.** Emotional eating is a common problem: people often use food to cope with stress. Most of us do this to some degree (I confess, I've got a little bowl of ice cream next to me right now). But if your emotional eating gets to the point where it makes you fat, you've got to tackle it—maybe even before you do anything else, according to psychologist Edward Abramson, author of *Emotional Eating* (1993, Lexington Books). But, writes Abramson, "It is not essential to curtail emotional eating completely before starting a weight-reduction program." He does urge that you get a handle on it and make some progress with it before embarking on the other diet changes. More on this and other emotional eating patterns in Chapter 9.

How to set a realistic weight goal

If you must set a weight goal, then make it attainable. The key here is to individualize. What's reasonable and attainable for your 5'4" frame will be different than what works for your 5'4" friend or colleague. Here are some questions to ask yourself, developed by obesity experts Kelly Brownell and Judith Rodin:

- Is there a history of excess weight in your parents or grandparents?

- What is the lowest weight you have been able to maintain as an adult for at least one year?

- What is the largest clothing size in which you feel comfortable and still can say, "I look pretty good considering where I've been?"

- Think of a time when you were at a lower weight. What degree of food restriction and/or exercise did it require to stay at that weight? Could you maintain the same degree of effort for the long term? If not, what level of effort do you feel would be reasonable?

- Think of a friend or family member with your frame and age who you feel looks normal. What does this person weigh?

It's not hard to see where these questions are leading: to discovering a body weight that you can stick with. And who knows, reading this book may direct you to a method, counselor, or program that will help you stick to an even lower weight. Ideally,

Watch Out! "Individuals interested in a specific do-it-yourself programs should search in the program literature for evidence that the program is successful; if information on success is absent or consists primarily of testimonials or other anecdotal evidence, the program should be viewed with suspicion." (Source: *Weighing the Options, Criteria for Evaluating Weight-Management Programs,* Institute of Medicine, Paul R. Thomas, Ed, National Academy Press, 1995.)

Unofficially . . .
A study of 267
commercial
weight loss pro-
gram participants
a year after they
left the program
found that 82
percent had
maintained their
weight loss with-
in 10 percent.
The key to their
success may have
been that these
people stayed
with the program
until they
achieved their
goal weight..

that body weight should put you at a BMI of 27 or less, the statistically healthier zone (see the BMI chart in Chapter 1). But if you're BMI is now, say, 32, and a BMI of 28 is what seems most attainable, go for it. It may not be your ultimate goal, but it's much better than where you are now.

Evaluating your options

Much of the $30 to $50 billion spent by people try-ing to lose weight this year went to questionable weight loss methods, but you can't complain that there's no choice: "fat burning" pills, cabbage soup diets, weird exercise contraptions hawked on infomercials, 30-pounds-in-30-days diets, plus all the legitimate stuff, like gyms and good counseling. I gave the word "weight loss" to an Internet search engine and got 294,517 matches; I put in "diet" and got 441,661 responses.

Chapters 6, 7, and 8 will help you sort out the "hype-ful" from the helpful. But remember, there isn't one guaranteed method for keeping weight off. In this book I'll direct you to the techniques consid-ered healthiest and most effective, but if a psychic who says she's a 2,000-year-old princess helps you keep the pounds off with a healthy diet, more power to her. When deciding on a weight loss "program," here are the major factors to take into consideration (The term "program" is used loosely here—it could mean a book, a counselor, or a commercial program like Nutri/System, among many other things):

- **State of readiness.** You should be at the "prepa-ration" or "action" stage in Table 2.1 before giv-ing your money to any program.

- **Your goals.** Either find a program that suits your goals or try to tailor the program that way. For instance, if you've decided the scale isn't going to be the way you measure success, don't pick a counselor or program that insists on weekly weigh-ins. (Many of the commercial programs do.) Or, say you know that the 1,200-calorie diets typically handed out at commercial weight loss programs are too low for you. If you still want to try out a commercial weight loss programs, make sure the counselor at the center will work with you on a higher calorie plan.

▪ **Your level of overweight.** In general, the less you have to lose, the less intensive (and usually less expensive) the program. However, there are exceptions. If you're not very overweight— say you've got 10 or 15 pounds to lose—but your diet looks like a fast-food version of the Pyramid, then some sessions with a nutritionist might be a good idea. And, of course, if you're not overweight or only barely over your optimal weight, but suffer from bulimia or anorexia, then you definitely need fairly intensive counseling.

▪ **Your physical health.** Some of the more drastic approaches can be dangerous; for instance, the medically supervised liquid diets can be hard on the heart. The diet drugs can cause—and worsen—hypertension and have other side effects.

▪ **Your pocketbook.** Of all the things you spend money on, weight loss has got to be one of the more important, especially if your health's at stake. But there's no need to go bankrupt in the process. Commercial weight loss programs run from $90 to $300 for the entire experience. For the ones that make you buy their food, figure another $50 to $80 a week, which may not be such a bad deal if you're single and are used to eating out and shelling out a lot for food. But if your food budget isn't large, and especially if you've got a family to feed, the Jenny Craig, Nutri/Systems, or Diet Center foods may be too expensive. So go with Weight Watchers. Private counseling varies in price, so shop around. Chapter 6 gives you an idea of how much various programs cost.

- **Past experience.** Don't go back to methods that you really couldn't stand. For instance, if you tried a very low-calorie, liquid diet program like Optifast and were miserable, don't repeat it again unless there's some pressing medical reason to do so. But remember, sometimes it's your attitude and stage of readiness, not the method, that's key. For instance, if you went to a nutritionist but didn't follow her advice, you may not have been ready to change. This time you might have greater success. Same thing with joining a gym—if you joined before you were ready to commit to exercise you probably ended up never going.

Use Table 2.2 to get yourself thinking about various options. You may fit into a different category than is suggested. Read more about all these options in greater depth in Chapter 6. As you can see from this chart, your body weight is sometimes, but not always, a factor in choosing a weight loss strategy. As I've been doing throughout the book, I'm using BMI, or body mass index, as a measure of overweight. Flip to Table 1.2 in Chapter 1 to find your BMI. In general, the less you have to lose, and the less complicated your medical/psychological issues, the simpler (and cheaper) your strategy.

TABLE 2.2   MAKING THE MATCH

Option	Best If BMI Is	Keep in Mind
Do-it-yourself. Simply cut back on the amount of food or follow a good diet book.	Under 28	Best if you're a self-starter and highly motivated with virtually no emotional eating issues.
Meal replacements (such as Slim Fast) plus "real meals."	Under 28	Not highly recommended, but if you must, it's best to work with a legitimate nutritionist (see Chapter 6) to learn how to wean off the shakes and onto real food.
Self-help groups (such as TOPS or Overeaters Anonymous).	Doesn't matter	A self-help group alone is usually not enough if your BMI is 32 and above.
Private counseling.	Doesn't matter	Prices and talent varies. See Chapter 6 for tips on choosing a good one. A nutrition counselor is enough if you don't have an eating disorder, otherwise, go to an RD as well as a psychotherapist specializing in eating disorders.
Commercial weight loss programs (such as Weight Watchers or Nutri/System) or similar worksite programs.	Under 28	Okay for higher BMIs as long as you don't have an eating disorder or serious medical complications such as an arrhythmia.
Hospital-based programs that are not very low-calorie (under 1,000) diets.	Over 31	Lower BMIs could do this as well, but unless it's got a great reputation, you might do just as well for less money on a commercial program. Those with BMIs over 31 are more likely to have medical complications that require a physician's monitoring, which you'll get at the hospital program.

continues

TABLE 2.2 (continued)

Option	Best If BMI Is	Keep in Mind
Hospital-based very low-calorie diets (under 1,000), such as Optifast.	Over 31	These should be used only if all other attempts have failed and there is a medical reason to lose weight. These diets can be risky, so people with certain conditions, such as a recent heart attack, an eating disorder, or substance abuse should exercise caution. Programs should involve intensive education and the best combine liquid meals with real food (see Chapter 6 for details).
Residential programs.	Doesn't matter	Since these are expensive, it's best to wait until you're ready to make a change. If you are very overweight or have medical conditions, go to one that's hospital-based, like the Duke Diet and Fitness Center (Chapter 6 has details).
Gastric surgery (making the stomach smaller and shortening the area where food is absorbed in the small intestine).	Double your healthy weight or more, or BMI over 40	It's still unclear who's the best candidate for this. The diet and exercise and/or psychological counseling should be tried first. Consider surgery only if all other weight loss techniques failed and obesity is severely impairing your quality of life. Details in Chapter 6.

Psychological support

While most decent weight loss programs or qualified counselors offer some sort of psychological insight into your weight problem and provide some psychological tools to keep you on track, for some of you that just isn't enough. If any of the following apply to you, you probably could benefit from seeing a psychologist or psychiatrist who specializes in eating disorders.

- You suffer high levels of depression and anxiety, which fuel binge eating.

- You feel as though you're addicted to food; you eat compulsively whether you're hungry or not and feel you can't say "no" to it.

- You're constantly preoccupied with thoughts of food and feelings of bodily dissatisfaction.

- You think that losing weight will solve all your emotional problems.

Rallying the troops

When making any big life change, use all the supportive relationships you can get. Now's the time to think about all the ways you can get support for your endeavor. Think of which friends and family members can help you. When you're ready, enlist them in your cause. Also, think about who's had a hand in sabotaging your past efforts and put an end to their negative influence (Chapters 9 and 11 offer suggestions).

Many people haven't built supportive friendships and strong networks. Obesity can be especially isolating, with lonely roots extending to the schoolyard teasing days of childhood. But in this era of dual-career parents, transient jobs, and home offices, everyone, overweight or not, is finding it harder to keep up their support networks. This lack of social support can itself become a cause of overeating if food is used to cope with the stress of

"
The new world
of intense,
but limited, rela-
tionships that
required a great
deal of effort to
establish and
maintain and the
decline of more
traditional sup-
portive relation-
ships that could
simply be taken
for granted put
an enormous
strain on the
individual and
were among the
main causes
of the nervous-
ness that so fre-
quently afflicted
middle-class
Americans before
and after the
turn of the cen-
tury. (Source:
*Habits of the
Heart,* by Robert
Bellah and oth-
ers, Perennial
Library, 1986.)
"

loneliness. If you find you don't have much of a support system, for whatever reason, then think
seriously about joining a support group. Support
groups such as Overeaters Anonymous, TOPS,
and ANAD (for anorexia and bulimia) can be
invaluable. These groups can make you feel a whole
lot better about yourself and about life. They can be
informative and interesting and lead to great friendships. Shop around until you find one you like.
(More on these in Chapter 6.)

In addition to human support, set up a supportive environment by stocking your kitchen and office
with healthy foods, making time for walking or other
exercise, or changing your walking route so you
don't pass the bakery. Check out Chapters 9 and 10
for more of these tips.

Finally, check out Mandee's weight loss saga. She
went through many of the issues discussed in this
chapter: lack of readiness, poor goal-setting, and
failure at weight loss maintenance. Don't worry if
the first time isn't the charm; it rarely is.

Success Story: Mandee S.

"I've been dieting a long time," sighs Mandee,
a law student. "I grew up with two obese
parents. When I was a kid, the whole family
would go on a diet." She lost (and gained)
many times: 15 pounds for a whole year,
37 pounds for six months, 40 pounds sopho-
more year of high school on Weight Watchers.
She gained it all back that summer. In college
she did bouts of Jenny Craig or Weight
Watchers. "I quit because I wasn't losing weight

fast enough. I was too young to understand it's really about permanent lifestyle change. I wasn't there yet." After college she spent a year in Israel and came back weighing 220 pounds, her highest weight ever (she's 5' 10").

Mandee entered law school and went to a nutritionist who balanced out her virtually all-carbohydrate diet with some protein. "Around then I started walking, 20 minutes a few times a week. I lost 15 pounds, so I was down to 205. I maintained that for a year." Her second year of law school she decided to lose more weight, mainly by jacking up exercise with a treadmill or by jogging three or four times weekly. "I decided to give myself a goal for the summer: the "Cure du Tour" diabetes bike ride. I worked out every day for it and rode it well. Next goal: a longer, 150 mile bike ride." Training for that involved spinning classes (a type of stationary bike) twice a week, running twice weekly, and riding her bike three times a week. She did well on the ride and by the summer's end was down to about 180.

Now, six months later, she fluctuates between 177 and 182. "My goal's 150 to 160. Now it no longer matters how long it takes me to get there." She's hired a personal trainer and faithfully spins, runs, or gets on the stair-climbing machine. While she denies herself nothing, her diet has become very low in fat. Even the splurges—fat-free chocolate pudding and Milky Way Lites—have replaced the

(continues)

full-fat versions. "If I try and satisfy a chocolate craving with anything else I'll go through half the kitchen." When she feels like giving up and "stuffing my face," she pulls a few motivators out of the hat. She tries on an old pair of too-big jeans and remembers what that was like. She looks at a photo of herself at 220. "And I remember what it was like to wake up in the morning without any energy. That expression 'Nothing tastes as good as thin feels' is absolutely true."

Just the facts

- Understanding your readiness can give you a sense of whether it's a good time to begin losing weight.

- Set reasonable goals and give yourself a chance at beating the odds.

- There's a wide world of weight loss options; think about which one will give you most bang for your buck.

- Start thinking about how to create a more supportive environment for your weight loss.

Nutrition You
Should Know

GET THE SCOOP ON...
Calories ▪ Fat genes? ▪ Your "set point" ▪
Future "diet" drugs

PART II

How Do You Get Fat?

Show a group of obesity researchers a fat lab rat and they'll tell you how it got that way, down to the last genetic mutation. Show them an overweight human and you'll see a lot of head-scratching. They've discovered six different genes that make rats and mice fat, and 55 potential "markers" or genetic regions that appear to affect body fat. But they've only come up with three genes that are linked to human obesity, and not nearly as neatly as the animal links. But scientists are doing a good job of uncovering the many maddeningly efficient ways some people's bodies store fat, even if they haven't yet nailed down the genes behind the trouble.

So, getting fat still boils down to taking in more calories than you burn. That's the simple part. It gets complicated when you try to figure out why some people can get away with eating twice as much as you, exercise less, and still stay skinny. That's where heredity, metabolism, and perhaps the type of diet you're eating come into play.

In a major shift in thinking, the health community now considers obesity a chronic disease, just like high blood pressure and diabetes. But, you might argue, why is it a disease when it can be cured by diet and exercise? Haven't you been listening to the news? A number of large-scale, scientifically solid studies have shown that with the right diet and exercise switches, about half of those with high blood pressure can chuck their medications out the window. Ditto for diabetes. It's just that society's sympathies lie with these diseases and they get the drug treatment nod. But obesity? Talk about judgmental . . . not only are overweight people expected to conquer it on their own, but they're made to feel like failures if they can't. Welcoming obesity in the disease club may seem like a dubious honor, but it means that the condition will get more research attention and increase the likelihood of a cure. As scientists start figuring out the physiology of obesity, they are developing drugs that should attack this condition at its very genetic and hormonal roots.

The calorie curse

It all begins with calories. Even though counting calories and even talking about calories has been downplayed in the last few years (replaced by fat grams or number of servings from each food group on the pyramid) calories are still your basic issue. Most of the research shows that overweight people do eat more calories than normal weight people. Why they do may be because of a physiological screwup somewhere in the body. And until they develop drugs to deal with that screwup, you've got to figure out how to eat less and burn more calories.

What the heck is a calorie?

Calories aren't molecules or any "thing," but units of measure, like inches or degrees Fahrenheit. Calories measure the energy in food and the energy your body needs to function. It's not that the 1,000 calories in a Big Mac and an order of fries will make you feel more energetic than the 260 calories in McDonald's plain hamburger (in fact, it's probably the opposite). In this case "energy" refers to the potential "fuel value" that food provides. The 1,000 calories are like a half a tank of gas; the 260 calories only about an eighth of a tank. If you were stranded on a desert island, that Big Mac meal would fuel you a lot longer than the plain burger. Some of that Big Mac might get stored as fat, to be used later, while you'd burn up the plain burger pretty quickly.

But unless you're planning to get shipwrecked, you've got to contend with a world brimming over with food, making it so easy to over fuel. And when that happens—when you take in more calories than your body needs—the rest gets stored as fat.

Only four things in food can be measured by calories: fat, carbohydrate, protein, and alcohol (see Chapter 5 for a more detailed explanation of these nutrients). Overdo any of these and you get fat. But it's easier to get fat eating fat because it's got more than double the calories of carbohydrate or protein. You'd have to eat nine cups of raw spinach (mostly carbohydrate) to reach the 104 calories in two tablespoons of cream (mostly fat) or one tablespoon of butter. Vitamins, minerals, cholesterol, water, and the thousands of other compounds in foods have no caloric value. A chart in Appendix D gives you calorie values of various foods.

Storing calories

Here's how those calories get transformed to your belly and thighs: Take last night's dinner—a turkey burger on a bun, a green salad with dressing, and a

Unofficially . . .
The reason fat is so fattening is that it's got more than double the calories per unit of weight as carbohydrate or protein. Here are the stats:

fat: 9 calories per gram

alcohol: 7 calories per gram

protein: 4 calories per gram

carbohydrate: 4 calories per gram

bowl of ice cream. It would have been reasonable had you not eaten way too much the rest of the day. Result: calorie overload.

Your body processes the meal by digesting it in the stomach, where harsh hydrochloric acid turns it into mush. The mush works its way down the small intestine, where it gets squirted with various enzymes that finally break it down into molecules of glucose, amino acids, and fatty acids that get absorbed through intestinal walls and wind up in your bloodstream. Cells grab some of the glucose for energy; use some of the amino acids to make muscle, enzymes, and other compounds; and use some of the fatty acids for energy or to make hormones and other substances. But the leftover fatty acids head straight to your fat cells. The excess glucose and amino acids get converted to fat (burning a few calories in the conversion process) then off to the fat cells. In men, and in post-menopausal women, the first fat cells to fill up are typically in the belly. In pre-menopausal women, fat prefers to reside in the hip and thigh area. While belly fat is more medically dangerous (see Chapter 1), it's also easier to get rid of; hip and thigh fat can be incredibly stubborn.

Burn, baby, burn

Okay, you've been tipping the balance for a while, and your body has become a very welcoming place for fat. To shed that fat, you've got to use it for energy, in the same way you use food. Let's say your body needs 1,800 calories a day to keep you at your current weight. Eat 1,600, and your body will have to reach into those fat stores for the extra 200. And, if you increase your exercise by burning 300 calories a day, and your body's got to dip even further into those fat stores. Now 500 calories of fat are being dragged out of storage. Keep this up and you'll lose a pound of fat a week (a pound of body fat is approximately 3,500 calories).

You don't just want to lose weight, you want to lose "fat weight." The trick is to shed fat and keep valuable muscle. That's why the combination of exercise and dieting is by far the ideal way to slim down. The exercise prevents you from losing muscle (in fact you may gain it) while drawing on fat stores to fuel your long walks, stints at the treadmill or bike, or whatever activity you're doing. So, how many calories does your body need? It's very individual; here are the factors that go into the calories you expend:

1. *Basal metabolic rate* (BMR) uses up about 60 percent of your calorie output. BMR is the number of calories the body needs to keep those important involuntary functions going, like heartbeat, breathing, and manufacturing thousands of enzymes and other chemicals and compounds. Your BMR is the rate at which you use up calories at rest when you're just lying around. What raises your BMR: being tall, being muscular (muscle burns up many more calories than body fat), being hot or cold (it takes energy to warm up or cool down), and exercising (BMR is elevated a few hours afterward).

   Although everyone's BMR is different, and those differences may be linked to obesity (some people are slower burners), a very rough rule of thumb is to assume you need 10 calories for every pound of body weight. That means a 160-pound person would need 1,600 calories daily just for BMR. Since BMR is about 60

Watch Out!
Drastically restricting your calories can be counterproductive because it slows your basal metabolic rate. Translation: You burn fewer calories and cling harder to the calories in your meals. For most people, going lower than 1,500 calories starts putting the brakes on metabolic rate; severe restriction (usually 1,000 calories or less) can reduce metabolic rate by as much as 45 percent.

percent of total calorie needs, the daily calorie requirement to keep up the 160 pounds of body weight is about 2,667 (to get that total I divided 1,600 by 0.6). This rule of thumb doesn't apply to infants and children, who need lots more than 10 calories per pound of body weight. And after age 25, metabolism declines by about 2 percent per decade, so as you get older you burn—and need—even fewer calories per pound.

2. *Physical activity* makes up about 30 percent of calorie output. As you can imagine, this is also a rough estimate and varies greatly depending on how much exercise you're getting. Although you can't jack up your basal metabolic rate by much, you can really make a calorie burning difference while exercising. In sprint running and swimming you burn up to 120 times as much as at rest; during a marathon, 20 to 30 times. The training involved in being a world class athlete nearly doubles the amount of calories burned daily. The more you weigh, the more you burn doing the same movements; so take heart—that exercise you do when you're overweight counts even more!

3. *Digesting food* uses up the final 10 percent of calories, too bad it's not more than that. And sorry, there are no foods that burn up more calories getting digested than they contribute. As you'll see, disturbances in the way you burn calories can contribute to becoming overweight.

Lean body mass

A happy side effect to gaining body fat is that you've also built up a structure of lean, muscular tissue

underneath to support the excess weight. You want
to hold onto as much precious muscle (also known
as lean body mass) as possible; it makes you look
better by giving your body definition, and, unlike
body fat, muscle mass burns calories, even when you
are sleeping. How to do this? Stay active. Lose
weight by exercising and eating less.

Research shows that people who lose weight by
dieting and exercising can actually gain muscle,
while those who only diet lose both fat and muscle.
That's because your body not only draws on fat
stores for fuel, but digs into muscle tissue as well.
But if you're working out and eating enough protein as you lose weight, you'll make muscle instead
of tearing it down. Any type of exercise will help preserve lean body mass, but a combination of aerobic
exercise (for example, fast walking, dancing, and
cycling) and weight lifting builds the most muscle.
And don't be fooled by ads for products that "turn
fat into muscle." The only way to build muscle is
through hard work (exercise). While you *can* burn
body fat to fuel exercise, you cannot skip the exercise step.

Did your genes make you do it?

Obesity is called a "multifactorial disease," caused by
both physiological and environmental factors.
Physiological as in basal metabolic rate and number
of fat cells; *environmental* as in a large order of fries.
On the physiological side, genetics seem to be most
important (seems, because as I mentioned, the
genes haven't been located yet in humans) but
other factors are also driving our "fat biology."

How big a role do genes play?

Obesity definitely runs in families, but it's hard to
tease out how much of the blame goes to genetics

Unofficially . . .
We're not the
only country in
obesity trouble.
In urban
Scotland, middle-
aged men are
suffering from an
epidemic of heart
disease. As the
Japanese diet
has gone from 7
percent of calo-
ries from fat to
24 percent,
heart disease and
obesity rates
have risen in
step. Still, we
win: The U.S.
has the highest
obesity levels in
the world.

> **"**
> Across the population, the amount of obesity that can be attributed to genetics is about one third. This is an average across populations. Clearly in some overweight people, it plays a huge role, in others no role.
> —Albert Stunkard, MD, Weight and Eating Disorders Program, Department of Psychiatry, University of Pennsylvania School of Medicine, and one of the country's leading obesity experts.
> **"**

and how much to the overeating and sedentary ways learned in the home. However in lab animal studies, where precise obesity genes have been pinpointed, it's very clear that obesity is genetic. As "fat genes" are starting to be uncovered in humans, we'll eventually find out the degree of genetic influence.

If both parents are normal weight, a child has a less than 20 percent chance of becoming obese. The odds increase to 40 percent with one overweight parent and shoot up to 80 percent when both parents are obese. But not everyone who's obese has obese parents. Other evidence for the genetic link: Identical twins are usually the same body weight, even when reared apart. Adoption studies do show that kids tend to resemble the body shape and weight of their biological parents over their adoptive parents, but the link isn't as strong as with identical twins.

In a powerful demonstration of the influence of genetics, researchers at Laval University in Quebec, Canada "overfed" sets of twins and watched to see how much weight they gained. Twelve sets of identical twins, age 19 to 27, were placed in a dormitory and fed their usual amount of food plus an extra 1,000 calories a day. For the 100 days of the study, researchers monitored their diet and exercise very carefully to make sure everyone was basically following the same protocol. As you might expect, they all gained weight. Interestingly, the members of a twin pair gained about the same amount of weight. But the differences between twin pairs were striking. One pair—let's call them Billy and Bob—gained about nine pounds each. Meanwhile, another set of twins, "Lester and Lowell," each gained about 29 pounds. Clearly, Lester and Lowell were storing

much more of that extra 1,000 calories daily than
Billy and Bob.

A peek into the fat factory

The research is divided on the question of whether
overweight people take in more calories than those
of normal weight. If and when they do, it could be
in response to hormones and other body chemicals
sending out powerful signals to eat more. So, it's not
always gluttony or emotional eating behind the calorie excess, in fact it may take an extraordinary act of
will power to not eat even more.

Fat storage is a major production requiring lots
of busy behind-the-scenes hormones and enzymes
to pull if off. How much of the hormonal and enzy-
matic workings are inherited is still not clear.
Having many fat cells, or a low metabolic rate, or
high insulin are all important factors in obesity, but
whether these are all genetically governed is still
unclear, according to Rockefeller University professor Jules Hirsch, MD.

Listed here are the major fat felons. You may
have just one of them, all of them, or a few of them.
Some may be genetically transferred; others may be
the result of something that went awry in the system
later in life.

Hunger, appetite, satiety (feeling of fullness),
storing and burning fat, and storing and burning
carbohydrates are all masterminded in the brain.
Like a general in a body weight command center,
the brain depends on intelligence from the ground
troops and CIA agents—signals emanating from
the intestines, pancreas, liver, taste buds, and blood
levels, to name some of the major sources. Disrup-
tions in those signals, or an inability of the brain to

Unofficially . . .
Most forms of
obesity are likely
to result not
from an over-
whelming lust for
food or lack of
willpower, but
from biochemical
defects at one or
more points in
the system
responsible for
the control of
body weight.
(Source: "The
New Biology of
Body Weight
Regulation,"
*Journal of the
American Dietetic
Association,*
January 1997,
Michael
Schwartz, MD
and Randy
Seeley, Ph.D.,
both from the
University of
Washington in
Seattle.)

receive the signals, may cause people to overeat and gain weight.

Here are some of the body's ways of favoring fat storage:

- **Low resting metabolic rate** (the number of calories you burn when you're lying at rest). Obese people start out with the same metabolism as normal weight people, burning the same amount per pound of body weight. But maddeningly, as they lose weight, metabolism slows, to try and conserve energy, to try and keep them fat. Even after losing the weight, a formerly obese person must take in 15 percent fewer calories to maintain the weight loss than a person of the same weight and height who's never been obese, according to research from Dr. Hirsch's team at Rockefeller.

- **More fat cells.** Some people are born with more fat cells than others, and during early childhood and then again at adolescence, your fat cells divide, giving you more. It's theorized that overeating during these stages may increase fat cell size. Also, in very obese adults, fat cells may also divide. Having a higher-than-normal number of fat cells makes it harder to lose weight because these fat cells want to stay filled, and they send out signals that favor fat storage. Also, some people have larger fat cells and must shrink the fat cells down to subnormal levels to keep body fat down.

- **Faulty hunger on/off switches.** You know that high you get when you're really hungry and sink your teeth into a burger or pasta dish or anything else you really love? Your brain actually produces opiates, brain chemicals similar to opium, in reaction to signals it gets from the taste buds and smell center sent up by nerves. Those brain chemicals are saying "Bring on the food; this feels great." Another eating trigger is the brain chemical neuropeptide Y, which urges us to eat more, burn less, and store more fat. Neuropeptide Y gets stimulated when we haven't eaten for a while, have exercised intensely, and when we lose weight.

Some time during or after a meal, the small intestine (where food is dumped out of the stomach) releases a hormone called cholecystokinin that signals to the brain, "Whoa, hold it right there . . . getting full, meal's over." Other compounds from the pancreas (glucagon) and stomach (gastrin releasing peptide) also send similar satiety signals. When researchers give people those compounds with a meal, people put their forks down sooner. It could be that obese people either don't produce enough of these "satiety compounds" or they don't register clearly in the brain. Talk about a great potential drug therapy; yup, it's being looked into.

Also, leptin, a hormone discharged from fat cells, tells the brain to lower appetite levels and increase physical activity. Since leptin levels are comparable in normal weight and obese people, it's thought that obese people's brains aren't as sensitive to the hormone. (Drug companies are experimenting with drugs that would increase leptin sensitivity.)

While researchers have seen bits and pieces of this faulty chemical signaling in humans, it's been clearly demonstrated in lab animals. For instance, one type of rat with a known genetic defect that causes obesity doesn't produce enough of the "stop

> 66
> We knew how to diet; what we didn't know was how to transfer that knowledge from our brains to our stomachs, our emotions, our genes, our will. I know rationally that the chocolate mousse I long for is not the only, the last, the best chocolate mousse in the world . . . but what if it is? I want it now. Maybe an air conditioner will fall on my head on the way home from this restaurant and I will die not having had the only last best chocolate mousse in the world. (Excerpt from *An Accidental Autobiography* by Barbara Grizzuti Harrison, copyright 1996. Reprinted by permission of Houghton Mifflin Company. All rights reserved.)
> 99

eating" chemical messengers. When these rats are given the chemical, they automatically, sponta-neously eat less and lose weight. A strain of obese mice with another genetic mutation do produce enough of the satiety chemicals, but they have faulty receptors in their brains that can't read the signals, so they just keep eating.

One other body mechanism involved in fat stor-age has become the current darling of the "low car-bohydrate" diet books (such as the *Zone* series or the Dr. Atkins' books). These basically tell you that if you keep blood insulin levels low, you won't get fat. While this particular spin on insulin is far from proven (and even discredited by many), there are other proven links between insulin and obesity.

Insulin is a hormone released from the pancreas in response to eating. Doesn't matter whether you eat carbohydrate, protein, fat or any combination of the three; insulin trudges out of the pancreas. In the bloodstream it helps the body cope with the influx of nutrients, greasing the wheels for glucose's and protein's entry into cells. Also, insulin ushers both fat and excess glucose into fat cells (glucose gets converted to fat). But unlike the picture of insulin portrayed by the fad diet books as the body's fat pad-der, insulin also indirectly signals the body to stop making body fat. There's a certain basic level of insulin that hangs out in the blood all the time; this level rises and falls according to the amount of body fat. As body fat goes up, insulin rises, warning the brain to cut back on eating. But some obese peo-ple's brains may not properly receive insulin's warn-ing because insulin receptors—landing sites geared specifically for insulin on brain cells—may be defec-tive. So the brain thinks the body is thin, and it con-tinues to send out those "I'm hungry" signals.

Can you fight your set point?

Many of the hormonal, metabolic, and chemical factors I just described conspire to keep your body fat at a certain level called the set point. That's why weight loss is so difficult; when you lose fat beneath your set point, your system springs into action to drive the level of body fat back up. Dieting, especially very calorie restrictive dieting seems to trigger the strongest set point defense.

But set point isn't all that set, points out Richard Keesey, Ph.D., a University of Wisconsin at Madison professor who has researched the phenomenon. "Set point slides up and down according to your age, a woman's menstrual cycle, and the amount of physical activity you get," explains Keesey. The good news is that you can turn the knob to a lower level of body fat, mainly through exercise and additionally perhaps by eating a low-fat diet. "Getting in about 30 minutes of physical activity three or four times a week can reduce body fat by 6 or 7 percent, in effect, resetting your set point," says Keesey. It seems to do this by regulating appetite, so you're hungry only when you really need the calories. It also builds up the lean, muscular part of your body, which can ever so slightly raise your metabolism. The low-fat diet may also help raise metabolic rate a tad because you burn more calories processing protein and carbs than fat.

Drugs like nicotine and some of the prescription and non-prescription weight loss drugs can rev up metabolism and, in effect, lower set point. Nicotine obviously is a counterproductive way to go, and the effects of long-term diet drug use are still unknown (see Chapter 8 for more on drugs). The bad news is that there is a natural tendency for set point to inch

Timesaver
Household chores steal time away from exercise. Do both at the same time:

■ An hour of window-washing = a half hour walk

■ An hour of car-waxing = a four-mile bike ride

■ An hour of gardening = a game of volleyball

Okay, they might not be equivalent in terms of fun, but you can say you spent your time wisely.

Unofficially . . .
Women have some great, natural metabolism boosters: Breastfeeding nudges metabolic rate up by about 6 percent and expends an extra 500 and 700 extra calories per day. Also, women's metabolism revs up premenstrually, burning between 150 and 300 extra calories daily.

up as we age. Declining levels of hormones such as estrogen in women and testosterone in men shift body composition to a higher percent fat and a lower percent lean. This means you simply have to fight back harder on the diet and exercise front. It also means that you may have to accept the changes to some extent.

Interestingly, Dr. Keesey doesn't consider a high set point a defect. "Overweight people are regulating their fat stores just as well as thin people, they are simply regulating at a higher level. It's like you went into your house and turned up the thermostat; everything still runs well, but at a higher temperature," he says. The conditions we evolved from determine our set point, speculates Keesey. For instance, "high regulators" probably evolved from ancestors whose survival depended on being able to store fat for times of scarcity.

All the discoveries regarding the hormonal and other mechanisms that drive obesity are not lost on the drug companies. In the same way that Type I diabetics (who don't make their own insulin) take insulin injections, drug companies would love to find a chemical that could signal the brain to slow down the fat factory. So far, no miracles—Chapter 8 gives you the info on what's available.

What Big Macs and sitting on your bum gotta do with it

But genetics and set point can't explain the rise in obesity rates in this country. Genetic changes take about 50,000 years. Over just the last decade, obesity rates rose by 30 percent. Now, a third of middle-aged Americans are obese. Our same old genes are flourishing in an environment of supersized fast-food "bargain" meals, muffins the size of small cakes, and door-to-door car trips that have made taking a walk quaint. You see, at any other point in history, your fat genes wouldn't get much of a chance at being expressed. Now they're having a field day.

Pima predicament

A fascinating, and somewhat tragic case in point are the Pima Indians, living in Arizona. Two generations ago they were farmers, burning lots of calories doing heavy manual labor and eating rice, beans, prickly pear, and plants unfamiliar to most people. If they had meat it was lean: jackrabbit, deer, or fish. Then the river they depended on for irrigation was diverted to developing the town of Phoenix and they stopped farming, became sedentary, and ate a typical American diet. While their traditional diet was 15 to 20 percent of calories from fat, they're now eating closer to 40 percent fat. And while obesity was rare and diabetes unheard of, the Pimas are now among the fattest people in the world, with a record-breaking diabetes rate of 50 percent. "You can't change genetics in three generations. The genetic tendency for diabetes was there, but it was the environmental factors—too many calories and not enough exercise—that allowed it to express itself," notes Frank Vinicor, MD, MPH, director of the Center for Disease Control's Diabetes Division.

In addition to diabetes, the Pimas have all the other baggage that travels with obesity: soaring heart disease rates and premature death. For decades scientists have been intensively studying the Pimas, hoping that this extreme case of obesity will provide the genetic and hormonal answers to the cause of obesity in all of us. Researchers speculate that the reason the Pimas are so genetically inclined

Watch Out!
TV can definitely make you fat. A 1996 study showed that people who watch more than five hours of television daily were nearly five times as likely to be fat than those who watched under two hours daily. The researchers concluded that 60 percent of the incidence of obesity could be linked to excessive television.

to being obese is because those with obese genes were the survivors in times of famine. Those who could hold onto their calories and store them as fat lasted longest.

Devious diet culprits

We're eating, on average, 6 percent more calories than we were 20 years ago. That's significant, but it can't explain the 30 percent leap in the obesity rate since that time; lack of exercise is the missing link. Ironically, we're eating less fat than we were 20 years ago. One of the reasons nutritionists have been shoving low-fat diets down our throats for the past decade is that research indicated that they were less fattening. In other words, even if you ate the same number of calories, you'd gain less weight on a low-fat diet compared to a high-fat diet. Compared to those used for protein and carbohydrate, the body spends as few calories as possible digesting and metabolizing fat. You burn only 5 calories processing a 100-calorie tablespoon of butter, while 100 calories' worth of jam (carbohydrate) "costs" 10 calories to process, and 100 calories of fat-free turkey breast (protein) costs 25 calories to process. In other words, you burn more calories processing a low-fat diet than a high-fat diet.

But researchers are divided on how meaningful that difference is. Some say that unless you're on an all-fat diet, this doesn't make much difference. But most agree that the main reason it's easier to lose weight on a low-fat diet is because of the safety net that catches you when you have a portion slipup. If you have two extra slices of lean turkey breast, you've only added about 100 calories to your daily tally. Try that with an extra Quarter Pounder, and you've just racked up 450 big ones.

The exceptions to this general low-fat-is-lower-calorie principle are low-fat and fat-free cookies, ice creams, and the like which are high calorie because they're packed with sugar. There are tales galore about people getting fat on portions they wouldn't dream of eating if the label didn't say "fat-free." Low-fat diets work when you eat lots of fruits, vegetables, and whole grains that are bulky and fill you up on fewer calories. Seems as though Snack-wells, reduced-fat Entenmann's danishes, and the like are partly to blame for our higher-calorie intake despite the reduction in fat.

Big-time blame also lies with supersized foods. Remember three-inch diameter bagels that weighed about 2 ounces? Those were about 160 calories. Now you're hard-pressed to find a bagel under 4 ounces and 320 calories. Why buy a plain burger when for just pennies more you can get a double cheeseburger, fries, and a soda? One Olive Garden pasta plate and one Big Gulp could satisfy an entire family for dinner. Portions have spun way out of control, skewing our notions of what's appropriate.

The slide into sedentary

If we walked a mile for an oversized muffin, things wouldn't be so bad. But most American adults—somewhere around 60 to 80 percent—don't get the amount of exercise it takes to lower their body weight and keep them even minimally fit. A survey by the Surgeon General's Report on Physical Activity and Health indicates that 25 percent of American adults are not getting any exercise at all; another 40 percent are nearly sedentary. Levels of activity decrease significantly with age. There's no one magic number of minutes or hours per week that's ideal for everyone, but many health experts

Moneysaver
Fast food "deals" on supersized meals are no health bargain. These are better deals:

■ Divide one supersized meal among two or three of you.

■ At McDonald's get a "My Size" meal, which still offers a discount even if you choose a small drink and small fries. Or, order a $2 kid's Happy Meal.

would be happy if we could all spend at least 30 minutes daily engaged in moderate-intensity activity. That's walking, dancing, housework, golfing, or other activities that involve moving the large muscles in your arms and legs.

When you look at the charts showing the number of calories burned for various exercises (see Chapter 13), it seems puny. A 30-minute walk might burn 160 to 200 calories—not even a bagel's worth. So how can physical activity be that important? Well, just imagine if you weren't getting even that bagel's worth of exercise; you'd be even heavier. So, if nothing else, getting a minimum of exercise can prevent you from gaining even more weight. But those ripple effects on your set point, described earlier, is why those 30-minute walks can also help you lose weight: by suppressing appetite and building calorie-burning lean muscle.

Finally, exercise is the bright hope in the frustrating area of weight loss maintenance. Both the studies of weight loss programs and the research examining the habits of successful maintainers come up with the same conclusions: If you stick with exercise, your chances of maintaining your weight loss go way up.

Booze and cigarettes

Hate to admit it, but yes, smoking does rev up your metabolic rate. One study found that metabolic rate rose by 10 percent; those in the study had to eat 200 fewer calories per day when they stopped smoking to maintain their body weight. So when you quit smoking (no, nowhere is there any evidence that cigarette's slimming effects outweigh its deadly ones), nicotine gum may help you keep your weight down.

That other drug—alcohol—should be particularly fattening because it's got seven calories per gram compared to four in carbs and protein. But there's something peculiar about the way the body metabolizes alcohol that makes its effects on body fat unpredictable.

An ongoing Harvard University study tracking 89,538 nurses showed that the more alcohol they drank, the more calories they took in, but the lower their body weight. The researchers statistically accounted for the effects of smoking (which helps keep weight down); still alcohol drinkers were thinner. However, once women started drinking 50 grams of alcohol daily (that's four beers, five glasses of wine, or five ounces of hard liquor) body weights started creeping up a little.

It may be that your body type affects the way you burn up alcohol calories, according to a U.S. Department of Agriculture study. Women were given a weight-maintaining diet deriving 36 percent of calories from fat, which included either 200 calories' worth of booze (two drinks a day) or Coke. Figure this: Leaner women who hit the sauce had to eat, on average, 212 calories more (in food) than they did when they were drinking Coke, otherwise they'd lose weight. But the heavier women who went on the diet that included alcohol had to eat 134 fewer calories to maintain body weight. (An example of a leaner woman in this study is 5'4" and 128 pounds; heavier is 5'4" and 145 pounds.) "This study supports the theory that alcohol calories may not be as caloric—at least for lean women. It also suggests that leaner and heavier people metabolize alcohol differently," says Beverly Clevidence, Ph.D., research nutritionist at the Beltsville Human Nutrition

Bright Idea
At parties and bars, have two glasses of seltzer for every alcoholic beverage. And make yourself weak drinks: wine spritzers cut with seltzer, mixed drinks with less than a shot of liquor. Even though alcohol itself may not be particularly fattening for some people, it can indirectly cause weight gain by removing your inhibitions. Just as that drink makes you more flirtatious than usual, it can also make you more calorie careless.

Timesaver
Fast food no
longer means
fat food. An
explosion of
"wrap" restau-
rants offer nutri-
tionally balanced
meals-to-go,
wrapped in a tor-
tilla or other
flatbread. While
there are high-
fat wraps, with a
little nutrition
savvy you'll wind
up with a great-
tasting low-fat
one. Choose
wraps based on
beans, chicken
breast, or fish
moistened with
salsa. Mango,
cranberry, and
other exotic sal-
sas in these
places really
liven things up.

Research Center, the leader of the USDA study. Since this is the only study of its kind, the connection between body weight and alcohol is still an open question. USDA researchers hope to come up with more definitive answers with upcoming studies. For now, make yourself an experiment of one; watch and see what happens to the scale when you drink.

Finally, what about a beer belly? Although there's no hard science behind it, one theory is that the carbohydrates in beer—over one-third of its calories—might be contributing to a gut. Hard liquor and wine have nearly no carb calories, just those from alcohol.

Outwitting your genes

In her book *Making the Case for Yourself: A Diet Book for Smart Women* (Putnam, 1998), Susan Estrich, a top-of-her-Harvard-class lawyer and television commentator says that her biggest accomplishment is losing weight. Her enviable career, her children, her marriage, are "blessings," but losing weight is what she takes most pride in. Look at it one way and it sounds incredibly superficial, but think about it as a battle won against the powerful forces of genetics, and you can see where she's coming from. (By the way, her diet plan is a little iffy, but some of her psychological strategies are worth checking into.)

Estrich is right; fighting your genetics, changing your environment and your destructive habits, and getting down to a reasonable weight is quite an accomplishment because it's really hard. But Estrich and so many others have done it, so it's well within all our grasps. It's just hard; for some, really hard. In this book, I equip you with all the techniques backed up by decent research and/or suggested by trusted

---

Success Story: Maye Musk

"Sure I'd love a box of cookies beside me right now, but I know that they'll cause me pain for the next week," says Maye Musk, a stunningly beautiful 50-year-old who's been a 150-pound, size 10 model for the past eight years. Before that she was a 200-pound, plus-size model. Her sisters and mother are all overweight, and sticking to a healthy weight doesn't come naturally. "I eat with models on shoots; they order cheeseburgers. They are genetically thin. I've got to work at it. Some days it's easy to eat well and exercise, other days are tough. On the tough days, you have to stay focused," she advises. Also a registered dietician for 23 years and author of *Feel Fantastic* (Macmillan, Canada), Musk shares her own strategies and experiences to help others lose weight.

---

experts. Chapters 9 through 14 will hone in on ways of thinking, eating, and exercise that can at least get you down to your set point, and, perhaps, break through it. Chapters 6 and 7 will point to programs that can help you through the process; some better than others.

Just the facts

- Although the reasons behind overeating and under "burning" are complex, getting fat still boils down to a calorie imbalance.

- Genes are very important in lab animal obesity; their importance in human obesity is still being tested.

- Set point—the weight and body fat levels your body defends—can be changed.
- All the research into the whys of obesity will certainly translate into drugs to stem it.
- You can't blame it all on genes; the rise in obesity rates shows that our diet and habits are big culprits in body-fat accumulation.

GET THE SCOOP ON...
What's really in that pizza ▪
Reading labels ▪ Food pyramids

Nutrition Basics to Keep You Basically Healthy

Time to hang up your food hang-ups for a chapter and discover some nitty-gritty important food facts. Like lower fat isn't always better, and some fats will make you smarter. Or, if you're eating a typical American diet, you're low in the fiber department, and fiber can do great things for your diet. This nutrition primer equips you with the facts about what foods are made of and shows you how two U.S. government issue nutrition tools—the food label and the Food Guide Pyramid—can help you construct a better diet.

What's in that pizza?

Eat a pizza, and you've covered three of the four sources of calories, also called *macronutrients*: fat (in the cheese), carbohydrate (in the crust, tomato sauce, and cheese), and protein (cheese again).

Unofficially . . .
The National
Cancer Institute
recommends you
get 20 to 30
grams (abbrevi-
ated *g*) of fiber
daily with
an upper limit
of 35 g; most
Americans meet
only a third of
their fiber needs.
The rule of
thumb for kids:
age + five, up
until age 18. For
instance, a six-
year-old should
take in 6 + 5, or
11 g daily.

Have it with beer, and you downed the fourth: alcohol (see Chapter 3 on how alcohol affects body
weight). Few foods are purely one type of macronu-
trient; most, like pizza, are a mixture. Read on to
learn what you need to know about macronutrients.

Carbohydrate complex

With all the fuss surrounding carbohydrates, you'd
think they were controlled substances. Diet books
such as *The Carbohydrate Addict's Diet* and *Dr. Atkins'
New Diet Revolution* severely restrict carbohydrates,
and we chide ourselves for giving into our "carb
cravings" (see Chapter 7 for more on low-carb
diets). I know a woman who won't let herself near a
loaf of French bread for fear she'll devour it all.
Let's get one thing straight: Carbohydrates, especially certain types, are not only healthy, but they are
the body's preferred fuel. Our cells run best on glucose (same thing as blood sugar), the building block
of most carbohydrates, and their eventual breakdown product. Carbs come in two basic varieties:

- Simple carbohydrates, which taste sweet and
  consist of one or two sugar molecules such as
  glucose and fructose (both found in fruit and
  honey), sucrose (table sugar), and the milk sugars lactose and galactose. Simple carbs sweeten
  soda, jelly beans, ice cream, and other sweets.

- Complex carbohydrates, which are like long
  Lego units of glucose linked together. In that
  form, they no longer taste sweet. The complex
  carbohydrates you eat are mainly starch and
  fiber. Since fiber can't be digested or absorbed,
  it has no caloric value.

Bread, any grain product (rice, barley, cereal),
and starchy vegetables such as potatoes and corn are

mainly complex carbs, with a little protein and a trace of fat. Fruits and more watery vegetables contain both simple carbs and complex carbs in the form of fiber.

Instead of avoiding them, we should make complex carbohydrates constitute the bulk of our diet, 55 to 65 percent of total calories, according to the leading health authorities (the U.S. government, the American Cancer Society, the American Dietetic Association, and the American Heart Association). There are certain situations when a slightly lower carb level is healthier (see Chapter 7's review of 40/30/30 diets). But otherwise, the consensus is that high complex carb diets are the healthiest. Why?

- **Energizers.** Remember the Lego glucose units? Well, they unlink slowly into your bloodstream, giving off steady energy. In contrast, sugar and other sweeteners flood the system with glucose, which, for many people, causes a short surge of energy followed by an energy lull.

- **Nutrient knockouts.** Grain-based foods, especially those made with whole grains such as whole wheat bread, oatmeal, and brown rice, are rich in B vitamins, which are critical for transforming food to energy and ensuring proper nerve function. Grains are also sprinkled with zinc, iron, calcium, and other minerals. And recent research has uncovered other disease-fighting compounds in whole grains, such as antioxidants (chemicals that ward off cancer, heart disease, and other age-related conditions) and phytoestrogens (plant compounds very similar to estrogen, which may help reduce estrogen-related cancers such as

66

Studies link whole grains to protection from colorectal, gastric, and endometrial cancers and heart disease. And the research looks promising for a protective effect against breast cancer protection and diabetes.
—Joanne Slavin, Ph.D., RD, Professor in the Department of Food Science and Nutrition at the University of Minnesota.

99

Timesaver
Forgot to soak dried beans overnight? Buy canned beans and rinse them quickly with water to get rid of the sodium (some come with very little sodium to begin with). Don't worry, canned beans are very nutritious, about equal to dried and cooked.

breast and uterine cancer). Processed grains, such as white flour, don't have antioxidants or phytoestrogens.

- **Fiber-filled.** Whole grains pack in dietary fiber, linked to reduced risk of heart disease, diabetes, and colon and other cancers. Also, dietary fiber is a dieter's best friend, making you feel full longer on fewer calories and trapping some of the fat you just ate and sending it out of the body before it can be absorbed. While sugar and other simple carbs have nothing to offer nutritionally except calories, they're fine in moderation.

Protein overload

Many of those same diet books that restrict carbohydrates jack up protein, making an unhealthy situation even worse, as you'll see in Chapter 7. And it doesn't take a fancy fad diet to tip the protein balance. Americans typically eat 60 percent more protein than they need, according to U.S. Department of Agriculture surveys. As you can see in Table 4.1, it doesn't take much to meet your daily protein needs.

Adults need→ about .36 g of protein per pound of body weight. Therefore a 150 pound person needs 54 g of protein daily. Watch how easy it is to get that amount from foods you'd typically eat over the course of a day; no wonder we overdo it.

TABLE 4.1   HOW MUCH PROTEIN DO YOU NEED?

Food	g Protein
2 glasses of milk	16
1 cup wheat flake cereal	5
2 slices bread	4
1/2 chicken breast (3 oz. cooked)	27
1 teaspoon peanut butter	2
TOTAL	**54**

Do you have to eat meat, chicken, or other foods of animal origin to get enough protein? No, you simply have to take in enough of the building blocks of protein, called amino acids, which you can get from plant-based foods, such as grains, beans, and vegetables. Your body will put them together into protein for muscles, organs, and enzymes. Protein's made of a combination of over 20 amino acids; different foods contain varying amounts.

- Complete, or high-quality, protein contains the nine amino acids that the body cannot make, called *essential amino acids*. Meat, poultry, chicken, fish, eggs, soy protein concentrate, and dairy products are complete proteins.

- Incomplete proteins, such as dried beans, nuts, bread, corn, and rice, are missing one or more essential amino acids. But combine them and you get the full complement. These foods are also high in carbohydrates.

"Incomplete" has a worrisome ring to it, but countless studies show that vegetarians, who rely mainly on incomplete protein, have a lower risk for many chronic diseases. With the exception of soy protein concentrate, complete proteins are all animal-based, and too much animal protein is linked to a higher risk of cancer. You'll keep your protein level under control if you stick with the pyramid guidelines outlined later in this chapter.

Fat flap

Fat's going from public enemy number one to, well, something more benign, although researchers are still not sure how much of what type of fat we should be eating. The "less fat the better" mantra of the past few decades turned us into a nation of fat phobics. In fact, a faction of experts saw the U.S. government's recommended 30 percent of calories from fat as a cop-out, saying you have to get down to

Unofficially . . .
Sugar has gotten a bum rap over the years, singled out as the cause of everything from hyperactivity to yeast infections. The science hasn't borne out any of the accusations, except that sugar does give you cavities. However, eating lots of ice cream, cookies, danishes, and the like is a good way to put on the pounds because of their double calorie whammy: simple sugars plus fat. And many of the fat-free versions of these foods are just as caloric thanks to an extra dose of sugar.

Bright Idea
You don't have
to eat your
beans and rice at
the same meal to
get a "complete"
protein. Simply
eating these
foods within the
same day is suf-
ficient. That also
works for bread
and beans or
bread and nuts.

20 percent to see health benefits. But recently the research has cut fat some slack, showing that more might be okay, as long as it's the right type of fat.

What's the "right" type? As you probably know, there are different types of fat. Fats are classified according to their level of saturation—a chemical term describing their structure. Usually, one type predominates in the fats we eat; for instance, about 74 percent of the fat in olive oil is monounsaturated, 11 percent is polyunsaturated, and 15 percent is saturated. The tricky part is that fat, no matter if it's the healthy or less healthy type, is still very high in calories, with over twice the calories per gram as carbohydrate or protein. So if you're watching your weight, keep fat to about 30 percent of calories (follow the pyramid guidelines below and you'll hit about 30 percent). But don't go lower than 20 percent—otherwise you may miss out on vitamins A, E, D, and K, called fat-soluble vitamins because the body absorbs them best when there's a little fat in the meal. When you do include fat in the diet, here's the healthiest strategy based on the current scientific knowledge (yes, I'm qualifying here—when it comes to fat, things do change . . .).

Choose more of:

- **Monounsaturated fat,** plentiful in olive oil, canola oil, almond and hazelnut oils, and avocado oil, helps lower LDL, the blood cholesterol carrier that clogs up your arteries without lowering levels of HDL—the blood cholesterol carrier that transports cholesterol out of your body. It appears not to increase cancer risk.

- **Omega-3s** are types of polyunsaturated fats, plentiful in fatty fish (the ingredient in fish oil tablets) and flaxseed oil. Omega-3s have been linked to lower risk of heart attacks, to improved mood, to smarter infants (if the mother ate fish during pregnancy and lactation), and to lessening of rheumatoid arthritis symptoms. Unless your doctor recommends fish oil tablets, get this fat from eating at least two fish meals a week (fatty fish such as salmon, haddock, sardines, or bluefish have the most).

Use moderately:

■ **Omega-6** polyunsaturated fat is the predominant fat in corn, safflower, sunflower, soy, and "vegetable" oils. Peanut oil is high in both poly and monos, so it's a better choice than these oils, but not as good as the high monounsaturated oils listed above. While this type doesn't raise blood cholesterol, when used as your staple fat it may raise cancer risk.

Use less of:

■ **Saturated fat,** found in fats of animal origin (butter, lard, chicken fat, red meat) and palm and coconut oils. Too much of this one raises blood cholesterol, much more than eating cholesterol itself.

■ **Trans fat,** formed when polyunsaturated vegetable oils become "partially hydrogenated" oils by undergoing a chemical process which hardens them into margarine or other shortenings. Main sources in our diet: hard, stick margarines (soft tub types have much less trans), fast foods, and packaged cookies, cakes, and crackers. Research has started to link this type of fat with increased risk for heart disease, and a few studies indicate a connection to breast cancer. While a little bit won't hurt, it's best to limit foods containing this fat. Don't avoid otherwise healthy,

> 66
> The dramatic shift in the last century away from omega-3 and toward omega-6 has caused a widespread, subclinical omega-3 deficiency which rarely produces overt symptoms, but seems to gradually take its toll on your health.
> —William Conner, MD, professor of medicine, Division of Endocrinology, Diabetes, and Nutrition at Oregon Health Sciences University in Portland.
> 99

low-fat foods just because they contain partially hydrogenated oil, for instance, whole wheat bread or a whole grain cereal.

Bright Idea
Since trans fat, implicated in raising the risk for heart disease and breast cancer, isn't listed on the nutrition label, you can figure out whether a food contains it by moving down to the ingredient list. The give-away: "partially hydrogenated" vegetable oil. You can find trans-free alternatives to cookies, crackers, and other baked goods in the health food store.

Two notes here: First, don't expect to see all these different fats on food labels. All the food label is required to tell you is the amount of total fat and saturated fat. If you're lucky, the company will voluntarily give you levels of monos and polys. But polys won't be further broken down into omega-3 or omega-6. And even though trans fat acts very much like saturated fat in your body, on a nutrition label it's included only under total fat, not under any of the specific fats such as saturated, monounsaturated, or polyunsaturated. As of press time for this book, the Food and Drug Administration is considering a petition to include trans on the label. Secondly, I didn't include cholesterol in this list because it's not a fat, but a waxy substance that our cells manufacture and that we get in the diet. But it belongs in the "Use less of" category because in excess it can contribute to high blood cholesterol, although not as potently as saturated fat. The recommended upper limit for cholesterol is 300 mg (.3 g) daily.

Food labels cut through the hype

Okay, now you know to minimize saturated and trans fats, to switch over to monounsaturates and omega-3, to eat more whole grains, and keep a lid on protein. But how the heck can you tell what levels of these nutrients are in foods? Fuhgeddaboudit! You've got better things to do than memorize the number of fat grams in an Oreo or the protein content of a chicken breast. And you don't have to—just nailing the basics of the Food Guide Pyramid (see Figure 4.2) will help keep your diet in order. But there is one instance when it's worth examining the minutia of food composition—when you're out buying groceries. That's when the nutrition label really comes in handy, pointing out the differences between products. Trying to decide between corn flakes or raisin bran? Wow, 8 grams of fiber in the raisin bran, only 1 gram in the corn flakes. And look, spaghetti sauce A has twice the sodium as spaghetti sauce B. Check out this sample label, and see how it relates to your diet goals:

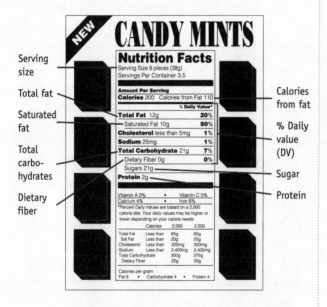

Figure 4.1 This sample label lists the required nutrients; some labels get more detailed, letting you in on the amounts of polyunsaturated and monounsaturated fat, and including more vitamins and minerals.

- **Serving size.** Scan this first to see what kind of portions they're talking. Eight little mints? See how easy it is to double and triple some of these servings?

- **Calories from fat.** Gives you a sense of the percentage. As long as the total diet is about 30 percent calories from fat, it doesn't matter if an individual food is higher.

- **% Daily value (DV).** In the case of fat, saturated fat, protein, and carbohydrate, these percentages are based on a 2,000-calorie diet. If you're trying to lose weight, you need fewer calories, somewhere between 1,400 to 1,800. Therefore this food will use up a bigger percent of your daily fat, carbs, and protein than the label shows. With all the rest of the nutrients, the DV is based on set standards for all calorie levels.

- **Total fat.** One high-fat food won't hurt you as long as you keep the overall fat level low, to 40 to 55 g daily (56 to 65 g if you're not trying to lose weight).

- **Saturated fat.** Here's one to watch. Saturated fat raises blood cholesterol, and high blood cholesterol increases your risk for heart disease. Have no more than 13 to 18 g daily (19 to 22 g if you're not trying to lose weight)—the less the better.

- **Total carbohydrates.** Includes complex (starch, fiber) and simple (sugars).

- **Dietary fiber.** Pay particular attention to this one when shopping for cereal (aim for at least 3 g per serving) and bread (aim for 2 g per slice). Your daily goal: 20 to 30 g, not to exceed 35 g.

- **Sugar.** It's sobering when you figure that 4 g of sugar equals one teaspoon. So your eight mints are the same as five teaspoons of straight sugar! The less the better when you're trying to lose weight.

- **Protein.** Remember, we don't need all that much.

On the front of the label you'll find other terms, like "light" and "reduced fat." It used to be that food manufacturers could slap these on whether they meant something or not. A few years ago the Food and Drug Administration came up with strict definitions for many of the terms, listed in Table 4.2.

Watch Out!
Don't choose one food over another just because it's labeled "no cholesterol." Only foods of animal origin contain cholesterol, so of course peanut butter and vegetable oils are cholesterol free. This claim on a naturally cholesterol-free food is just a marketing ploy.

TABLE 4.2 FEDERAL DEFINITIONS FOR NUTRITION CLAIMS

Claim	Definition
Fat free	Fewer than 0.5 g of fat per serving
Low fat	3 g of fat or fewer per serving
Reduced or less fat	At least 25 percent less fat than the regular version of that food
Cholesterol free	Fewer than 2 mg of cholesterol and 2 g or fewer of saturated fat per serving
Low cholesterol	20 mg or fewer and 2 g or fewer of saturated fat per serving
Reduced or less cholesterol	At least 25 percent less and 2 g or fewer of saturated fat per serving than the regular version
Sodium free	Fewer than 5 mg per serving
Low sodium	140 mg or fewer per serving
Very low sodium	35 mg or fewer per serving
Reduced or less sodium	At least 25 percent less per serving than the regular version
High fiber	5 g or more per serving
Good source of fiber	2.5 to 4.9 g per serving
More or added fiber	At least 2.5 g more per serving than the regular food

Be as careful with reduced-fat or fat-free foods as you would with the regular version: In many cases the calories are nearly identical. That's because the food is injected with extra sugar or other carbohydrates, bringing calorie levels back up. For instance:

Unofficially . . .
It's still contro-
versial, but you
can get a num-
ber of experts to
agree that one
or two eggs a
day are okay if
your diet is vir-
tually vegetarian
with some nonfat
dairy thrown in.
But that drops
to three to four
eggs *weekly* if
you regularly eat
high-cholesterol
or saturated-fat
foods such
as burgers
and poultry
with skin. Egg
whites are okay
anytime; it's the
yolk that carries
the cholesterol.
Remember,
much more
than dietary
cholesterol, it's
too much satu-
rated fat that
raises blood
cholesterol.

2 Tbsp. regular peanut butter	190–200 calories
2 Tbsp. reduced-fat peanut butter	190–200 calories
2 regular Fig Newtons	110 calories
2 fat-free Fig Newtons	100 calories
3 Oreos	160 calories
3 reduced-fat Oreos	140 calories

So if you want to buy reduced-fat or fat-free, go ahead, but keep portions moderate.

The pyramid: substance versus sensationalism

It's not sexy or exciting, hanging out in elementary school classrooms instead of the pages of best-selling diet books, but it's actually a pretty good weight loss tool. It's just that The U.S. Department of Agriculture's (USDA) Food Guide Pyramid doesn't get your hopes up the way *The 5-Day Miracle Diet* or *30 Days to Swimsuit Lean* can. It's kind of like a date with a nerdy scientist; at first you wish you were listening to sweet nothings from that sexy hunk, but by the end of the night the scientist has grown on you—he's someone you can stick with. Stick with the guidelines on that pyramid, and you'll not only lose some weight, but get your diet back in balance.

The USDA pyramid and the other pyramids presented in this chapter weren't designed as a weight loss program, but as a model for nutritionally balanced diets. But tweak them a little and you get some very good weight loss diets for those who like their diets as unstructured as possible. No menu plans, no recipes, just a loose framework that you can plug your own foods into.

The USDA's pyramid

As you can see in Figure 4.2, the USDA's Food Guide Pyramid is based on servings of food, not on calories, fat grams, or other forgettable numbers. With a few exceptions, the food groups make sense, offering similar nutrients in each category. These divisions aren't perfect—for instance, cheese went into the dairy group when it also fits into the protein group (meat, poultry, fish, dry beans, eggs, and nuts). And beans and nuts, although high in protein, are in other ways very different nutritionally from animal protein.

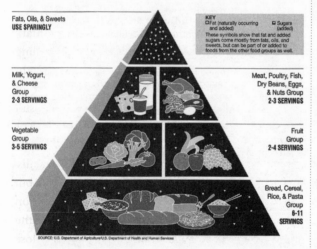

Figure 4.2
The Food Guide Pyramid. Drawing from all five food groups increases your chances of getting all the nutrients your body needs. But if you're a strict vegan (eating plant-based foods only), you can safely skip the dairy group as long as you have calcium-fortified soy or rice milk. Otherwise, as you can see from Table 4.3, each food group contributes a different set of vital nutrients.

The Pyramid talks a good talk, but if you are in deep calorie denial, it leaves room for dangerous interpretations, especially if you don't read the fine print on the accompanying brochure. Sorry, you won't lose weight if croissants are your bread, cereal, rice, and pasta group staple and whole milk and fatty steaks constitute the dairy and protein groups. Table 4.3 shows how to turn it into a pyramid you can get healthy on.

TABLE 4.3   MAKING THE MOST OF THE PYRAMID

Food Group	Nutrition Highlights	Make It Better
Bread, cereal, rice, and pasta	Grain products are good sources of B vitamins and critical for converting food to energy and for a healthy nervous system.	Choose whole grains (whole wheat bread, more fiber and more bran, and pasta) for more nutrients than processed grains. Also, choose lower-fat foods in this category—bread, english muffins, and bagels instead of croissants, danishes, doughnuts, and biscuits.

A serving is: one slice bread; $1/2$ cup cooked pasta, rice, or other grain; 1 oz. cold cereal or 1 cup hot; or any 80-calorie complex carbohydrate.

Food Group	Nutrition Highlights	Make It Better
Vegetables	Excellent sources of vitamins A and C and hundreds of disease-fighting compounds called phytochemicals. Also good sources of fiber.	All vegetables are nutritious; some seem particularly so. Brussels sprouts, broccoli, cauliflower, water watercress, yams, carrots, onions, garlic, and dark leafy greens contain potent health-producing compounds. Limit french fries and other fried vegetables to twice a month; when sautéeing, go easy on the oil.

A serving is: 1 cup of raw leafy vegetables; $1/2$ cup other vegetables, chopped or cooked; $3/4$ cup vegetable juice.

Food Group	Nutrition Highlights	Make It Better
Fruits	Stellar sources of vitamin C and fiber, and rich in phytochemicals.	Limit juice to once a day. Go with whole fruit, which is much higher in fiber and lower in calories. Good bets: citrus, cantaloupe, strawberries, kiwi for vitamin C, and oranges for folic acid (helps prevent birth defects).

A serving is: one medium apple, orange, or banana; $1/2$ cup chopped, cooked, or canned fruit; $3/4$ cup fruit juice.

Food Group	Nutrition Highlights	Make It Better
Milk, yogurt, and cheese	Our major source of calcium, the mineral critical for making and maintaining strong bones and helping stave off osteoporosis, a debilitating bone-thinning disease.	Save over a teaspoon of fat per cup by working your way down from whole milk and 2 percent to $1/2$ percent or nonfat milk or yogurt. Add your own fruit and a little honey to plain yogurt for fewer calories and more nutrients.

A serving is: 1 cup milk or plain yogurt, $1 1/2$ oz. cheese.

Food Group	Nutrition Highlights	Make It Better
Meat, poultry, dry beans, eggs, and nuts	The pyramid has been criticized for lumping together these nutritionally diverse foods. What they have in common are good sources of protein. But beans are high in fiber and carbs, red meat is iron-rich, poultry has more of the B vitamin niacin, and nuts are much higher in fat.	Go vegetarian a few times a week, using beans or tofu for protein. Otherwise stick with lean red meat (round, sirloin, or skirt steak), skinless poultry, or lean (5 per-cent or less fat) ham. Have fish at least twicea week to help prevent heart disease, and limit nuts—they're wildly caloric.

A serving is: 2 or 3 oz. cooked lean meat, poultry, or fish (about the size of a deck of cards). Foods that count as 1 oz. meat: $1/2$ cup cooked dried beans, one egg, 2 Tbsp. peanut butter, $1/3$ cup nuts.

Food Group	Nutrition Highlights	Make It Better
Fats, oils, and sweets	We need about a teaspoon of fat daily for "essential fats," those our bodies can't make. Then we need a little more to help us feel full longer and make things taste better. Sorry, no such justification for sugar or other sweeteners.	Compare labels, picking the lower-sugar and lower-fat items. Remember, 4 g sugar = 1 tsp. (so that's 10 tsp. in a can of soda!). Use olive and canola oil in cooking (they're healthier), and limit foods containing trans fat (those made with hydrogenated or partially hydrogenated oil) and saturated fat.

No serving size given. A good rule of thumb: Keep added fats (those you smear or drizzle on like butter or salad dressing) between 4 and 6 tsp. daily and added sugar between 1 and 5 tsp. daily. And limit foods that are loaded with fat (french fries and other fried foods, fatty meats, and high-fat dairy, for example) or fat *and* sugar (like ice cream, cookies, and cake).

Keeping the pyramid low cal

Now, to lose weight on the pyramid, you have to stick with the lower-fat foods in each food group (refer to Table 4.3 for guidelines), and for some groups, go with the lower range of servings. Table 4.4 shows what 1,500 and 1,700 calories look like on a low-fat pyramid plan . . . pretty generous, huh?

TABLE 4.4 LOW-FAT PYRAMID PLAN SERVINGS AND CALORIES

	1,500 calories	1,700 calories
Bread group servings	6	8
Vegetable group servings	3	3
Fruit group servings	2	3
Milk group servings	2–3	2–3
Meat group servings	2	2
Added fat (in teaspoons)	5	5
Added sugar (in teaspoons)	4	4

Here's how that translates into food on a 1,500-calorie day:

Breakfast

Bowl of cereal with skim milk (one "bread," one "milk")

with a sliced banana (one fruit)

$3/4$ cup orange juice (one fruit)

coffee with a teaspoon of sugar (1 tsp. sugar)

Lunch

Tuna salad (3 oz. tuna, 1 tsp. mayo) (one "meat," 1 tsp. fat) on whole wheat bread (two "breads")

with sliced tomatoes ($1/2$ vegetable)

apple (one fruit)

three Hershey's kisses (equivalent to 2 tsp. sugar, 1 tsp. fat)

Snack

Low-fat nachos:

$^3/_4$ ounce fat-free tortilla chips
(one "bread")

with $^3/_4$ ounces low-fat cheese melted
($^1/_2$ "milk")

$^1/_3$ cup salsa ($^1/_2$ vegetable)

Dinner

1 cup spaghetti (two "breads")

with tomato sauce ($^1/_2$ vegetable)

and shrimp (one "meat")

1 Tbsp. parmesan cheese ($^1/_2$ "milk")

1 cup mixed vegetables stir-fry (in 2 tsp. oil)
(1 vegetable, 2 tsp. fat)

The "other" pyramids

A variety of organizations have come up with a whole slew of pyramids, including ones for Latin food and Asian food. I've chosen the vegetarian and Mediterranean pyramids because there's so much research showing these ways of eating are healthy and generally slimming.

A pyramid vegetarians can call their own

As you can see, the major points of departure between this pyramid and the good ol' USDA standard are the addition of fortified alternatives (that means rice or soy milk fortified with calcium and other nutrients) in the "milk" group, and, of course, the complete exclusion of any animal/fish/bird meat in the "protein" group. Also, the vegetarian pyramid calls for whole grains up front, not in the fine print.

Moneysaver
Buying in-season fruits and vegetables from a farmer's market can save a bundle. For instance, while supermarket apples are selling for $1.40 a pound, you can buy fresher, way-crisper, much more delicious ones for 60¢ a pound from the farmer's stall.

Figure 4.3 The
Vegetarian Food
Pyramid. I like
this vegetarian
pyramid, put out
by The Health
Connection, a
health consult-
ing group based
in Hagerstown,
Maryland,
because you can
plug it into all of
the healthy diet
plans that use
food exchanges.

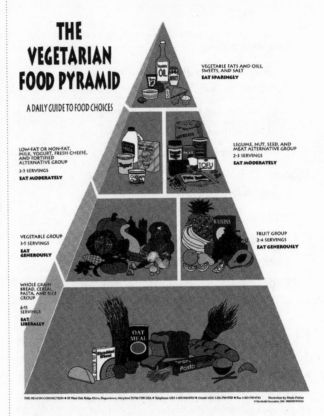

For the most part, the serving sizes are the same as those listed in Table 4.3, "Making the Most of the Pyramid." Here's some additional info to help you use this pyramid:

- If you don't eat dairy foods, for each glass of milk or yogurt substitute soy or rice milk forti-fied with at least 25 percent of the daily value (DV) for calcium per cup (reduced fat is best). Otherwise, your diet could run low on this vital mineral.

- For this pyramid, servings sizes in the protein group are:

$^{1}/_{2}$ cup cooked dried beans or peas

$^{1}/_{2}$ cup tofu

$^{1}/_{4}$ cup seeds, such as sunflower seeds

$^{1}/_{4}$ cup nuts

2 Tbsp. nut butter, such as peanut or almond butter

$^{1}/_{4}$ cup meat alternative (such as soy-based ground meat substitute)

2 egg whites

▪ To keep fat and calories low, choose nuts no more than four times a week.

Bright Idea
Carotenoids are the plant pigment that give carrots, squash, and yams their orange color and are present (though masked by all the green chlorophyll) in dark green vegetables, such as broccoli and kale. In the body, carotenoids, such as beta-carotene, battle disease-promoting compounds called free radicals. Since carotenoids dissolve in fat, you'll absorb more from vegetables if you sautée them in oil. Don't go overboard with the oil—just a thin coating in the pan is all you need.

While vegetarian diets are generally healthier than the typical American diet (because they're lower in saturated fat and animal protein and higher in fruits and vegetables), done wrong, they can actually be more unhealthy. Think about it— a teenager can call herself vegetarian and subsist on french fries and milkshakes. But follow this pyramid, and you're covered. Well, almost. If you are a vegan (eating only plant-based foods) and avoiding dairy and eggs, you run the chance of not getting enough of two vitamins: B12 and D. B12 is critical for proper red blood cell formation and is found in all foods of animal origin, such as meat, poultry, dairy, and fish. The main dietary source of vitamin D—which helps put calcium in bone—is D-fortified milk. Vitamin D is also made in the body in reaction to sunlight hitting the skin, so if you get 15 minutes of sunlight daily (just arms or legs is enough) you probably don't need to get D from milk. But in many parts of the country, it's hard to get enough sunlight in winter months. Two easy vegan solutions: fortified cereals and fortified soy or rice milk (check labels for at least 25 percent of the DV per cup of both D and B12).

Mediterranean eating

Piles of research papers show that people living in Greece, Southern Italy, and other Mediterranean countries have lower risks of heart disease and cancer. They are also thinner than we are. Though other lifestyle factors come into play, researchers are convinced that the Mediterranean diet, rich in fruits and vegetables, low in saturated fat but rich in monounsaturated fat (from olive oil) deserves much of the credit. Oldways, a society of scientists (including prominent Harvard researchers) interested in the Mediterranean diet and other traditional diets came up with this Mediterranean pyramid.

Figure 4.4 The Mediterranean Diet Pyramid. If you love Greek and Southern Italian food, here's a pyramid tailored to your tastes. Research shows that this way of eating is linked to reduced risk of heart disease and certain types of cancer.

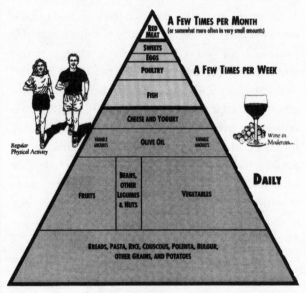

A FEW TIMES PER MONTH (or somewhat more often in very small amounts)

RED MEAT

SWEETS

EGGS

POULTRY   A FEW TIMES PER WEEK

FISH

CHEESE AND YOGURT

Regular Physical Activity   VARIABLE AMOUNTS   OLIVE OIL   VARIABLE AMOUNTS   Wine in Moderati...

FRUITS   BEANS, OTHER LEGUMES & NUTS   VEGETABLES   DAILY

BREADS, PASTA, RICE, COUSCOUS, POLENTA, BULGUR, OTHER GRAINS, AND POTATOES

If you're looking gleefully at the lack of serving sizes for olive oil and cheese, remember, you eat more of the foods that get the biggest blocks. The blocks for olive oil and cheese aren't so big. One reason this pyramid doesn't specify number of servings is that it wasn't created for weight loss. However, with a little tinkering it makes for a great way to eat while you're losing weight and forever after. Here's how to make the Mediterranean pyramid more low-cal:

- Keep the bottom "grain" block to about six servings daily (use serving sizes in Table 4.3).

- Eat even more than five servings total of fruits and vegetables.

- In the "Beans, Other Legumes and Nuts" category, choose beans frequently, nuts rarely (just once or twice a week, no more than 1/4 cup).

- Use no more than 4 to 7 total teaspoons of olive oil daily (includes sautéeing, dipping, salad dressing, and so on).

- If you eat cheese more than three times a week, make it reduced fat (no more than 5 grams fat per ounce). For any cheese, try to keep portions down to one to two ounces.

- For the "A few times a week" foods, use common sense with portion sizes. For instance, three Hershey's kisses a few times a week won't put on pounds, but a big slab of cheesecake four times a week will.

- Alcohol is pretty high in calories (seven calories per gram, a little more than carbs or protein, a little less than fat). A good rule of thumb: limit alcohol to four drinks a week.

Watch Out!
Drinking alcohol is good for your heart; that's why it's on the Mediterranean pyramid. But more than three drinks a day and alcohol starts becoming less healthy. And even one drink a day raises breast cancer risk for women. Bottom line: If you've got a family history of breast cancer, don't drink—or stop at four drinks a week. If heart disease runs in the family, don't go beyond three drinks a day (no more than one if you're trying to lose weight).

Just the facts

- All carbs and all fats are not created equal; whole-grain complex carbs and monounsaturated and omega-3 fats are healthiest. And hey, watch that protein.

- Forget about fat grams or any grams until you get to the market; then ruthlessly compare products using the food label.

- Much more than a Home Ec yawn, the food pyramids—all three of them—make for a happening diet, especially if you tweak them the right way.

GET THE SCOOP ON...
Using supplements ▪ All about vitamins and
minerals ▪ Other disease fighters

Vital Nutrients

If you're cutting calories, you probably need to supplement. But with the thousands of options out there, trying to figure out which vitamin or mineral supplements to take home with you can drive anyone to a Stresstab. But don't do it! Stresstabs don't make any difference; they're just one example of many, many, misleading or implied claims that show up on supplement labels. Manufacturers get particularly creative—and amoral—when it comes to selling you fake weight loss supplements.

Still, there *are* good supplements out there. Use this chapter to pick a good vitamin and mineral supplement, so that you leave the drugstore or health food store with a worthwhile value instead of a gimmicky rip-off. The info here will help keep you at tiptop health. Supplements that claim to do more, to "melt fat" or in other ways promote weight loss, are a different kettle of fish. To see just how fishy that business is, turn to Chapter 8.

Why supplement?

Do you even need a supplement? If you're eating about 2,000 calories and your diet looks just like those pyramids in Chapter 4, you may not need one. However, studies show that even then it's hard to get 100 percent of the recommended levels of vitamins and minerals. So if you're on a reduced calorie diet, you can forget about getting all the nutrients you need through diet alone.

But here's the catch: Supplementing is still no guarantee that you'll be adequately protecting yourself from killer diseases like cancer. You still have to eat a good diet to make all those reduced calories count as much as possible. Because, as labs around the world are discovering, it's much more than the vitamins and minerals in foods that are keeping you healthy, it's also the hundreds, perhaps thousands, of other naturally occurring chemicals, mainly found in grains and fruits and vegetables. Over 200 studies confirm that people who eat the most fruits and vegetables have a third to half the risk of getting cancer and heart disease as those who eat the fewest. Vitamin C, beta-carotene, or other known vitamins and minerals in oranges, broccoli, and other types of produce are protective, but credit also lies with recently discovered—and yet-undiscovered— food substances and in the way nutrients interact in foods. So your first line of defense is to eat a pyramid-style diet (see Chapter 4) rich in fruits, vegetables, whole grains, and low-fat dairy foods.

But now the evidence is trickling in that supplementing with pills is also protective. Some preliminary findings: multivitamin and mineral tablets may boost immunity (making you less susceptible to colds and other respiratory infections), improve mood, and slash your risk of heart attack. The case for supplementing with folic acid enjoys rare, universal support among scientists because of solid research showing that it lowers the risk of having a baby with a type of birth defect called neural tube defect. Getting lots of calcium and vitamin D seems to help ward off osteoporosis, a debilitating bone-thinning disease; it's hard to get all that calcium and D without a supplement. And while the government health authorities and some researchers are still reluctant to recommend supplementing with vitamin E, many other leaders in the nutrition field wholeheartedly support it.

Buying a decent supplement

Once you've checked out the vitamin and mineral tables (Tables 5.2 and 5.3 and the end of this chapter) and taken a good hard look at your diet, you may make the decision to supplement. If so, take a deep breath, and read on. Your purchasing decision is about to get a lot easier. Despite the overwhelming variety, picking one that fits in with current scientific thinking isn't that hard. Just go for a multivitamin/mineral ("multi") tablet at levels close to 100 percent of the Daily Value. At this point in the research, herbs and other substances haven't been proven useful, so I'd skip them; they just make things pricier. That's the basic advice. To make sure your pill is good quality and you're not overpaying for unnecessary nonsense, read on.

When selecting a multi, look for safe levels of vitamins and minerals. What's reasonable? Multis that hover around 100 percent of the DV. Some brands give you all that in one tablet; others crowd out the important stuff with unproven herbs and other substances so you end up taking two to six tablets to

Watch Out!
Vitamins A and D and some minerals are lethal in high doses. (Those doses are usually at minimum 10 times higher than the recommended levels.) Less serious, but still harmful: slightly higher than recom-mended levels of some nutrients can block the absorption of other nutrients. So, stick with the recommended levels of nutrients by making sure levels on your multivitamin hover around 100 percent of the daily value (DV). Vitamin E is the exception; higher levels seem beneficial (see Table 5.2 for details).

get 100 percent of your DV levels. Here are some of the claims you'll encounter on the label of a multivitamin:

- "High Potency": Currently it can mean anything, but under the new FDA ruling to go into effect March 1999, it will mean that two-thirds of the vitamins and minerals in the multi are at levels of 100 percent or more of the DV. On a single nutrient pill, it means there's at least 100 percent the DV of that nutrient.

- "Including the Complete Antioxidant Group": Complete according to whom? There are potentially hundreds of substances out there that act as antioxidants: compounds that may help protect us from cancer, heart disease, and other age-related conditions by destroying cell-damaging molecules called "free radicals." In normal label usage it means beta-carotene, vitamins C and E, and selenium. The FDA plans to evaluate whether this claim is misleading on a case-by-case basis.

- "%Daily Value": Often listed as "%DV," these are levels set by the Food and Drug Administration as a rough guide to nutrient needs of the general population of men and women. For some nutrients, it's a little more than an adult woman needs (for instance the recommended level of zinc is 15 mg for men, 12 mg for women; the FDA chose 15 mg for the DV), but the levels are still within a very safe range. Buy tablets that don't exceed 100 percent of the DV for any nutrient; higher doses are gimmicky.

- "Vitamin A (As acetate and beta-carotene) 5,000 IU, 100% DV": Acetate is vitamin A, and beta-carotene is a plant pigment that your body converts to vitamin A as needed. Also, beta-carotene has its own benefits as an antioxidant. Ideally, the label should plainly tell you what percent of vitamin A comes from beta-carotene. (A good ratio is 50/50.) When the new FDA regulations go into effect, labels must state the percent of vitamin A that's beta-carotene if somewhere else on the label a claim is made about beta-carotene (for instance, saying it's an antioxidant). Preg-nant women shouldn't get more than 5000 IU (International Units) of vitamin A daily from all sources; more than that may harm the fetus. However, beta-carotene in high doses does not appear to be harmful to pregnant women.

- "Iron 18 mg, 100% DV": Men and post-menopausal women need only 10 mg of iron; if that's you, then buy a "senior" vitamin to avoid iron overload (for details, see Table 5.3 at the end of this chapter).

- "Thiamin 1.5 mg, 100%; Riboflavin 1.7 mg, 100%; Niacin 20 mg, 100%; Vitamin B6 2 mg, 100%; Pantothenic Acid, 100%": A label listing 100% the DV for this group of vitamins (all B vitamins) is a tip-off to a responsible tablet. Gimmicky brands jack up levels of these inexpensive vitamins. Stick with no more than 200% the DV of Bs until research tells us otherwise.

- "Molybdenum, Chloride, Nickel, Tin, Silicon, Vanadium, Boron": Research shows these keep lab animals healthier, but there hasn't been enough research to tell whether or not these are essential to humans. Just in case, supplements include them in minute amounts.

Unofficially . . .
Research shows
that taking more
than 20 mg of
zinc daily starts
to cut into cop-
per absorption.
So stick close
to the recom-
mended 12 to 15
mg of zinc daily.

- "Expiration Date": The date by which you should have swallowed the last tablet, usually set about three years from the day the tablets are manufactured. Don't buy a tablet that's expiring in a month or two; a year or more is best—and *don't* buy tablets that lack an expiration date.

Congrats—you've found one or more multis that meet the basic guidelines just outlined. Now before opening your wallet, run down this checklist:

- **Expiration date.** It should be there, and at least a few months away.

- **USP.** Many of the supplements sold in drugstores and supermarkets (but virtually none in health food stores) are marked "USP," which stands for U.S. Pharmacopeia. This organization sets standards of quality for drugs and supplements. Since the Food and Drug Administration doesn't regulate supplements as strictly as drugs, it's up to the manufacturer to voluntarily comply with standards set by the USP. These standards ensure the following:

  1. The tablet will disintegrate into small pieces in the stomach and gut so that your system can absorb it.

  2. By the expiration date, it will contain at least 90 percent of the levels of nutrients stated on the label.

  3. The ingredients are pure, with a minimum of contaminants such as lead.

  While "USP" on the label doesn't guarantee a better pill, it's the best assurance we've got at the moment. If the whole tablet is "USP" (for instance it may read "Oil- and Water-soluble

Vitamins with Minerals Tablets USP") it means every vitamin and mineral has met USP standards. Sometimes the label indicates that only specific nutrients meet USP standards. If your supplement isn't marked USP, it still might meet the standards; call the manufacturer to find out. In other words a supplement not marked USP may be fine, but since supplements are so unregulated, seeing "USP" on the label raises the comfort level a notch.

- **$$$.** More expensive isn't necessarily better, especially if they're all marked "USP."

Here's what manufacturers tell you in hopes of impressing you and scaring you away from other brands. It's not that a supplement making these claims is necessarily a bad one, it could be high quality. It's just that supplements that don't try to fool you with this double-talk can also be of excellent quality.

TABLE 5.1 SPOTTING GIMMICKS ON MULTIVITAMIN LABELS

Claim	Why It's Hokey
A "woman's" multi	I've found that a regular multi is usually better. Women's multis tend to be high in iron, over 18 mg, which may be too high for most women (see Table 5.3 at the end of the chapter). These tablets may give you more than the standard 200 mg of calcium in most multis, but often at the expense of other minerals. That's because the tablet would look like a horse pill if they tried to fit in all that calcium on top of a complete roundup of everything else. Or, they do offer a complete array by having you take two to six pills. This works out to be way more expensive than buying a standard multi and taking a calcium tablet along with it.

continues

Moneysaver
Drugstore label vitamins are much less expensive than name brands and brands sold at health food stores and may be better quality. That's because many of them are marked "USP," meaning they have complied with voluntary standards set by the U.S. Pharmacopeia, the same organization that sets standards for drugs (explained earlier). It doesn't mean that brands that don't say USP are worse, but since supplements are so unregulated, it raises the comfort level a notch.

TABLE 5.1   (continued)

Claim	Why It's Hokey
Timed release	Drug manufacturers must prove that timed-release pills gradually release into your system, but supplement makers do not. So, you can't be sure this works; if it doesn't, the nutrients may get released too late, way down your intestines where they can't be absorbed.
No sugar, no starch	If a tablet did contain sugar, the minute amounts wouldn't make any difference calorie-wise. As for starch, it's actually a good thing because it helps the tablet disintegrate in your stomach. Gimmicks, gimmicks!
No artificial colors or flavors	Big deal, you eat these all the time and in these small amounts they haven't been shown to harm anyone except those rare people who have a sensitivity or allergy to them.
No preservatives	It's not as if other brands are poisoning you with preservatives; in fact, most don't have any. The vitamins themselves act as preservatives.
Sodium free	Sodium does appear in some tablets, sometimes bound to minerals, but in tiny amounts that don't make a difference, even if you're on a low sodium diet.
No wheat, no corn, no starch, no dairy	If there's no starch, then naturally there's no wheat, corn, or soy, all starch-based foods. Only those rare people allergic to these foods or to dairy benefit from this claim.
Yeast free	As if other manufacturers go around adding yeast to tablets! This statement is probably for the benefit of people who've been indoctrinated by a popular quacky misconception that an excess of yeast in the body is the root of many diseases.
Natural source of vitamin "whatever"	Even most vitamins labeled "natural" contain some synthetically derived vitamins—it would be prohibitively expensive to squeeze out all the vitamins and minerals from food sources. Both work equally well.

Claim	Why It's Hokey
Chelated minerals	Most pills bind their minerals to sodium or another element to form a salt; once swallowed the salt dissolves, freeing up the mineral. Chelated minerals are bound to other types of molecules, supposedly forming a looser bond, which frees the mineral more easily. Maybe—I've found no evidence that chelated minerals perform any better.
Bee pollen, herbs, and other oddities.	They'll stick anything into these tablets; I still can't get over the powdered ground bull testicles I saw in a "men's" supplement. As if. By the way, bee pollen is dangerous to those of you allergic to bee stings. Look, the science is just beginning to support taking vitamins and minerals; I'd wait for decent research before putting some of these other things in my mouth. (To read about ingredients in weight loss supplements, see Chapter 8.)

Bright Idea
Since minerals compete for absorption into your system, take them at different times of the day if possible. For instance, if you're taking a separate calcium supplement, take it at least two hours apart from your multi. Ditto for an iron supplement (which you should be taking only if you've been diagnosed with iron deficiency anemia).

Getting the most from your multi

You are now more informed about buying supplements than most nutrition professionals. You went out and bought a great tablet and now . . . there's still more to learn! Not much more, but a few tips that will help you make the best use of your supplement.

Housebreaking your supplement

These tips will help you absorb more nutrients:

- **Swallowing pills.** Tablets are the hardest, and capsules and gel caps are smoother and easier. If swallowing's difficult, there's nothing wrong with grinding up your pill and drinking it down with some juice. Just do it immediately—if the ground-up pill sits around some of the vitamins will be lost. Or find a chewable multi (some of the children's chewables are pretty complete). C comes in both chewable and effervescent that dissolves in water, and E also comes in chewable. Chewable C is designed not to hurt tooth enamel, but don't try biting down on regular C. Finally, you can opt for a liquid vitamin, but don't expect as much coverage as a tablet. Liquids have to leave some nutrients out because they won't stay intact in a liquid environment.

- **Timing.** Take supplements with a meal; fat in the meal will help you absorb the fat-soluble vitamins (A, E, D, and K), and digestive juices that are triggered by food also improve absorption. Take calcium supplements two hours before or after your multi; otherwise calcium can interfere with iron absorption.

- **Storage.** Keep in a cool, dry place (perhaps next to the sugar bowl). Worst places: in the fridge or bathroom cabinet—both way too moist.

Special cases

The levels recommended in the vitamin and mineral Tables 5.2 and 5.3, appearing at the end of this chapter, cover the vast majority of readers. But if you smoke, take medications, or eat special diets, your nutrient needs may be different. Since in many of these cases it's unclear just how much more of the nutrient you need, make sure you get at least the recommended levels and ask your doctor if you need even more.

- **Smokers.** You need more vitamin C, perhaps twice as much. But don't take too much C because it can drive nicotine out in the urine, bringing on the urge for the next cigarette that much faster. And you need more calcium, as nicotine reduces the body's ability to use this mineral. Female smokers are at higher risk for developing osteoporosis, a debilitating bone-thinning disease.

■ **Birth control pill takers.** May need more C.

■ **Vegetarians.** Since vitamin B12 is only in animal products, strict vegans need to supplement with daily value levels of 2 micrograms (mcg).

■ **Over 60.** Vitamin B12 absorption depends on stomach acid, which declines with age. In fact, 30 to 50 percent of the elderly have some form of atrophic gastritis (deficient stomach acid production). Check with your doc—a mild form of this condition warrants two times the DV of B12 (DV is 2 mcg)—a severe form warrants five times the DV.

■ **Chronic drug users.** These common drugs interfere with vitamins and minerals. If your drug isn't on this list, ask your physician about its possible interactions with nutrients.

> Antihypertensives based on hydralazine deplete B6.
>
> Anticonvulsants based on phenytoin, such as Dilantin, deplete folate and vitamin D.
>
> Anticoagulants, such as warfarin or coumarin, work by depleting vitamin K, which acts as a coagulant (blood clotting aid). While you need some vitamin K for bone health, don't supplement with more than the RDA, or you'll derail the action of these drugs.
>
> Antacids based on aluminum hydroxide deplete phosphate, vitamin D, and folate. Don't overcompensate—too much

Unofficially . . .
A Harvard University study suggests that getting recommended levels of folic acid and doubling the recommended levels of vitamin B6 through foods and supplements may reduce heart disease risk. These B vitamins lower blood levels of homocysteine, an amino acid that is associated with heart disease if present in high levels in the blood.

Moneysaver
Buying antacids
made with calci-
um carbonate
instead of
tablets marketed
as "calcium sup-
plements" saves
up to half your
money. And,
admits antacid
manufacturing
giant, Tums,
they're exactly
the same stuff.
Take it with a
meal to avoid
the antacid
action.

phosphate and D can be harmful, so just
make sure to get 100 percent DV amounts
from your multi. As for folate, aim for at
least 400 mcg. And taking antacids of any
kind on a daily basis may lower stomach
acid levels to the point of interfering with
B12 absorption, especially if you're over
60 years old (follow advice for "Over 60,"
listed earlier).

Cholesterol-lowering drugs based on
cholestyramine bind with fat and deplete
the fat-soluble vitamins A, E, D and K in
addition to B12 and folate. Make sure to
get at least 100 percent DV levels of these
in your multi.

Diuretics based on thiazide or furosemide
deplete potassium, zinc, and magnesium.

Glucocorticoids decrease calcium absorption and increase excretion into urine.

▪ **Laxative users.** Mineral oil depletes fat-soluble
vitamins as well as calcium and phosphorus—
it's not a good idea to use this. Stimulant laxatives such as bisacodyl and phenolphthalein
deplete calcium and vitamin D. You're better off
using a fiber-based bulk-forming laxative that
doesn't interfere with nutrients.

Phyto-what?

Research consistently shows that people who eat the
most fruits and vegetables have half the risk of developing cancer as those who eat the fewest, and they
get less heart disease. What is it in fruits and vegetables that's so protective? The protective nutrients are both the familiar-sounding nutrients like
vitamin C and fiber and other naturally occurring

plant compounds called phytochemicals. One way they work is through their anti-oxidant action. Antioxidants, such as vitamins A, C, and E, and the mineral selenium, attack cancer and heart disease triggers called free radicals, which are formed in the body in the presence of oxygen. Labs the world over are uncovering these compounds: Stay tuned. Here are a few examples of phytochemicals that show promise as potent disease-fighters:

- **Sulforaphane,** found in broccoli, cabbage, Brussel sprouts, and cauliflower (the smelly ones), stops the cancer process at its very inception. Sulforaphane raises levels of the body's own "detoxifying" enzymes, which disarm potentially cancer-causing chemicals before they can initiate cancer.

- **Lycopene** gives tomatoes and watermelon their red color and is also found in carrots and some of the dark, leafy green vegetables. People who eat diets rich in lycopene (usually because they eat lots of foods with tomato sauce) seem to have extra protection from prostate cancer and heart disease.

- **Allylic compounds** contribute to the strong taste and smell in garlic, onions, leeks, shallots, and chives. A rich body of scientific literature shows that eating raw, cooked, or powdered garlic, or garlic pills reduces blood cholesterol. Lab animal research shows that garlic and it's allylic compounds also reduce cancer risk.

Vitamins and minerals at a glance

Tables 5.2 and 5.3 sum up the whys and hows of vitamins and minerals. The scientific body that develops the recommended levels has recently come up with new values. So, if my numbers don't jibe with your old books, that's why. They used to be called RDAs, or Recommended Dietary (or Daily) Allowances. There are still RDAs for certain nutrients; others are given AIs (Adequate Intake) or EARs (Estimated Average Requirements). All these definitions are under the umbrella term Dietary Reference Intakes. Don't worry about it; it's too confusing. On the chart, I didn't bother with the terminology; I just gave you the values.

Why you might need a vitamin C supplement. Leading multivitamins have about 60 mg of C, a standard most experts believe to be out of date. Recent studies by the National Institutes of Health suggest as much as 200 mg to keep cells saturated. There's no evidence that taking more than 500 mg is helpful, and it may increase your risk for kidney stones.

Why you might need a separate vitamin E supplement. Most multivitamins supply only about 30 IUs of E—much less than levels shown by research to be effective. Your supplement should have between 200 and 400 IUs, and best taken with a meal containing at least some fat.

Just the facts

- If you're restricting calories, you probably should supplement.

- The labels are persuasive, but don't get duped: Buy a standard multivitamin with reasonable levels of nutrients.

- Once you've got it, use your supplement to its best advantage, taking it with food and avoiding interactions.

- Phytochemicals make fruits and vegetables potent disease-fighters.

TABLE 5.2   VITAMIN BASICS

Vitamin	Why You Need It	Rich Food Sources	Recommended Daily Level
A	Necessary for healthy skin and tissues lining the digestive tract, lungs, and urinary-genital areas. Plays a role in vision and has been shown to reduce the risk of cancer in lab animals and in some human studies.	Eggs, liver, vitamin-A fortified milk and cereals; also from the plant pigments beta-carotene and alpha-carotene, which the body converts to vitamin A as needed. See next entry for sources of beta-carotene.	Women: 800 RE* or 4000 IU**. Men: 1,000 RE or 5,000 IU.
Beta-carotene	A plant pigment that our bodies convert to vitamin A as needed. Also an antioxidant. Countless studies show that people with higher blood levels of beta-carotene are at lower risk for cancer and heart disease. But two studies of long-term smokers show that those taking beta-carotene supplements developed more cases of lung cancer.	Orange-fleshed vegetables such as carrots, yams, butternut squash; dark leafy greens such as kale and broccoli; cantaloupe and papaya.	No formal recommendation established. 2 to 6 mg is considered safe.
B1 (thiamin) B2 (riboflavin) B3 (niacin)	These B vitamins help convert carbohydrates, protein, or fat into energy. Deficiencies are very rare, causing nervous system and skin disorders. High levels of niacin may help lower high blood cholesterol, but there are side effects, so do this only under a doctor's supervision.	All three are in enriched and forti-fied bread and other flour-based foods, meat, and organ meats (but these are high in cholesterol and fat, so limit them). Milk's a good source of riboflavin; nuts and dried beans are niacin-rich.	Thiamin: Women, 1.1 mg; men, 1.2 mg; pregnant women, 1.4 mg; lactating women, 1.5 mg. Riboflavin: Women, 1.1 mg; men, 1.3 mg; pregnant women, 1.4 mg; lactating women, 1.6 mg. Niacin: Women, 14 mg; men 16 mg, pregnant women, 18 mg, lactating women, 17 mg.

continues

TABLE 5.2   (continued)

Vitamin	Why You Need It	Rich Food Sources	Recommended Daily Level
Biotin, Pantothenic Acid	More B vitamins, also involved in transforming food into energy.	Both are found in a wide variety of foods, such as meat, eggs, and whole-grain cereals.	Biotin: 30 mcg for both women and men, 35 mcg for pregnant women. Pantothenic Acid: 5 mg for women and men, 6 mg for pregnant women, 7 mg for lactating women.
B6 (pyridoxine)	Helps the body make protein, hormones, and other substances. Helps convert tryptophan (a building block of protein) into niacin and into serotonin, a brain chemical.	Chicken, fish, pork, and whole grains.	1.3 mg for women aged 19–50, 1.5 mg for women 51 and older, 1.9 mg for pregnant women, 2 mg for lactating women. For men 19–50: 1.3 mg, 1.7 mg for men 51 and older.
B12 (cobalamin)	Helps make red blood cells and maintain a healthy nervous system.	Only in foods of animal origin, such as meat, chicken, and milk. Some grain-based foods (cereals) are fortified with B12.	2.5 mcg for both owmen and men, 2.6 mcg for pregnant women, 2.8 mcg for lactating women.
Folic Acid (folate or folacin)	Cuts down on a woman's chance of bearing an infant with a neural tube defect. Also appears to protect your heart by reducing blood levels of a substance called homocysteine, which is associated with heart disease. Helps form red blood cells. Preliminary research shows it plays a role in preventing colon cancer. Large-scale surveys show most Americans aren't getting enough.	Leafy vegetables like spinach, dried beans, orange juice, wheat germ, and fortified flour.	400 mcg for both women and men, 600 mcg for pregnant women, 500 mcg for lactating women.
Choline	This B vitamin plays a role in keeping cells structurally sound, in communication between nerve cells, and in transporting fats around the body.	It's in many foods, but particularly concentrated in milk, eggs, and peanuts.	425 mg for women, 450 for pregnant women, 550 mg for lactating women, and 550 mg for men.

Vitamin	Why You Need It	Rich Food Sources	Recommended Daily Level
C (ascorbic acid)	Involved in the production of collagen (connective tissue that holds together muscle, bones, and so on) in wound healing; keeps gums healthy; helps the body absorb iron from non-animal food sources; improves immunities; linked to reduced risk of cataracts; acts as an antioxidant.	Citrus fruits and juices, cantaloupe, strawberries, mangoes, papaya, broccoli, cauliflower, tomatoes, and potatoes with skin.	Evidence suggests that we need at least 200 mg of vitamin C daily, instead of the 60 mg that had previously been recommended.
D	Gets calcium and phosphorus into bones and teeth, prevents bone disorders like rickets (bone softening causing bow-legs in children) or osteoporosis (brittle bones). Early research shows it plays a role in preventing colon cancer.	Exposure to sunlight and from fish oils and vitamin-D enriched milk and cereals. Hard to get enough from food sources.	5 mcg (200 IU) up to age 50; 10 mcg (400 IU) from ages 51–70; 15 mcg (600 IU) after age 71. D can be toxic—never go beyond 50 mcg (2000 IU).
E	Antioxidant. Seems especially protective against heart disease. May also counter the natural age-related slump in immune function. Role in cancer prevention is unclear.	Vegetable oils, nuts, seeds, and wheat germ. But you'd have to eat too much fat to get the levels recommended for staving off heart disease.	Health organizations recommend no more than 30 IUs, but many scientists recommend 100 to 400 IUs, requiring a supplement.
K	Makes a variety of proteins, including blood-clotting compounds needed to stop bleeding.	Greens like spinach and broccoli, also found in eggs and wheat bran/wheat germ. Also formed by bacteria in your intestines.	Women: 60 mcg for ages 19–24; 65 for age 25. Men: 70 mcg for ages 19–24; 80 after age 25.

*RE: retinol equivalents
**IU: international units

TABLE 5.3   MINERAL BASICS

Mineral	Why You Need It	Rich Food Sources	Recommended Daily Level
Boron	Appears to help body retain calcium and magnesium; may play a role in preserving bone.	Fruits and vegetables are good sources; animal-derived foods are poor sources.	None yet established.
Calcium	Integral part of bone. Builds bone and slows rate of bone loss as you age. Involved in muscle contraction (including heart beat) and nerve function. Helps prevent osteoporosis. May help reduce blood pressure.	Milk and yogurt (about 300 mg per cup); collard greens, spinach, turnip greens (about 250–350 per cup, cooked); hard cheese (about 200 mg per oz.); calcium-fortified soy or rice milk (200–300 mg per cup); calcium-fortified orange juice (300–350 mg per cup).	Ages 19–50: 1,000 mg. After 50: 1200 mg. 1,300 for pregnant women 18 and under. Safe upper limit: 2,500.
Chromium	Critical to proper functioning of insulin, a hormone that helps regulate blood sugar. May help prevent and treat Type II diabetes by improving insulin function.	Meat (11–45 mcg per 3 oz.), eggs (26 mcg per egg), and whole grains (65 mcg in 2 oz. shredded wheat).	50–200 mcg. No safe upper limit has been established for this.
Copper	Helps body make hemoglobin (which carries oxygen to red blood cells), part of many enzymes. Helps body convert fuel to energy.	Seafood, nuts, and seeds.	3 mg. No safe upper limit has been established, but don't go much beyond 5 mg daily.
Iron	Essential part of hemoglobin. Too little causes iron deficiency anemia, which makes you tired and dizzy and reduces concentration. Too much is linked to	Animal-source iron (from meat and chicken) is better absorbed than iron from plant sources. Vitamin C and a little meat enhances iron absorption	Women under 50: 15 mg. Over 50: 10 mg. Men: 10 mg. Safe upper limit is 50–75 mg, but be careful—too much iron can poison children.

Mineral	Why You Need It	Rich Food Sources	Recommended Daily Level
	increased risk of heart disease and cancer.	from plant sources; tea and coffee reduces it. Spinach is a rich source, but naturally occurring compounds called oxalates reduce the body's ability to absorb iron from spinach.	
Magnesium	Part of the bones. Involved in over 300 enzymes in the body that help regulate muscle and nerve function. Linked to protection from diabetes, osteoporosis, atherosclerosis, hypertension, and migraine headaches.	Tofu, raw spinach, pumpkin seeds, dried beans, beet greens, okra, high-fiber cereals, oysters, and some fish.	Women 19–30: 310 mg. Over 30: 320 mg. Men 19–30: 400 mg. Over 30: 420 mg.
Manganese	Part of many enzyme systems; essential for normal growth and bone formation.	Whole grains and, to a lesser extent, fruits and vegetables.	2–5 mg for adults. Safe upper limit: 5 mg.
Molybdenum	Works with the B vitamin riboflavin to make red blood cells.	Milk, beans, whole grains.	75–250 mcg. Safe upper limit hasn't been established, so don't supplement with more than 250 mcg.
Phosphorus	Helps generate energy in cells. Is a major component of bones and teeth and part of DNA.	Dairy, fish, beans, and tofu.	Adults: 700 mg. Pregnant and lactating women age 18 and under, 1,250 mg; 19 and older, 700 mg.
Selenium	Works with vitamin E to form an antioxidant complex that protects from heart disease, cancer, and other age-related conditions.	Beef, chicken, turkey, seafood, and wheat germ. Whole grains are generally rich sources, but amounts vary widely depending on the soils in which they were grown.	Women over 19: 55 mcg. Men over 19: 70 mcg. Safe upper limit hasn't been established. Stick with the recommendations, going no further than doubling them.
Zinc	Essential for growth and wound healing. Helps the body use protein. Plays	Oysters, zinc-fortified cereals, wheat germ, and crabmeat.	Women: 12 mg. Men: 15 mg. Safe upper limit: 15 mg. More may interfere

Weighing the Options

GET THE SCOOP ON...
Hiring a counselor ▪ Commercial weight loss
programs ▪ Doctor-supervised weight loss ▪
Support groups ▪ Residential program ▪
Weight loss surgery

PART III

Getting Good Help

W hile joining a weight loss program or hiring a dietician is no guarantee of success, the helping hand they provide works well for some people. About half the successful weight maintainers in the National Weight Registry Study or mentioned in Anne Fletcher's *Thin for Life* (see Chapter 1 for details) used programs or one-on-one consultations while losing the initial weight and some still use them occasionally for maintenance. Quite a few of the weight loss success stories interviewed for this book started off at a weight loss program, and some still go back for a "booster" when they find their weight starting to creep back up. And, if you can afford it, there are some decent residential weight loss facilities out there that give you a good running start into your weight loss. Finally, you've got a few surgical options to consider if the diet and exercise route doesn't do the trick. But as you'll see, surgery is not for everyone and is usually best avoided.

No matter what route you take, your chances of success will improve if there is a focus on:

- Long-term weight management
- Healthy eating
- Increasing activity
- Improving self-esteem

Finally, the sidebars in this chapter all come from the weight loss programs mentioned. Don't take them as an endorsement of any particular program. When I especially like a program, you'll know.

Consulting a nutritionist

Anyone can hang out a shingle and claim to be a nutritionist, although states are starting to regulate the practice. Its not like an MD, where you either went to medical school and passed or you didn't. The guy in the white lab coat at the health food store who's never taken a nutrition course in his life can call himself a nutritionist and recommend all sorts of nutritional supplements. (I've had more than one narrow escape from a health food store after I've taken aside desperate overweight customers about to hand over $100 for unproven pills and powders.)

Now, as I mentioned earlier, if your favorite psychic can help you lose weight and keep it off while you're eating a nutritious diet, stick with her. And just because someone has the right credentials, it doesn't mean he or she is a good weight loss counselor. Just like doctors, lawyers, and other professionals, some are better than others. But unless you've got satisfied friends who've gone to the psychic or the health food store guy—or any other noncredentialed person—and lost weight and kept it off on a healthy diet, then credentials had better be your starting point.

Who's legit?

Again, it's not straightforward as in the case of an MD. Here are the most legit credentials:

- **Registered Dietician (RD).** An RD holds a degree conferred by the American Dietetic Association, the largest nutrition organization in the country. RDs have at minimum a bachelor's degree in nutrition or a related field from an accredited college or university program approved of by the American Dietetic Association. In addition, they must complete a supervised internship program in some field of nutrition—often conducted in a hospital. Finally, they must pass an exam that tests their knowledge of a wide variety of nutrition areas (I know, I took it). By this point they certainly have at least the theoretical knowledge about the weight loss process, if not the counseling experience.

- **Licensed Nutritionist (LN).** Some states require that people practicing nutrition to be licensed; in that case, they'll have an LN after their name. But enforcement is negligible.

- **Nutritionist with an advanced degree.** Even if your counselor doesn't have an RD, a master's (MS) or Ph.D. in nutrition certainly equips him or her with a sound nutrition background. Also, an M.Ed (Master of Education), a Sc.D. (Doctor of Science), or an MD with a specialty or extensive coursework in nutrition at an accredited college or university usually means they have enough training. But don't be sold just because someone has an MD. Most medical schools don't require even one nutrition course! So that

Bright Idea
The next time you slip up, take these four steps: 1. Forgive yourself, 2. Analyze what happened, 3. Plan for next time, and 4. Rehearse your plan. (Source: Jenny Craig's *Little Survival Guide,* Jenny Craig International, 1996.)

MD has still got to prove to you that he or she has taken extensive coursework in nutrition. Some of the most notorious nutrition quacks out there are MDs.

- **Dietetic Technician, Registered (DTR).** A DTR is someone who has at least an associate's degree from an accredited college or university and has completed a program approved by the American Dietetic Association. DTRs do not have as much formal nutrition education as RDs, but if they've done internships in weight loss counseling they may have good practical experience. But keep in mind that choosing a DTR is more of a gamble than the other options on this list.

- **Certified Lifestyle Counselor.** A nutritionist with this credential has—on top of a background in nutrition—some training in the exercise and psychological aspects of weight loss. This means that they are trained to spot problem areas beyond their nutritional scope and can refer you to other health professionals, such as psychotherapists or exercise specialists, if needed. The certifying body is the American Association of Lifestyle Counselors (AALC), an organization which includes many of the field's luminaries from institutions such as Yale, Harvard, and the University of Pennsylvania. Since this is a relatively new certification, don't expect too many to have it. To find a Certified Lifestyle Counselor in your area, call (800) 736-7323 or check the AALC website (www.aalc. com). Please note that MDs, exercise specialists, and other health professionals can also become Certified Lifestyle Counselors. If it's mainly nutrition work you need, rather than exercise, I'd go with a Certified Lifestyle Counselor who is also an RD or one of the other qualified nutritionists mentioned here.

What to expect from a good nutritionist

Whether they have a Ph.D. or an RD with a bachelor's degree, here are tip-offs that you are getting sane and safe counseling:

- You're asked about your medical history, your history of weight loss and gain, and about any history of eating disorders.

- You're consulted about your weight loss goals and the counselor helps you form realistic goals based on your past experience.

- Counselor focuses on lifestyle changes, including exercise, and doesn't hand out "miracle" cures.

- Together, you and the counselor come up with a weight loss program that uses foods you will actually eat and a way of eating that you're comfortable with. Or, you choose from a variety of pre-printed diet plans that you can individualize, and you walk away with something you're comfortable with.

- You keep a diet record. Some counselors may ask you to keep a diet record of everything you eat for three to seven days before you even come in for the first visit. This helps the nutritionist get a handle on your likes and dislikes and your eating habits. Throughout the counseling you should keep a diet record for at least part of the time so the two of you can chart your progress and pinpoint problem areas.

- The counselor recommends losing no more than $1/2$ to two pounds a week (the heavier you are, the faster you'll lose). When you first start cutting calories, especially if you've got lots of weight to lose, you lose more than this per week (much of it's water weight, which returns). But by the third week, you shouldn't lose more (for reasons, see Chapters 1 and 3).

- The counselor doesn't push pills.

"Chain" weight loss programs

When you've got Fergie hawking Weight Watchers and Jenny Craig commercials on prime time you know commercial weight loss programs are big business. That doesn't mean they are uncaring factories—people do lose on these programs. For instance, published reports show that Weight Watchers does help people lose weight. How many keep the weight off on any of these programs is anyone's guess because there is little research on that issue. However, a few studies of Weight Watchers and Jenny Craig clients show that people who stick with the program until they reach their goal weight have a better chance of keeping it off. Here are some program "pros and cons":

- **Pros:** Commercial weight loss programs are fairly inexpensive. Also, group sessions, if included, can be supportive and motivating. If you need lots of structure, the prepackaged meals are helpful for the initial weight loss.

- **Cons:** You don't get the individualized attention of a private counselor. Also, it may be difficult to wean yourself off programs that hinge on prepackaged foods, making weight maintenance

> **❝**
> Changing the way you think about food can lead you to healthy eating. It's not impossible. The ability to 'de-powerize' the role food plays in your life is a skill that can be practiced and acquired. In the same way competent women master other areas of their lives, eating well can be learned. (Source: Green Mountain at Fox Run program materials.)
> **❞**

more difficult. (But not necessarily—these programs do have maintenance components.)

You may have heard that the commercial weight loss programs have been investigated by the Federal Trade Commission (FTC). They have—all of them—but most have settled the cases. The FTC's quibble isn't with their techniques, but with exaggerated claims of weight loss and weight maintenance. Among other things, the FTC settlement requires the programs to include the following statement in their literature: "For many dieters, weight loss is temporary." Also, if the companies claim that their programs help you maintain weight loss, that claim must be backed up by a two-year follow-up study of their clients.

Shopper's guide to weight loss programs

Before you put your money down for any program, try to talk to someone who's been through it. And make sure of the following:

- That your weight loss needs are appropriate for the program. Some, like those using very low-calorie diets, should be used only if you have a lot of weight to lose and are in dangerous medical straits requiring fast weight loss.

- That the program is suitable for your age group: adolescent, adult, or older adult.

- That you understand the program's approach to weight loss, such as whether they encourage physical activity and provide a maintenance plan for after you lose the weight.

- That the program is run by qualified people. That means registered dieticians or other

Watch Out!
When exercising, it's *not* okay to feel any of the following:

- An irregular heartbeat

- Pain or pressure in your chest, neck, jaw, or arms

- Unusual or extreme shortness of breath

- Nausea, dizziness, cold sweating, or fainting

If you experience any of these symptoms, stop exercising and sit or lie down. Contact your physician promptly. (Source: Adaptation of Weight Watchers 1-2-3 Success Plan.)

Watch Out!
It is not advisable to drop your calorie level below 1,000 calories per day. It is extremely difficult to pack in the necessary nutrients into fewer calories than this, so by eating fewer than 1,000 calories you may be losing weight at the expense of good nutrition. Diets of less than 1,000 calories should be supervised by a physician. (Source: the LEARN® Program for Weight Control, 7th edition.)

health professionals should be running the hospital- or medical center–based programs, and MDs should run the very low-calorie diet programs. For franchise weight loss programs such as Jenny Craig, make sure the staff has been trained by health professionals.

You should also make certain that the program is safe and sound. This is easier said than done, but here are features that a good program will include:

1. It measures your body weight, BMI (see Chapter 1), and waist-to-hip ratio.

2. It encourages a balanced, pyramid-style, low-fat diet (see Chapter 4) that stresses moderation and variety.

3. It asks about any medical conditions that might make dieting risky.

4. It asks about your level of physical activity. A good program will encourage exercise and check back with you periodically, or at least at the end of the program, to see how you're doing on the exercise front.

5. It offers guidance on behavioral changes—like coping with food cravings, reducing stress, or improving self-esteem—that not only help you lose weight but also help keep it off.

On the other hand, a questionable program has its own set of distinguishing features:

1. It strongly urges you to take herbal supplements or vitamin and mineral tablets other than a standard multivitamin/mineral tablet.

2. It does hair or blood analysis to measure nutrition deficiencies (for more on why this is bogus, see Chapter 8).

3. It forbids certain categories of foods, offers a high protein diet, advocates food combining, or pushes any of the other fad diets listed in Chapter 8.

4. It is not up-front about costs and hidden costs.

5. It has no health professionals, such as registered dieticians, Ph.D.s in nutrition, or MDs involved on any level (even the corporate level, where the materials are designed).

6. It advocates losing more than $1/2$ to two pounds a week (unless it's a medically supervised low-calorie program like those discussed under "Medically supervised very low-calorie programs," later in this chapter).

The three biggies

Jenny Craig, Nutri/System, and Weight Watchers are the "Three Biggies" of the commercial weight loss programs. (We should include a "Fourth Biggie"—Diet Center, but executives of that program refused to be interviewed, saying they've been maligned too many times by the media. For info on Diet Center, go to their website at www.dietcenterworldwide.com.) Jenny Craig, Nutri/System, and Weight Watchers all use a variation on the theme of a reduced calorie diet coupled with one-on-one or group counseling, with exercise factored in, or at least recommended. Most use their own prepackaged foods, and one of them—Nutri/System—has an option for people who are taking a prescription weight loss drug. None use health professionals as counselors, but all three programs were designed by MDs, RDs, and Ph.D.s in nutrition. The counselors are trained by program staff or by other trained counselors.

Bright Idea
Plan your response to an insistent host or hostess. Practice saying "No thank you, I've had enough" or "I can't eat another bite." Your last resort? "I can't, I'm allergic." It works every time. (Source: Nutri/System *Handling Special Occasions & Holidays Guide*.)

WHAT EVERY PROGRAM SHOULD DISCLOSE

You have a right to get the following information from the people running the weight loss program. This list is reprinted with permission from *Weighing The Options* (National Academy Press, 1995), a report by the prestigious National Academy of Sciences:

- A truthful, unambiguous, and nonmisleading statement of the approach and goals of the program. Part of such a statement might read, for example, "We are a program that emphasizes changes in lifestyle, with group instruction in diet and physical activity."

- A brief description of the credentials of staff, with more detailed information available on request. For example, "Our staff is composed of one physician (MD), two registered nurses (RNs), three registered dietitians (RDs), one master's-level exercise physiologist, and one Ph.D.-level psychologist. At your first visit, you will be seen by the physician. At each visit you will be seen by a dietitian and exercise physiologist and after every five visits by the psychologist. Resumes of our staff are available upon request."

- A statement of the client population and experiences over a period of nine months or more. For example, "To date, we have seen 823 clients for at least three visits each. Although only 26 clients have participated in this program for more

CHAPTER 6 ▪ GETTING GOOD HELP

than one year, they have maintained an average weight loss of 12 pounds." [*Author's note: this is ideal, but since some reasonable programs don't have this, don't discount them on this point alone, but try to get some sense of this.*]

- A full disclosure of costs. For example, "If you avail yourself to all our facilities with one weekly visit for a period of one year, the total cost to you will be between $2,000 and $2,500." Costs should include the initial cost; ongoing costs and additional cost of extra products, services, supplements, and laboratory tests; and costs paid by the average client. Programs may also wish to provide information on the experiences clients have had in recovering their costs from third-party payers.

- A statement of procedures recommended for clients. For example, "We urge that each of our clients see a physician before joining our program. If you have high blood pressure or diabetes, you should see your physician at intervals of his or her choosing while with our program."

To see whether commercial weight loss programs are for you, shop around a little and talk to the counselors before you sign on the dotted line. Since counselors and groups can vary so much, you might have to shop around even within programs. For instance, you may not like the lunchtime Weight Watchers group in your office building, but feel really good about the 8 p.m. meeting near your home.

Right off the bat, there are two big differences in these plans that can help you make your decision.

- **Prepackaged foods.** Can you eat prepackaged frozen or shelf-stable meals and snacks for weeks or months? If that appeals to you, then go with Nutri/System, Jenny Craig, or Diet Center. It's easier if you don't have a family to feed because cooking for others gets tempting. If you like to cook and the thought of microwavable frozen dinners turns your stomach, better go with Weight Watchers. Weight Watchers is the only one that lets you have complete freedom to choose your own foods.

  On the other hand, prepared foods do make for a very uncomplicated weight loss: Unless you stray outside the plan, you can't screw up. Also, these prepackaged meals teach portion control, which may be valuable for those of you who really pile it on. The criticism often leveled at these programs is that they don't teach you to eat in the real world. Facing the kitchen or restaurant menus again can be tough and lead you to slip back to your old ways. However, if you stick with these programs to the bitter end, they do help you re-acclimate to the real world of food.

- **Drugs.** Only Nutri/System offers a plan that gives you the prescription appetite suppressing drug Sibutrimine, brand name Meridia. To qualify for the use of the drug you've got to have a BMI of at least 27, and you should have medical risk factors such as diabetes. (See Chapter 8 for more on this drug.)

Unfortunately, it's impossible to judge how successful these programs are, as they haven't kept adequate records on the percent of members who've kept weight off over the long haul. But they definitely help some people. Here's the basics on the top three programs (costs may change by the time you read this):

Weight Watchers
(800) 651-6000
website: www.weightwatchers.com

- **Approach:** A diet and lifestyle change program that promotes a pyramid-style approach to eating. Exercise gets particular emphasis in this new plan as you earn more points if you're more active. The program was designed by registered dieticians in consultation with MDs and nutrition Ph.D.s.

- **Diet plan:** The new "1-2-3 Success"™ plan assigns points to every food; you get a daily point range that corresponds to your current body weight. You can eat anything you want as long as you stay within your point range. You could, of course, use up all your points on chocolate, but you could also wind up with a very balanced diet if you follow their five nutrition guidelines (such as eat five fruits and vegetables and limit sweets to two to three times a week). You get more points if you exercise. High-fat and high-calorie foods cost you more points; lower-fat, lower-calorie, and high-fiber foods cost fewer points. Someone weighing between 150 and 174 pounds would wind up eating somewhere between 1,150 and 1,500 calories.

Moneysaver
Make your own cooking spray and cut the fat by filling a regular spray bottle with vegetable oil (such as canola) and lightly spray it on the pan when browning meat or sautéeing vegetables. (Source: Adaptation of Weight Watchers 1-2-3 Success Plan.)

Unofficially . . .
Watchdogs are very proud of you and tell you how good you look. They also make you feel like you're being supervised instead of supported. They say things like, "Are you sure that's okay to eat?" Tell the watchdogs you appreciate their support, but those comments about what or how much you eat aren't helpful. Explain how they *can* help you. (Source: Adaptation of Weight Watchers 1-2-3 Success Plan.)

- **What you do:** Your counselor weighs you, helps you pick a weight goal, and assigns your diet "points." Then you attend weekly group meetings, led by a Weight Watcher's–trained leader, which cover nutrition, exercise, and psychological aspects of losing weight. Each week you get weighed. There are no one-on-one counseling sessions, but it's okay to have the leader phone you to answer questions. To help you figure out how many points are in various foods, you carry around a guide listing point values for 1,500 foods. Also, a little cardboard slide "calculator" helps you figure out points.

- **Expected weight loss:** $1^1/_2$ to 2 pounds per week. If you're losing more, have a consultation.

- **Cost:** A \$30 registration fee, then a weekly charge of \$10 to \$14 depending on the center. Ask about special promotions.

- **Comments:** Of the three programs, this is the only one that doesn't push the company's brand of food or supplements. From what I've gathered from the experts I consulted for this book, Weight Watchers has the best reputation of the lot. One of the principle reasons is because the program is so flexible, thereby teaching you how to cope with real foods. However, this 1-2-3 Success is new, so it's hard to tell how effective it is. Weight Watchers is launching a two-year study at six different sites to test the program's effectiveness. Be assertive about your calorie level; ask how many calories your points translate to and if it seems too low, go higher. Try not to dip below 1,200 daily.

Jenny Craig

(800) 435-3669

website: www.jennycraig.com

- **Approach:** A diet and lifestyle change program that uses a balanced low-fat weight loss diet with calories varying according to weight loss needs. The pyramid-style diet is based on Jenny Craig foods. "It's not so much about the weight as about lifestyle choices learned," according to Lisa Tallamini Jones, a registered dietician at Jenny Craig headquarters.

- **Diet plan:** The "ABC Program" consists of weight loss and "weight stabilization" (maintenance) menus, including special menus for vegetarians and adolescents. The weight loss menus range from 1,000 to 2,300 calories daily (adolescent menus go from 1,400 to 2,200 calories). Weight stabilization menus range from 1,200 to 2,600. For the first half of your weight loss: Jenny Craig frozen and "shelf stable" entrees, snacks, and diet bars, available only at the weight loss center. For the second half of weight loss: both Jenny Craig and regular foods. According to a friend who just completed the program, you'll quickly learn which foods are tasty and which are "inedible," and you can choose accordingly.

- **What you do:** With the help of a computer and a counselor you figure out your goal weight and daily calorie level. Then you're in for two weeks of tightly structured, preplanned menus, eating Jenny Craig entrees and snacks along with store-bought fresh fruits and vegetables, dairy, and

Moneysaver
Don't have your own five-pound weights? Start out holding a 16-ounce can of vegetables in hand and work your way up gradually increasing the can size. (Source: Jenny Craig's *Little Survival Guide*.)

Bright Idea
If your hotel
doesn't have a
fitness room,
find some stairs.
Go up and down
as many flights
as you can for a
terrific workout!
(Source: Jenny
Craig's *Little
Survival Guide*.)

bread. You can loosen things up a little starting at week three, where you can choose among several Jenny Craig Cuisine breakfasts, lunches, and dinners (these are categorized within A, B, or C levels, but don't worry about what that means; I'm just letting you know where the ABC comes from). When you reach half your goal weight you move into "Five/Two:" five Jenny Craig food days, two days of regular food. If you go for the maintenance program, you'll get help weaning yourself completely off of the Jenny Craig food after you hit your goal weight. During the entire process, you meet weekly for individual consultations with Jenny Craig–trained counselors, and you can attend 12 weekly group classes and use exercise tapes and videos. If you bought the "Platinum program," you then segue into maintenance, which focuses on preventing relapse. Maintenance means unlimited weekly sessions with a counselor and access to group classes focusing on maintenance.

- **Expected weight loss:** 1 to 2 pounds per week.

- **Cost:** The weight loss program only, called the "Gold Program," costs $148 for a year of consultation and classes. In addition, the Jenny Craig cuisine averages $72 per week during the first half of the weight loss. The "Platinum Program" (weight loss plus maintenance) costs $296 for an unlimited time period. Platinum also offers 25 percent discounts for family members and a rebate of 50 percent of the enrollment fee if, one year later, you are still within five pounds of your desired weight.

- **Comments:** Since the meal plans are fairly rigid in the initial phase, this would work best for those of you who need lots of structure and don't want to make food decisions. This program offers lots of support, which will be great if you get a decent counselor and group. Unless you absolutely can't lose weight on more than 1,000 calories (which means you've decided to forego exercise), then insist on eating at least 1,200. And with anything under 1,500, take a multivitamin/mineral tablet.

Nutri/System® and L.A. Weight Loss Centers
(800) 321-THIN®
website: www.nutrisystem.com

- **Approach:** A diet and lifestyle change program that uses a balanced low-fat weight loss diet with calories varying according to weight loss needs. The pyramid-style diet is based on Nutri/System foods. Nutri/System also offers a "Medical Program:" the regular program with the addition of the prescription drug Meridia (see Chapter 8 for info on this drug). Medical Program centers are staffed with a physician. To qualify, your BMI must be at least 27, and you must be at least 18 years old and have medical conditions that respond to weight loss such as high blood pressure.

- **Diet plan:** Three meals and a snack based on Nutri/System's "NuCuisine™" foods. Calories vary from 1,000 to 3,500 based on your needs; typically women end up eating 1,200 calories, men 1,500. While getting down to your goal weight, you eat NuCuisine shelf-stable foods and snacks supplemented with store-bought

> **"** Our focus is very much on practical problem solving. You're going to a banquet this week? You and your counselor will work out a strategy.
> —Mary Gregg, a registered dietician working at Nutri/System corporate headquarters. **"**

fruits, vegetables, and milk. During maintenance you slowly wean yourself off Nutri/
System foods.

▪ **What you do:** Using a computer, you and the
counselor come up with a goal weight. Then it's
weekly meetings with a counselor who monitors
your weight and measurements, readjusts meal
plans, and helps you work on your particular weight loss issues. Very few centers offer
group counseling. It's seven days a week of
NuCuisine foods plus store-bought fruits, vegetables, and milk until you reach your goal
weight. On the Medical Program, you'll also
receive a physical exam at your first meeting,
complete with an electrocardiogram (EKG) to
detect arrhythmia (abnormal heart beats).
Meridia can be dangerous if you have arrhythmia; this condition excludes you from the
Medical Program.

On either the medical or regular plans, you
can opt for a maintenance program after reaching your goal weight. For the first eight weeks of
maintenance you eat Nutri/System meals
four days a week, and your own meals the rest of
the week. After that, you move down to two days
of NuCuisine meals weekly and gradually wean
off. They want you to meet with a counselor
weekly for the first eight weeks of maintenance,
then bi-weekly for the following four months.
After that, it's an "open door" policy: You come
in when you need a booster.

▪ **Expected weight loss:** 1 to 2 pounds a week.

▪ **Cost:** New member: $159 for a year's worth of
weight loss consultations; $259 for a year's worth

of the maintenance plan. Former members can come back for weight loss (and maintenance) for $119. NuCuisine foods cost $49 to $79 per week, depending on the center's markup. The Medical Program costs $270 for three months or $500 for a year, which includes maintenance.

■ **Comments:** Rigidly relying on their own products makes this best for out-of-control eaters that need, and work well with, structure. But talk about structure. . . . Depending on how much weight you've got to lose, you'll be getting very familiar with NuCuisine offerings. Again, try not to go under 1,200 calories daily.

Please note: Nutri/System is in a state of transition having sold their corporately owned centers to a company called Complete Wellness Weight Management. The centers still under the "Nutri/ System" logo are all franchises, which get their direction from the corporate office. Complete Wellness sells the same foods (under the NuCuisine brand name) and follows similar practices. During transitions, things like training can get lax; I would question my counselor very carefully to see how much training he or she has received.

In addition to these well-known programs, hospitals and or medical centers often have their own versions, of varying quality. Use the same criteria for judging these as you would for the commercial programs.

Four stellar programs

These top-of-the-line programs don't fit into any of the categories mentioned in this chapter. All were developed by leaders in their respective fields, and, unlike most programs, three of them have been scientifically tested with the successful outcomes published in well-respected medical or nutrition journals.

The LEARN® Program for Weight Control

(800) 736-7323

website: www.learneducation.com

Call the 800 number to order the manual. Locating a LEARN group isn't easy; check the American Association of Lifestyle Counselors (the same organization that developed LEARN). Go to the website www.aalc.com for a directory of certified Lifestyle Counselors. It's worth calling a few in your area to see whether any of them are running a group.

- **What it is:** Developed by Yale University psychologist Kelly Brownell, considered a leader in the weight loss field, this well-rounded program covers the psychological, nutritional, and exercise components of weight loss. (LEARN stands for Lifestyle, Exercise, Attitudes, Relationships, and Nutrition.)

- **What you do:** There are two approaches— you can do it yourself or join a group. The entire "program" consists of a 16-lesson workbook, which you follow at your own pace. Brownell's research found that people usually take 12 to 20 weeks to finish it. The engaging material forces you to closely examine your habits through quizzes, food diaries, and other "self-monitoring" devices. These tools also become ways to assess your progress. You can purchase cassettes that reinforce the principles learned and are helpful in dealing with crisis situations.

For those of you who have decided to take the diet drug Meridia, there is a separate "Special Medication Edition" of LEARN. It's basically the same program plus it monitors your reaction to the medication. (See Chapter 8 for information about weight loss drugs.) The first 16 lessons should take about four months, then there are eight monthly lessons to get you through the year. You'll probably lose a lot more weight combining this type of program with the medication than just taking the medication alone. A University of Pennsylvania study of people taking a similar diet drug to Meridia found that those who received 26 weeks of lifestyle counseling lost 34 pounds compared to the 13 pounds lost by people who received no counseling.

With either the regular or medication version, doing it in a group setting means that you and others follow the exact same manual and meet once a week or so with a trained counselor to discuss what you've read and deal with issues that come up. Groups *can* be motivating and supportive, but they aren't necessary; the LEARN program has been proven effective for those working alone.

- **Expected weight loss:** 1 to 2 pounds a week. Both the regular and medication LEARN program produce an average weight loss of 20 to 30 pounds.

- **Cost:** $22.95 for the manual, $24.95 for the Special Medical Edition, and $25.95 for the cassettes (not required).

Timesaver
No time for breakfast? Take it to go. Pack yourself a breakfast-to-go the night before, and eat it the following morning when you have a few extra minutes. Try celery stuffed with cheese, fresh or dried fruits, canned juice or milk, breakfast bars, a bagel, or English muffin. (Source: Adaptation of the LEARN manual, 7th edition.)

The Solution

(415) 457-3331

website: www.weightsolution.com

- **What it is:** A confident name for a program that inspires confidence because it's backed up by good research. It's the product of 10 years of development and 10 years of testing, the brainchild of University of California at San Francisco's Laurel Mellin, who also developed the highly acclaimed "Shapedown," a weight loss program for adolescents. "There are two main factors in weight loss: genetics and developmental skills. You can't do anything about your genes, but my program will teach you the skills that will take you down to your genetic comfort zone of body weight," says Mellin. Her published research showed that people not only lost weight during the 18 weeks they attended the program, but continued to lose afterward (the opposite trend from most programs). Two years later, on average, people were 17 pounds lighter than when they began and improved in other areas such as depression and financial responsibility. This is a good program for those of you willing and ready to put a substantial chunk of time and thought into the process.

- **What you do:** For nine months you attend weekly group meetings that follow the Solution workbook. The meetings are led by a registered dietician and a certified mental health counselor, both of whom have completed a 50-hour Solution course. During the sessions, the group practices the following six skills: strong nurturing, setting effective limits, developing body pride, maintaining good health, balanced eating, and mastery living. Outside of sessions, participants spend about two hours a week working on journals, another two hours practicing the skills through phone conversations with other members. To get a good idea of the program, check out the book *The Solution* (HarperCollins, 1997), coming out in paperback as *The Diet-free Solution* (HarperCollins, 1998).

- **Expected weight loss:** Varies with participant.

- **Cost:** Ideally, you follow through for nine months. You pay $400 to $500 (depending on where you live: Urban areas are more expensive) for three months at a time. So the whole nine months winds up costing $1,200 to $1,500.

Choose to Lose Weight Loss/Healthy Eating Program
(888) 897-9360
website: www.choicediets.com

- **What it is:** A weight loss program based on a low-fat diet and increased physical activity. This program is much more generous with calories than most; a 5'5" woman can take in up to 2,000 calories daily if she exercises regularly. That's because, say developers Ron and Nancy Goor, you can eat that much and still lose as long as your diet is low in fat (and they don't mean Snackwells and the like, but foods naturally low in fat such as fruits, vegetables, whole grains, and lean meats). However, high-fat splurges can be worked in as long as you stick within your fat budget. Ron Goor has a Ph.D. in biochemistry and a Masters in public health nutrition and used to head the government's National Cholesterol Education Program. His research specialty was heart disease. In the 1980s the

Bright Idea
Ground turkey usually contains 20 fat calories per ounce. A 5 oz. turkey burger contains 100 fat calories. Although better than a 5 oz. extra lean hamburger (220 calories), a 100-fat calorie turkey burger is not a low-fat food. If ground turkey is not labeled, don't buy it. It may contain a lot of turkey fat and thus be very high in fat. To be sure your ground turkey is only 2 fat calories per ounce, buy unadulterated turkey breast and grind it yourself. (Source: Ron and Nancy Goor, *Choose to Lose* skill-builder workbook.)

husband-and-wife team wrote the popular *Eater's Choice* (fourth edition, Houghton Mifflin, 1995), a low-fat diet book for heart disease prevention. Their second book, *Choose to Lose* (Houghton Mifflin, 1995), adapts the low-fat diet for weight loss.

- **What you do:** Attend eight weekly meetings where you practice low-fat eating skills and become a whiz at figuring out the fat calories in foods. For instance, one skill is maneuvering through restaurant menus for low-fat choices. Some groups practice this skill with a night out on the town (lucky waiter). To bone up on low-fat cooking techniques, participants bring in snacks made from the *Choose to Lose* recipes. The group leaders, usually registered dieticians, take a course and are tested before earning their certificates. In addition to a workbook, both the Goor books, a motivational tape, and a video tape, you get a nifty fat "Balance Book" that looks like a checkbook and which you use to keep a running tally of the day's and week's fat calories.

- **Expected weight loss:** 5 to 10 pounds during the eight weeks, with continued weight loss expected if you keep following the guidelines.

- **Cost:** Depends on the site. Worksite programs may be free; at YMCAs, clinics, hospitals, and other sites it ranges from $60 to $200.

The Program for Reversing Heart Disease
(415) 332-2525
website: still under development at press time

- **What it is:** This is the state-of-the-art program for those of you who are overweight and have heart disease or are at high risk of developing it (based on family history or medical clues). Although the focus here is much more than weight loss—stress management and group support are as important as diet and exercise—if you're overweight, you'll certainly lose on this program. It was developed by Dean Ornish, MD, famous for being the first researcher to prove that changing your lifestyle can actually reverse heart disease. Until Ornish, they thought that once you got heart disease it could only get worse, progressing to a heart attack or heart surgery. But Ornish took patients awaiting heart surgery, whose arteries were so clogged that they could hardly walk across a room from the strain, and turned them into healthy, active, people—without heart surgery. His electronic images of starved heart muscles transformed into healthy hearts transfixed the scientific community, and his books and PBS series have inspired thousands. Ornish has taken his "Program for Reversing Heart Disease" to hospitals around the nation.

▪ **What you do:** Attend an outpatient program run by hospitals. This includes light exercise classes, nutrition instruction on a very low-fat vegetarian diet, stress management (yoga and meditation classes), and support groups. You go in several times a week for exercise classes, support group meetings, low-fat cooking demonstrations, and meditation and yoga classes.

▪ **Expected weight loss:** Since the focus is not primarily on weight, there is no "expected" weight loss. However, if you follow the program faithfully, you'll lose weight.

▪ **Cost:** Varies according to hospital and according to which program you choose: the eight-week "core" or the year-long program. I found prices ranging from free (part of an insurance plan) to $6,000 for the year-long program, less for the eight-week "core" program.

▪ **Where:** At press time, these were the participating hospitals; more are on the way:

1. FLORIDA:
   Broward General Medical Center,
   Wellness Center
   Fort Lauderdale
   (954) 355-4386

2. NEBRASKA:
   Alegent Health, Alegent Immanuel Medical
   Center
   Omaha
   (402) 572-3300
   Alegent Health, Alegent Bergen Mercy
   Medical Center
   Omaha, NE
   (402) 398-5655

3. IOWA:
   Iowa Heart Center
   Mercy Hospital Medical Center
   Des Moines
   (515) 235-5147

4. CALIFORNIA:
   University of California San Francisco/
   California Pacific Medical Center Heart
   Disease Reversal Program
   San Francisco
   (415) 353-4278

Scripps Health, Shilley Sports and
Health Center FC2
La Jolla
(619) 554-9282

5. SOUTH CAROLINA:
   Richland Memorial Hospital, Cardiac
   Ancillary Services
   Columbia
   (803) 434-3852

6. PENNSYLVANIA:
   Highmark Blue Cross Blue Shield
   Pittsburgh
   (412) 447-1352

7. OHIO:
   Franciscan Health System of the Ohio Valley
   Cincinnati
   (513) 853-5987
   Franciscan Health System of the Ohio Valley
   Cincinnati
   (937) 229-6202

8. ILLINOIS:
   Swedish American Health System
   Rockford
   (815) 391-7033

Medically supervised very low-calorie programs

While quick weight loss is generally frowned upon, it does have its merits in certain dire situations, like a very dangerous heart disease profile. Or, you may need to lose weight quickly to lower risk for an operation.

To the rescue: very low-calorie diets (in medical jargon, VLCD) ranging from 450 to 850 calories a

day. As you can imagine, there's no way to get a balanced diet eating real foods on so few calories.
While some of these programs offer real meals, they
also require vitamin-injected liquid meals and bars.
Another name for these diets is "protein-sparing
modified fasts" because they keep the level of protein as close to normal as possible, thus encouraging
you to lose more fat than muscle. This is tricky business; done wrong you could get imbalances of blood
sodium and potassium (electrolytes), which can
cause heart attacks. That's why these programs are
medically supervised.

While people do drop pounds quickly on these
programs, most gain them back within a year or
more. However, if you get good lifestyle change
instruction as you're losing the weight and stick with
the maintenance program (they'd better offer
one!), you may beat the odds.

- **Leading programs:** Optifast, Medifast, New
  Direction, and Health Management Resources
  (HMR), usually conducted out of your local
  hospital, medical center, or physician's office.
  Some also offer higher calorie programs (1,000
  to 1,500).

- **Overweight criteria:** Depending on the program, you need to be at least 40 to 50 pounds
  overweight or have a BMI of 30 or above to go
  on the very low-calorie regimens.

- **What you do:** Occasionally, in cases where the
  obesity has put you in grave medical danger, you
  check into the hospital to go on the program.
  But usually, you go to your doctor to pick up the
  liquid formula and snack bars and check back
  once a week for counseling. The counseling prepares you for coping with real food once the

liquid diet part ends. Some programs also offer exercise instruction.

- **Expected weight loss:** You often lose more in the first two weeks, but after that, depending on your metabolism and the calorie level, expect to lose about 3 to 5 pounds a week. Optifast says on average, their clients lose 52 pounds.

- **How long you can stay on them:** 12 to 24 weeks.

- **Risks:** Do this only if you really need to. Side effects include fatigue, constipation, and nausea, which usually goes away after a few weeks. Losing weight at this fast pace can bring on gallstones, which can be painful (see Chapter 1 for more on gallstones). And in very rare cases, these diets can cause heart attacks, even under medical supervision.

Non-profit support groups

If you always assumed support groups were too touchy-feely for you, think again. A good support group can provide stimulating, useful conversation and the comfort of knowing you're not alone. Studies of women who've had breast cancer show that those participating in support groups stayed in remission significantly longer and had a lower risk of death. The emotional support you can derive from a good group can help keep you motivated to stay on track. And these programs take very different approaches, so if you can't imagine yourself working through 12 steps, you might feel very comfortable with a group that reinforces healthy lifestyle habits. And remember, each group is different; you might have to attend a few before finding people you can relate to. Look them up in your local Yellow Pages or call the headquarter numbers given here.

TOPS (Take Off Pounds Sensibly)

(800) 932-8677

website: www.tops.org

Designed to offer support to anyone losing weight and to promote an unfaddish, healthy approach to weight loss, TOPS strongly encourages you to consult with a physician before embarking on your weight loss.

Your one-time $20 fee gives you access to unlimited weekly meetings and a year-long subscription to their magazine, and it contributes to obesity research. Group leaders are untrained volunteers who use a TOPS curriculum; health professionals are invited to speak at meetings. You can opt to participate in social events not related to weight loss such as volunteering at local charities or attending retreats.

Overeaters Anonymous (OA)

(505) 891-2664

website: www.overeatersanonymous.org

This group views compulsive eating in the same way Alcoholics Anonymous views alcoholism: as an addiction. Their literature states very clearly that they are not nutrition experts; they deal with the psychological aspects of overeating. They believe that compulsive eating is a physical, emotional, and spiritual disease, which, like alcoholism and drug abuse, can be arrested, but never cured. While this approach is very useful for some people, others take issue with the idea that you're never cured. For instance, eating disorders expert Christopher Fairburn, MD, believes that the addiction model does not apply to binge eating, and that people can be cured. My advice: Try it out and see if it helps you. As of press time, you couldn't locate a meeting

Unofficially . . .
Take each party or special occasion one at a time. Let "just for today" be your standard. "Just for today, I'll make a deliberate decision on what to eat . . . savor my choices . . . and stop before I feel stuffed." "Just for today, I'll skip the snack table and concentrate on other party guests." (Source: TOPS Special Hints for Guests.)

on the website, but this information should be accessible soon.

Residential weight loss programs

These are places where you get away from it all and focus entirely on your weight loss. More serious and rigorous than spas, you go not only to lose weight but to learn how to keep it off. There are a number of good ones; I chose these three to give you a sense of what to expect.

Duke Diet and Fitness Center, Durham, North Carolina

(800) 362-8446

website: www.mc.duke.edu/dfc/home.html

The thing that sets this one apart is its medical emphasis. Affiliated with the Duke University Medical Center, if you have any medical conditions that might affect your diet or ability to exercise, they can handle it. Also, they can prescribe diet drugs or antidepressants. But the program is also for perfectly healthy people trying to lose weight or get in better shape. Staffed by MDs, registered dieticians, psychologists, and exercise physiologists, they use a multi-pronged approach to helping you change your lifestyle. This one isn't really residential in that it has no housing on the premises. However, there are hotels nearby, and people fly in from all over the country.

- **What you do:** At the outset you get a complete physical, a treadmill test, a psychological assessment, and a nutrition assessment. All this feeds into an individualized diet and exercise plan for the remainder of your stay. Then it's off to classes in nutrition, life skills, goals, and lots of exercise for one to four weeks. (You can stay longer; that's the typical stint.) The emphasis is on developing weight loss–inducing skills you can take back home with you, and you leave with a diet plan that suits your lifestyle. You can opt for the "Aftercare" plan, in which you check in regularly with a counselor by phone when you return home.

■ **Expected weight loss:** On average, over four weeks, women typically lose 12 to 15 pounds; men, 17 to 20 pounds.

■ **Cost:** Fees for the program and meals (excluding housing) are $2,500 for a week, $4,500 for two weeks, and $5,600 for four weeks. Stay any longer and prices fall to $650 per week, and return visits are also $650 per week. Aftercare is $325 for weekly telephone sessions for six months.

Structure House, Durham, North Carolina
(800) 553-0052
website: www.structurehouse.com

Gerald Musante, a Ph.D. in psychology, left the Duke Fitness Center but stayed in town to start up his own retreat. Like Duke, the program approaches weight loss from every angle, but it's less medically oriented, and the clients have fewer health problems. Structure House's claim to fame is its strong psychological orientation, reflecting Musante's research specialization in behavior modification. Structure House is also equipped to deal with binge eating disorder. Everything happens in the 21-acre campus: your living quarters (apartments), the classes, the cafeteria, and the exercise areas.

■ **What you do:** You initially see an exercise physiologist, a nutritionist, and a psychologist who set up your individualized strategy. Days are filled

Bright Idea
Structure in three healthy meals a day at a regular time and a regular place—"slow, satisfying, sit-down meals." Chaotic eating, meal skipping, starving, or snacking is considered "unstructured" and will sabotage long-term weight control. (Source: Structure House Tips for Weight Control.)

with nutrition and stress management classes, workouts, and friendly group meals ranging from 1,000 to 2,000 calories daily. (I know they're friendly because I've visited Structure House.) Registered dietitians and psychologists teach the classes. Weather permitting (and it usually does) you can go on nature trail hikes. The average length of stay is 28 days, but you can stay as long as you can afford to.

- **Expected weight loss:** 3 to 5 pounds per week for women, 5 to 10 pound per week for men. This is high, but it's okay because the program is supervised. Research tracking clients anywhere from six months to five years later shows that two-thirds of the clients maintain their weight loss.

- **Cost:** A private apartment is $1,800 for one week, $3,600 for two weeks, $4,800 for three weeks, and $6,400 for four weeks. After four weeks the price drops 40 percent and remains 40 percent lower for return visits.

Green Mountain at Fox Chase
(800) 448-8106
website: www.fitwoman.com

Sorry guys, this is for women only. Besides its location—a gorgeous mountain retreat in Vermont—what sets this program apart is it's focus away from dieting (they don't dip below 1,400 calories) and toward becoming more active and better able to cope with emotional eating. "Our clients have read every diet book in the world, they know what to do. They come here when they're serious about doing it. We teach problem solving, ways of managing, developing behaviors that keep your

> We have significantly greater depth and intensity to our psychological component. Ours is a place to focus and seriously deal with the problem of overweight,
> —Gerald Musante, director of Structure House.

Unofficially . . .
Good, reputable, programs can take very different approaches. Case in point:

▪ "The scale has created more obesity than moved people down in weight. It's a reminder of failure." —Alan Wayler, executive director of Green Mountain.

▪ "Weigh every day—just like brushing your teeth, this is a health behavior to make a habit. Weighing provides feedback. Don't avoid the scale." (Source: Structure House Tips for Weight Control.)

weight down over the long haul," says Executive Director Alan Wayler, Ph.D. The program was founded by his wife, Thelma Wayler, a registered dietitian. With a maximum enrollment of 42, you get more personalized attention than at most places.

▪ **What you do:** Days are spent walking and hiking outdoors, attending "workshops" on topics such as "Managing Food Cravings," "De-powerizing Food" and "Fitness Planning for Back Home." You can take a number of exercise classes including "Water Toning" yoga and Tai Chi, all taught by credentialed health professionals. Daily calories are adjusted to your needs but never drop under 1,400. There's a separate two-week "Body Image" program consisting of a step-by-step approach to decreasing body dissatisfaction while helping you lose weight.

▪ **Expected weight loss:** Since the average stay is one week, this isn't measured.

▪ **Cost:** Varies according to season (winter is least expensive) and whether you take a single apartment or a duplex (you still get your own room). For instance, a week in spring or autumn runs $1,225 to $1,825 depending on your apartment.

Spas

There are so many spas, using so many different techniques, and so many books written on them. Here are a few things to consider:

▪ Go for the fun of it, not for a crash weight loss session. You'll just come home and gain it back.

▪ Some are more serious about diet and exercise than others. If you're considering one that emphasizes weight loss, go over the program by phone before you commit, making sure the diet is sound (no fruit juice fasts!) and that the exercise people are credentialed.

■ Think of a spa week or weekend as a great jump-start. It can reintroduce you to exercise, show you that low-fat food isn't so bad, and even knock off an encouraging pound or two.

■ Going for a little destressing, to begin yoga or learn stress management techniques, may be more valuable than going to lose weight. You can use those valuable techniques to help you cope without turning to food.

Surgery

Surgery should be used only as a last resort, after years of trying the diet/exercise/behavioral approach. But if nothing else truly works, don't be intimidated. Although complicated with life-altering side effects, these surgeries are relatively safe.

Gastric surgery

The idea behind gastric surgery is to limit the amount of food your stomach can hold and/or limit the opportunity for food to get absorbed in the small intestine.

Normally, food takes the path shown in Figure 6.1. You swallow, it goes down the esophagus and lands in the stomach, where it gets attacked by hydrochloric acid to help digest it down to small particles. Then off to the small intestine, which has three sections. In the first section, the duodenum, it gets further broken down with a shower of bile acids and pancreatic juice. Iron and calcium in food is absorbed through the duodenum walls and into the bloodstream. The remainder of the caloric and non-caloric nutrients get absorbed in the next sections,

Figure 6.1
Here's what a
normal digestive
tract looks like.
Food goes down
the esophagus,
lands in the
stomach, then
particles travel
to the duodenum
where certain
nutrients get
absorbed. More
absorption takes
place in the next
areas of the
small intestine,
the jejunum and
ileum. Waste is
stored in the
large intestine
before being
excreted.
(Source: National
Institutes of
Health.)

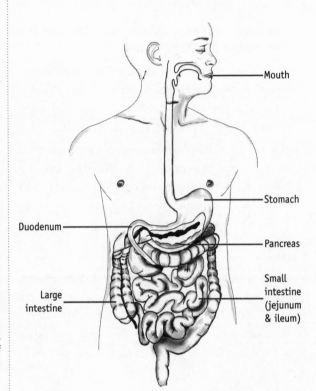

the jejunum and ileum, which are about 20 feet long. Any remaining undigested particles get stored in the large intestine, turning into feces, which get eliminated. Surgery restricts this process.

Do this only if your BMI is over 40 (see BMI chart in Chapter 1) and the obesity is endangering your life. Don't do it unless absolutely necessary; changing eating habits and increasing exercise are by far better ways to lose weight and keep it off. Although this is a serious operation with side effects, if your doctor strongly recommends surgery as your best option, then take note that a recent government report concluded that this operation is not excessively risky. "[I]t is puzzling that this treatment [gastric surgery] is not more widely used for severely obese individuals at very high risk for obesity-related morbidity and mortality. It is possible that health-care providers and individuals fail to fully understand the severity and costs of obesity in terms of both increased morbidity and mortality and its impact on the quality of life. Perhaps there is an intrinsic fear of the dangers of surgery due in part to lack of knowledge. In fact, mortality associated with gastric surgery for obesity is less than one percent." (Source: *Weighing the Options,* Institute of Medicine, 1995.) Gastric surgery involves one or both of the following operations:

In gastric banding (see Figure 6.2), a band or staples is used to almost completely close off most of the stomach, leaving only a small pouch connected to your esophagus. The procedure involves wrapping a band around the top part of the stomach. In vertical banded gastroplasty (see Figure 6.3) both a band and staples are used to make the pouch. In both, a narrow passage right under the band connects the pouch to the rest of the stomach.

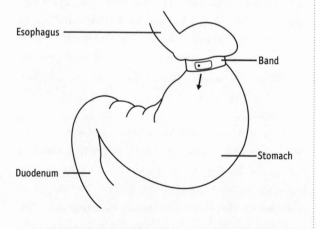

Figure 6.2 A band ties off most of the stomach, leaving just a small pouch to hold food. (Source: National Institutes of Health.)

After the operation, your stomach can hold only a half cup to a cup of food, whereas normally it can

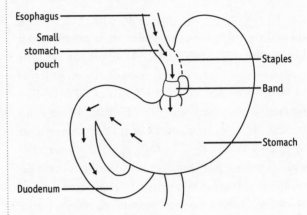

hold three pints. There's a tiny opening from the pouch to the rest of the stomach, where food drips down very slowly, making you feel full longer. As you can imagine, unless you eat pure fat all day, it's hard to consume enough food to make you fat.

Payoff: About 30 percent achieve normal weight, while 80 percent achieve some degree of weight loss.

Risks: Overeating causes the stomach to over-stretch, which causes vomiting. Also, the band can erode or the staples loosen. In a small number of cases stomach juices leak into the abdomen, requiring an emergency operation. In less than 1 percent of cases, there's infection or death from complications. Compared to many other surgeries, this is fairly safe.

In a Roux-en-Y gastric bypass, first you do the pouch operation described earlier. Then, instead of letting the food go from the stomach to the duodenum, the duodenum is circumvented. Instead a section lower down in the small intestine (in the jejunum) is attached directly to the stomach pouch, as you can see from Figure 6.4. By bypassing entire

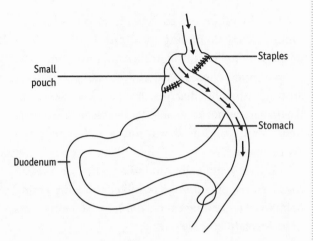

Small
pouch

Staples

Stomach

Duodenum

Figure 6.4 In order to minimize absorption of calorie-containing nutrients, an entire section of the small intestine, from the duodenum into the jejunal area of the small intestine, is bypassed. Instead, a section from the further reaches of the intestine is sewn onto the stomach pouch. As the arrows show, food goes directly into the sewn-on section. (Source: National Institutes of Health.)

sections of the small intestine, less calorie-containing particles get a chance to be absorbed. There's also a more complicated version of this operation called "extensive gastric bypass" where parts of the stomach are cut out and even more of the small intestine is bypassed.

Payoff: In general, people lose two-thirds of their excess weight within two years.

Risks: Somewhere between 10 to 20 percent of patients require follow-up operations to correct complications. One-third develop gallstones (clumps of cholesterol and other matter that form in the gallbladder).

In addition to all the risks described for the gastric surgery, nearly 30 percent develop nutrition deficiencies because food isn't as well absorbed. As I mentioned earlier, the duodenum is where we absorb iron and calcium. Lack of iron and calcium can lead to anemia and osteoporosis. However, taking vitamin and mineral supplements can partially or completely offset the deficiencies (if you have enough of the nutrients traveling through, some will get absorbed by the lower small intestine).

The operation can cause an uncomfortable sensation called "dumping syndrome," where food moves too quickly through the small intestine. The symptoms are nausea, weakness, sweating, faintness, and, occasionally, diarrhea after eating. Sweets in particular can make people feel so weak and sweaty that they have to lie down until the dumping syndrome passes.

Not very appealing-sounding stuff. I repeat: Avoid either operation if possible; changing eating habits and increasing exercise are, by far, better ways to lose weight and keep it off.

Liposuction

Liposuction isn't about weight loss, it's about contouring the body: vacuuming out fat from specific areas, usually the abdomen, thighs, and back. Most doctors use the Tumescent technique, which involves infiltrating the area to be suctioned with a saline solution containing anesthetic to minimize pain and epinephrine, which constricts blood vessels and minimizes bleeding. A probe, called a cannula, is inserted through the skin and into the fatty tissue. The cannula is connected to a vacuuming device that sucks out the fat cells. Some hospitals and clinics are starting to use ultrasound as an adjunct to the traditional liposuction operation. It involves inserting a special ultrasonic cannula into a small incision to destroy the fat cells, literally liquefying them. Then the traditional cannula is inserted and the fat is vacuumed out, making for an easier operation.

I repeat, liposuction is not a way to lose weight. In fact, you should have lost weight and kept it off before even considering liposuction, according to Saeed Marefat, MD, of the Metropolitan Plastic

Surgery Center in Fairfax, Virginia. "The ideal candidate for liposuction is someone who is normal weight, but has localized areas of fat that do not respond to diet and exercise," says Marefat.

While this is a piece of cake compared to the gastric operations, it's still surgery, and any surgery has risks. So if you decide to do it, make sure your physician has been certified by the American Board of Plastic Surgery; certification from other boards may not be legitimate. If you opt for ultrasound liposuction, make sure your surgeon has been trained in the procedure and has experience performing it. Ultrasound is tricky—if not done properly the waves can damage the skin.

Watch Out!
"Liposuction is definitely no substitute for diet and exercise. And even after surgery, you've got to stick with a good diet and exercise program to maintain the results."
—Saeed Marefat, MD of the Metropolitan Plastic Surgery Center in Fairfax Virginia.

Just the facts

- Commercial weight loss programs are a relatively inexpensive way to get weight loss help, but they're not the same, so understand what you're getting into.

- LEARN and Dr. Ornish's program are well researched and, depending on your needs, well worth investigating.

- Don't go on the very low-calorie liquid programs unless you've got to, and then only under an MD's supervision

- Residential programs are crash courses in weight loss—the good ones can teach you a lot.

- Last-resort surgery is just that, but if you need it, don't be intimidated about seriously considering it.

GET THE SCOOP ON...
Tip-offs to quack diets ▪ Diet claims ▪
A few good not-very-diet diet books ▪
Why we buy the con

Diets that Deliver,
Diets that Deceive

N eed a few laughs? Try searching "diet" on the Barnes and Noble bookstore website. Some 600-plus eye-blurring titles later, you'll see how the stiff competition has prompted so many ridiculous or implausible titles. The variety was astounding; you could spend a busy lifetime losing weight in every imaginable way. Somehow *The Chocolate Lovers' Diet: Enjoy Chocolate and Say Goodbye to Fat* sounded much more enticing than the *No-Cellulite Cookbook: The First Cookbook/Menu Planner to Help You Fight Those Lumps, Bumps, and Bulges.* And equally intriguing in completely different ways were *God's Answer to Fat, Lose It,* and *The Fabulous Sex Organ Diet: On the Leading Edge of the Science of Weight Loss.* Until it showed up on my screen I'd almost forgotten about an old classic in empty promises: *The Rotation Diet: Lose up to a Pound a Day and Never Gain It Back.*

171

Do any of these work? Well . . . yes—whether you rely on chocolate or God, you'll lose weight on *any* diet that reduces calories from the level you normally eat. Are any of these diets going to help you keep the weight off long term? Only those that offer a way of eating that you can stick with long term. And you can't tell nutritional soundness by the title of the book—some of the more official sounding books, complete with a doctor's name and photo on the cover, are the worst. (Two cases in point are *Dr. Berger's Immune Power Diet* and *Dr. Atkins' New Diet Revolution.* Meanwhile, perfectly decent diets may be hyped with lighter-weight titles—*Eat More, Weigh Less.*) To give you an idea of what these books are saying, check out this chapter's sidebars for excerpts from both the good and the questionable ones.

With all the zillions of diets out there, really there are only a few that are taken seriously in the nutrition community. And really only one is widely promoted in professional circles: the low-fat, USDA pyramid-style diet, abundant in fruits, vegetables, and whole grains. Others that are starting to gain a following are the Mediterranean diet—also rich in fruits and vegetables but higher in fat because of all the olive oil—and the traditional Asian diet. (Chapter 4 describes the USDA and Mediterranean pyramids.)

Even those on opposite sides of the obesity-as-a-health-hazard debate agree that we should adopt one of these diets (and get regular exercise). Those who see obesity as a health risk think we should lose weight on these diets; members of other camps, who believe that you can be fit and fat, recommend these same diets for health, but not necessarily for weight loss.

Evaluating diets

Here are the important questions you should ask yourself before following *any* diet:

- Is it healthy? Take a look at a typical day on the diet and compare it to the Food Guide Pyramid in Chapter 4. If it closely matches up then the diet's healthy.

- Is it at least 1,200 calories? Believe me, you'll lose weight on 1,200 calories. You'll probably lose on 2,000 or more if the diet's low in fat and you exercise regularly. Even on 1,200 calories you can't get the recommended levels of all the nutrients you need, so you'll still need to take a multivitamin/mineral tablet for insurance. Under 1,200, forget it; your metabolism will slow, and you'll be miserably hungry and too weak to exercise.

- Does it advocate a half- to two-pound-a-week weight loss? Any more than that and the diet's too low in calories (or the exercise recommendations are too high for the calorie intake). Lose more than a pound or two a week and you'll probably gain it back just as quickly, and it could take a toll on your health. But even on 1,200+ calories, expect to lose up to five pounds a week the first few weeks of the diet—it's water weight, which eventually comes back.

- Does it forbid certain foods? Diets based on single foods (like fruit, or juice), and diets that eliminate whole categories of food (such as dairy or wheat) limit you nutritionally. It's hard enough trying to get the recommended levels of vitamins and minerals from our regular food supply. Crossing out a whole category—such as wheat—could result in nutrient deficiencies. Or, eliminating sugar could set you up for a major cookie and candy binge when you can't take it any more.

▪ Does it recommend that you increase physical activity? Research shows that most people need to get regular exercise to keep off the weight they lose. Diet alone usually doesn't cut it over the long haul. (A very good diet book that spotlights exercise with a detailed plan is *Strong Women Stay Slim* by Miriam E. Nelson, Ph.D., Bantam, 1998.)

▪ Does it require supplements such as herbs, amino acids, or high doses of vitamins and minerals? No supplements have been proven to help you lose weight, except ephedra (in the herb Ma Huang), which is dangerous (see Chapter 8). As mentioned earlier, a standard multivitamin/mineral supplement is good insurance for health—not weight loss—when you're taking in only 1,200 to 1,500 calories. Also, there's a case to made for taking separate calcium and vitamin E tablets (presented in Chapter 5). If the diet plan calls for higher levels of supplementation than this, I smell a gimmick. Compare the plan's recommendations to the appropriate levels of vitamins and minerals in the charts in Chapter 5.

▪ Does the author criticize well-known experts and trash the scientific establishment? While it's true that the medical/nutritional establishment hasn't been able to stem the obesity problem, neither has anyone else. The "underdog vs. the big, bad, establishment" marketing ploy implies that there is a conspiracy to keep out good information. Nonsense. First of all the "establishment" is breaking down. Nutrition researchers are not a monolithic group; there's debate within the scientific community on how to treat obesity. Second, even if they wanted to, nutritionists and doctors couldn't suppress a new technique, food combination, or supplement that conquers obesity; overweight people would be beating down doors for it.

If you come across any of following buzzwords, be skeptical:

- **Breakthrough.** If it were a real breakthrough we'd be seeing a lot less overweight people out there.

- **Melt fat.** Sounds like it has something to do with a blowtorch and high pain tolerance. . .

- **Revolutionary.** Look carefully, it's probably the same old thing cleverly repackaged.

- **Miracle.** Uh huh.

- **Easy.** For most people, making the type of changes that will take off body fat *isn't* easy. But it can be easi*er* with a plan that's caloric enough so that you're not hungry and promotes a gradual increase in doable exercise. And, depending on your mind-set, the experience can be challenging, interesting, exciting, tortuous, difficult, or painful.

- **Detoxifying.** If you truly ate something toxic—like arsenic, lead, or another poison, or megadosed on selenium, vitamin A, or another nutrient—you'd better get to the hospital pronto, not wait for some diet plan to not work. Of course they never mean *real* toxins. They're talking about vague, never-scientifically-defined

Unofficially . . .
"Books that served up . . . provocative dieting advice rang up an estimated $141 million in sales in 1997. Almost a dozen new ones appear each year. But best-seller status has more to do with the marketing of the book—publicity, a novel gimmick, talk-show host appearances by the author—than with content. The boring truth is that a sensible diet, in combination with exercise, has always been the way for most people to lose weight." (Source: *Consumer Reports*, January, 1998.)

substances that supposedly have built up because of your old diet. This is just one more unsubstantiated marketing gimmick.

▪ **Food combining.** This should be your unequivocal signal to drop the book immediately (later in the chapter I explain why food combining is so meaningless).

▪ **30 pounds in 30 days.** Anything that promises rapid weight loss is either extremely dangerous or extremely untruthful.

What's out there

Most of the 600-plus diet books in the Barnes and Noble website are variations on a few themes. The following sections list the themes: types of diets that you'll run into again and again. There are so many books that fit under the following categories; I can give only a few examples.

Healthy diets

Whether you can stick with a particular diet or not depends on how skillfully the authors lead you into change, how easy it is to follow the plan, and how motivated you are. But at least you can be sure that the following are good for you:

▪ **Low-fat/high-carbohydrate diets.** According to U.S. Department of Agriculture surveys, the average American derives about 37 percent of calories from fat. According to many experts I spoke with, the number is probably closer to 42 percent. In any case, the government wants us at 30 percent, while other experts say 20 percent. The rest of the diet: 55 to 60 percent should come from carbohydrates and 15 to 20 percent from protein.

Pros: At this stage in the science, these seem to be the best diets for weight loss. It's easier to lose weight on a low-fat diet because low-fat foods are usually low-calorie, so boo-boos aren't such a big deal. Also, there's evidence that you expend more calories digesting carbohydrates and protein than fat. Storing butter, salad dressing, fatty meat, and all the other high-fat foods on your belly and thighs is a cinch for your body, whereas it takes a lot more effort to convert protein and carbs into body fat. These are all reasons to go low-fat if you can possibly stand it. And it's getting easier to stand; many books offer truly delicious recipes and it's easier than ever to get a tasty low-fat meal in a restaurant.

If the plan follows a low-fat pyramid approach (nonfat dairy; plenty of fruits, vegetables, and whole grains; and little animal protein) it's very healthy. Low-fat diets also seem to have an edge over others for long-term weight maintenance; people who've successfully kept their weight loss often report eating a low-fat diet.

Cons: If you've been living on fried foods and creamy desserts, going low-fat can be such a shock that you drop out. However, a gradual approach works and is worth it. Another drawback: If done wrong, low-fat diets are not necessarily low in calories. I've heard it countless times: "I got fat eating fat-free cookies, fat-free ice cream and fat-free Entenmann's cakes." These diets only work if you stick with naturally low-fat foods, such as beans, fruits, cereals, and grains. Sugar-pumped fat-free sweets are still loaded with calories and can undermine the whole thing. Also, even a well-balanced low-fat diet can dip so low in fat (under 15 percent of total calories) that you miss out on beneficial fats,

Timesaver
This beautiful, quick dessert feels so much more luxurious than plain fruit: Peel three oranges with a knife, removing with pith. Slice oranges crosswise, into rounds. Soak for 15 minutes up to 24 hours in a mixture of 1 Tablespoon honey, 2 teaspoons fresh lemon juice, and a teaspoon of orange or citrus liqueur.

such as omega-3s in fish oil (more on omega-3s in Chapter 5).

Examples: Eat More, Weigh Less, by Dean Ornish (HarperCollins, 1993) and all the other Dean Ornish books. Dr. Ornish developed his virtually vegetarian, under-10-percent-of-calories-from-fat diet for people with heart disease (recently, he's added flax seed oil tablets to ensure that you get essential fats). Ornish, widely respected in the research community, showed for the first time that heart disease could be reversed with a combination of his diet, exercise, and meditation. Clogged arteries opened, and people who were scheduled for heart surgery canceled their appointments. But you'd probably have to be facing a life-threatening illness to make the radical lifestyle changes required in this book and in his first book, *Dr. Dean Ornish's Program for Reversing Heart Disease.* If you're good at keeping fat low but don't want to go Ornish low, then you can stick with the basic principles of the book but increase the fat a little by adding such healthier fats as olive and canola oils and fatty fish. This way, you'll get a very healthy weight loss plan. But remember, if you want to reverse heart disease, you really need to follow his diet (and his exercise and stress reduction strategies). If some of the book's 250 recipes developed by celebrity chefs are a little too involved (but yummy-sounding), you might do better with *Everyday Cooking with Dr. Dean Ornish* (HarperCollins, 1996).

Choose to Lose, by Ron and Nancy Goor (Houghton Mifflin, 1995) presents a three-pronged strategy for staying within a fat limit, eating (ironically) enough calories, and getting daily aerobic exercise (walking is fine). All foods are fair game as long as you stay within your "Fat Budget," which is individualized according to your sex and goal weight. One of the nice things about this plan is that it's not hung up on calories. The authors believe that if you keep fat low; stick with whole grains, fruits and vegetables, lean dairy, and meats; limit high sugar foods (even fat-free ones); and get some exercise, you can pretty much eat what you want. Unlike the health-foody or wan, fat-free versions of rich American favorites found in many diet books, the 50 recipes here seem both interesting and easy.

Two Not-Necessarily-Weight Loss Diets. In addition to the standard low-fat, high-carb, USDA pyramid-style diets, the traditional Mediterranean and Asian diets are also considered very healthy. At this point, you'll find more cookbooks than diet books on these ethnic ways of eating. The diet books may come. For now, you can adapt these diets to a weight loss plan by keeping calories reasonable:

▪ *The Mediterranean Diet:* Greeks, Southern Italians, and Spaniards have about half the risk of nutritionally linked cancers, such as colon cancer, and a lower risk of heart disease than we Americans. Many researchers, including the head of Harvard's School of Public Health, are convinced it has something to do with their diet. (However, as their diets are getting more Americanized, their risk for our diseases are increasing. So, this Mediterranean diet I'm referring to is the traditional diet.) What this diet shares with the healthy diet recommended by leading health authorities in the U.S. is that it's high in complex carbohydrates, fruits, and vegetables and moderate in meat. Interestingly, the diet is not low-fat—in fact at about

Moneysaver
"[W]hat you gain in convenience you often sacrifice in taste, health, and your weight. The price is also steep in terms of dollars. For that little box called dinner, you are paying at least five times what it would cost you if you were to purchase the ingredients separately and make the dish yourself." (Source: A critique of frozen dinners from *Choose to Lose* by Ron and Nancy Goor, Houghton Mifflin, 1995.)

Unofficially . . .
Fat intake as percent of caloric intake in the U.S. and Japan:

Year	U.S.	Japan
1950	40.0	7.9
1960	41.5	10.6
1970	42.3	18.7
1980	41.8	23.6
1985	43.5	24.5

Source: A scientific paper in the *Japan Journal of Cancer Research,* 1992–83 by E. L. Wynder, E. Taioli, and Y. Fujita.

40 percent of calories, the Greeks eat more fat than we currently do. But the quality of their fat is very different from ours. Ours comes mainly from vegetable oils, such as corn and soybean oil, that are rich in a type of polyunsaturated fat called omega-6. Most of the fat in the Mediterranean diet is olive oil. This is predominantly monounsaturated fat, which has been shown not to elevate blood cholesterol in humans or increase cancer risk in lab animals. But it's not just the fat; the abundant fruits and vegetables eaten in these sunny climes impart lots of protective compounds. Then there's speculation that their regular but moderate wine intake may be protective. Besides diet, other lifestyle factors also seem to be protective—like afternoon siestas, closer families, more social support, and walking instead of taking the car.

- *The Asian Diet:* Two of the leading cancer killers in this country—cancers of the colon and breast—used to be rare in Japan. But rates of these cancers are now rising among Japanese, and scientists are pointing fingers at the change in diet as one of the culprits. More specifically, they note an increase in fat consumption, from about 8 percent of total calories in the 1950s to 25 percent or more nowadays. In a study of Asians who emigrated to California, breast cancer rates rose up to American levels in just one generation. The traditional Asian diet is based on rice, noodles, breads, and other grainy foods and is rich in fruits, vegetables, tofu, and beans. Oil is the main fat, and it's used sparingly (think of Chinese food cooked in a minimum of oil). Meat is an occasional condiment, sweets and eggs are eaten only a few times a week. The one amendment I'd make to this diet would be to include more dairy, which is rarely eaten in Japan.

Meals out of the blender

Slim Fast is probably the best known of the "meal replacement" bunch, followed by such rivals as Nestle's Sweet Success Booster and Ensure Lite and a few health food store variations. The standard prescription: that you have a shake (it comes either in powdered form that you mix with skim milk or in a ready-to-drink can) for breakfast, lunch, and snack, then have a healthful "real meal" for dinner.

Pros: This portion-controlled system can help rein in an out-of-control eating situation. Still unpublished results of long-term studies using Slim Fast suggest that it can also help maintain weight loss. (Normally, I don't report on unpublished research, but parts of this study have been released to fellow scientists in meetings.) The Slim Fast study is led by George Blackburn, MD, an associate professor of medicine at Harvard Medical School and chief of the nutrition and medicine clinic at Beth Israel Deaconess Medical Center at Harvard. Five years ago, Blackburn recruited 109 women and 49 men and put them on the three-shakes-a-day-plus-one-real-meal plan for 12 weeks. Going into the experiment, the average age of the group was 40, with an average weight of 195. Over the 12 weeks, women lost 7.5 percent of their body weight (so a 195-pound woman would have dropped to 180), and men lost 9 percent (going from 195 to $177^{1}/_{2}$ pounds, for example). After the 12-week weight loss phase, the group was given a workbook teaching them how to incorporate the shakes into a healthy

Bright Idea
Make room on your healthy, low-fat diet to include even junky favorites so you don't wind up binge-ing. A 100-cal portion daily, or a larger portion three times a week is fine. A sure fire way to develop a food craving is to go on a diet that restricts the food. On a low carb diet you'll dream of pasta, on a no-sugar diet you'll be sneaking Snickers.

eating plan. Blackburn dubs it "10-and-10"—over the course of a week you eat 10 real meals and 10 shakes. The participants have been tracked for the past five years, coming in to be weighed twice a year. Almost everyone is leaner than when they first started the experiment, but the average weight loss is not quite as good as when they ended the initial 12-week phase. On average, women have remained at 5 percent below their starting weight; men, 7 per-cent below. Even though this weight loss may seem minor, it's better than the weight gain that typically happens over five years. And, says Blackburn, it's enough to have made significant improvements in levels of blood cholesterol and blood sugar, thus lowering these risk factors for heart disease and diabetes.

Cons: The shakes can get pretty monotonous and hard to stick with. Even though the better brands include the full complement of vitamins and miner-als, unless you pack your real meals with fruits and vegetables, you may be missing out on the hundreds of other beneficial compounds such as lycopenes (compounds that give tomatoes their red color) or the allylic compounds in garlic and onions. Without counseling (or a big effort on your own) to make the eating and exercise lifestyle changes necessary to keep weight off, you'll be stranded when you go off the shakes, setting up a weight regain situation.

What to Look For: The sanest, healthiest choices are those offering the following per ready-to-drink or powdered shake mixed with milk:

- 180 calories
- About 33 percent of daily value (DV) of 19 to 21 vitamins and minerals
- 4 g fiber

- About 10 g of protein
- About 6 g of fat
- About 19 to 22 g carbohydrate

Herbs and the like are not proven to help and may even be harmful.

Out of the scientific mainstream

"The Zone Diet": It's called a 40/30/30 diet, and it's spawned lots of copycats. That's 40 percent from carbohydrates, 30 percent from protein, and 30 percent from fat (meanwhile 55-65/15/20-30 is generally considered healthiest). In other words, not quite as low-carb as the diets just described and not quite as high-protein as some of them. So you don't have the problem of ketosis or the strain of too much protein on the kidneys. The main claim: This configuration will keep insulin low, and since insulin favors fat storage, you'll store less and burn more body fat. "It's excess insulin that makes you fat and keeps you fat," writes Barry Sears, author of the best-selling "Zone" books.

Pros: There are a few research reports indicating that this type of diet might help Type II diabetics lose weight, but there's really not enough evidence to know whether this approach is more effective than losing weight on higher-carb diets, or whether it's safe, long-term. Also, if for some reason you decide to go on a very low-calorie diet (around 1,000 calories), 30 percent protein is okay because it's the amount you need to keep up lean body mass. And, if the diet is "Zone"-like, with a decent number of fruits and vegetables, it's as reasonable as low-cal diets get.

Cons: The three problems with the Zone diet are too few calories, too much fat if you try to increase

Watch Out!
Try a "Lose
30 Pounds in
30 Days" diet
and you might
spend some of
those days in a
hospital.

calories, and, possibly, too few carbohydrates for optimum health. Sears has you figure out how many "blocks" of protein, carbohydrate, and fat you should eat daily, based on your weight and an estimate of your lean body mass. It's all pretty complicated, and I wonder how many of the hundred thousand plus people buying the book got through these initial calculations. After plugging in both my and my mother's numbers I saw immediately why everyone's losing weight on the Zone: Our daily allotted protein, carb, and fat blocks came to about 900 calories! So, whether Sears' insulin theories prove legitimate or not, anyone's going to lose weight on this low a level.

So what happens if you try to make the Zone higher in calories? Since protein is fixed, and carbs are closely tied to protein (one carb block is allowed for every protein block), something's got to give, and that's fat. To his credit, Sears does push the healthier fats described in Chapter 4, but there's always the danger with a high-fat diet, even one high in healthier fats, that you'll easily overdo calories and gain weight.

Then there's the whole question of Sears' scientific rationale. He brings a mind-boggling set of biochemical theories to the weight loss table—theories that most mainstream scientists find interesting but unproven at best and quacky at worst. For instance, while it's true that many obese people are insulin resistant (often one step before diabetes), the prevailing viewpoint is that obesity *causes* insulin resistance, not the other way around. So losing weight on any diet will reverse the insulin resistance. And cutting carbs back to 40 percent is a little restrictive both nutritionally and psychologically. Nutritionally, you may end up skimping on magnesium, B vitamins, fiber, and other nutrients rich in grain-based foods. Psychologically, especially for you carb lovers, that little bit of pasta, bread, and rice may leave you feeling deprived.

Examples: The Carbohydrate Addicts LifeSpan Program by Richard and Rachel Heller (Dutton, 1997) (see sidebar). And of, course the best-selling "Zone" books by Barry Sears, Ph.D.

The only circumstance under which I could possibly recommend a diet that allows fewer than 50 to 60 percent of calories as carbohydrates is in the case of high blood triglycerides (blood fat is different from cholesterol but still heart damaging). Diabetics are prone to this condition, and the American Diabetic Association suggests trying a 45 percent carb, 40 percent fat (using mainly monounsaturated fat, still keeping saturated fat low), 15 percent protein diet. But, recommends diet and diabetes researcher Thomas Wolever, MD, Ph.D., associate professor of Medicine and Nutritional Sciences at the University of Toronto, "Usually just losing weight is enough to lower blood triglycerides. First try the high-carb, low-fat diet because it's more likely to help you lose weight." If follow-up blood tests in one month show that you still have high triglycerides on the high carb diet, then slightly lower the amount of carbohydrates and slightly increase the fat level, using olive oil and canola oil, he advises. But, as you can see, this diet is not high in protein. The lower-carbohydrate levels are replaced by monounsaturated fat, not protein.

Low-Carbohydrate/High-Protein Diets: Imagine never eating pasta, bread, or rice again. That's basically what you'd have to do to bring your carb

> " If you, like millions of Americans, are carbohydrate addicted, frequent snacking on "healthy" high-carbo, low-fat foods such as breads, pasta, fruits, and juices—even carrots, cottage cheese, and yogurt—may increase your chances for weight gain and ill health." (Source: The inside jacket cover of *The Carbohydrate Addict's LifeSpan Program* by Richard and Rachel Heller Dutton, 1997—an example of how diet-book authors can make manistream science look suspect.) "

consumption down to the 6-to-25 percent of calories that these diets demand. Meanwhile, your fat intake can soar to 65 percent of calories, and protein consumption generally runs from 30 to 50 percent of calories. You're eating a lot of meat, cheese, and eggs. Sounds heavenly? Read on and think again.

Pros: The only one I can think of is that you'll lose more weight the first few weeks than you would on high-carb diets of the same calorie level. But it's all smoke and mirrors. Those extra pounds you're shedding are water weight, lost as a result of the

---

Want to see how unhealthy the Atkins' diet really is? Check out this prototype menu plan from *Dr. Atkins' New Diet Revolution* 1995, (M. Evans and Co.):

Breakfast

Eggs, scrambled or fried, with bacon, ham, sugarless sausage, or Canadian bacon

Decaffeinated coffee or tea

Lunch

Bacon cheeseburger, no bun

Small tossed salad

Seltzer water

Dinner

Shrimp cocktail with mustard and mayo

Clear consommé

Steak, roast, chops, fish, or fowl

Tossed salad (choice of dressings)

Diet gelatin with a spoonful of whipped, artificially sweetened heavy cream

diuretic (water excreting) action of all that protein. Water weight *always* comes back.

Cons: Let me count the ways.

1. Diets high in animal protein are linked to cancer.

2. You skimp on all the nutritional goodies packed into complex carbs like fiber, B vitamins, magnesium, and other minerals.

3. Years of eating high levels of protein could cause kidney damage because of all the protein by-products that will have to be processed by this organ.

4. Lowering carbs below 20 percent of calories means the body can't make enough blood sugar and is forced to produce *ketones* as an alternate source of fuel for the cells. Ketones can make you feel dizzy and make your breath stink like rotten apples—and a by-product of ketone production are fat-like "remnant particles" which may have a role in clogging up arteries. Ketones, however, do suppress appetite, which is one reason these diets "work."

5. Diets like Atkins', loaded with steak, eggs, cheese, and other saturated fat, can do a number on your cholesterol level. Even though, in some cases, cholesterol may drop a little if you lose weight on his diet, that's because cholesterol usually drops with weight loss. But if you're prone to high cholesterol, you'll most likely see a much bigger drop on a high-carb/low-fat diet).

6. No one can stand these diets for long—sooner or later, the urge for something healthy like a piece of bread or a bowl of cereal gets the

Unofficially . . .
Warning: "This diet will cause your body to lose so much weight so quickly, that you should only stay on it 14 days at a time because it is not healthy to get too thin too quickly. Some people stay on it longer than 14 days at a time, but we don't recommend it unless you want to get too thin." (From the website of a company called Modern Methods.) Oh no, none of us wants to get too thin now do we? From the pseudo-sciencemumbo-jumbo of this website, the Modern Methods diet sounds like another low-carb/high-protein clone.

better of you, and then you're left where you began, not having picked up any good rest-of-your-life slimming eating habits.

Examples: These diets were all the rage in the 1970s, with *Dr. Atkins' Diet Revolution* and *The Scarsdale Diet* leading the pack. They've recently made a big comeback with *Dr. Atkins' New Diet Revolution* (basically the same stuff as the original), *Protein Power,* and *Healthy for Life.*

Macrobiotic Diet: At its strictest, this diet can be lethal. At its most lax, it can be fairly healthy. Not necessarily for weight loss, macrobiotics is a philosophical system founded by George Ohsawa in the early part of this century. Ohsawa credits a diet based on brown rice, miso soup, sea vegetables, and other Japanese foods with curing his tuberculosis. He advocated a 10-step Zen macrobiotic diet. The steps get progressively stricter until a person is eating just grains. Scientifically unsubstantiated claims for this diet include preventing and treating cancer, AIDS, and other diseases. The Kushi Institute in Brookline, Massachusetts is a leading center of macrobiotics.

Pros: The least rigid approach to macrobiotics, done very carefully, could be healthy. You eat certain whole grains (30 to 50 percent of intake), cooked vegetables (30 to 50 percent of intake), beans and seaweed (5 percent each), a little oil and nuts, some fermented foods such as soy sauce and miso, and a few cooked fruits. So you'd be getting a high-fiber, low-fat vegetarian diet (some macrobiotic systems allow a little chicken or fish).

Cons: Even at its most lax, this diet allows no raw foods; fruits and vegetables must be cooked.

Most fruit, many vegetables, and some grains are excluded, which makes absolutely no scientific sense at all. While you could still fashion a nutritious diet from the permitted foods, you'd have to devote a huge part of your life to thinking about and preparing food. And forget about doing it at its strictest, unless you want to wind up with scurvy (vitamin C deficiency, which causes gum and skin disease and eventually death) and other deficiencies. Also don't get bamboozled by the non-science found in much of the macrobiotic literature: Among other things, this literature links heart disease to "too much fruit," and claims that cold drinks cause kidney stones.

Single Food Diets: These diets focus on a single food type because of (you guessed it) its "amazing fat-burning qualities." Remember the grapefruit diet where you had to eat grapefruit before each meal? Somehow they had people convinced that enzymes in the grapefruit would burn up the fat in the meal.

Pros: None

Cons: Even if the food is healthy, like grapefruit, too much of one food means exclusion of others, and, voilà! a nutritionally unbalanced diet. For instance, on the cabbage soup diet, you have no dairy all week except for the day when you drink eight glasses of skim milk. Ugh! And, of course, these diets leave you with no life lessons to help you keep off the weight, although they may instill in you a new food aversion.

Examples: The New Cabbage Soup Diet by Margaret Danbrot (St. Martins Mass Market Paper, 1997) has you eating unlimited cabbage soup every day, plus a few other foods.

66

Let's face it, everyone wants the quick fix. We think, 'If they can find a cure for dread diseases, isn't there an easy solution to this weight I've been struggling with?' Faddish diets are marketed extremely well, whereas diets that bring long-lasting results aren't exciting, and are hard work.
—Polly Fitz, MA, RD, CD/N, past president of the American Dietetic Association and Co-Owner, Health Training Resources.

99

Bright Idea
Vary your diet and it will probably be healthier. A study in the *Journal of the American Dietetic Association* found that people who averaged 71 to 83 different foods during the course of the 15 days of the study ate diets much higher in vitamin C, lower in sugar and sodium, and a little lower in saturated fat than those who ate 37 to 58 different foods.

Typing Diets: That's my name for diets that are geared, supposedly, to your particular physical "type."

Pros: None.

Cons: These diets have a high potential for being nutritionally unbalanced because they exclude foods that don't match your "type." And your "type" may be a figment of the author's imagination.

Examples: Dr. Abravanel's Body Type Diet (Bantam, 1993) divides us into gonadal, adrenal, thyroid, or pituitary types. *Eat Right 4 Your Blood Type* by Peter J. D'Admano (G.P. Putnam's Sons, 1997) recommends that you avoid or go for certain foods depending on whether you're a type O or A (no eggplant, but go for those snails), or B or AB (for you guys, tofu sardine fritters). All I can say is . . . "the gall of some people."

Herbal or Botanical Diets: These are either the whole shebang, with meal replacement shakes and herbal supplements, or just a bunch of herbal supplements that "enhance" your weight loss regimen. According to Varro E. Tyler, Ph.D., Emeritus Professor of Pharmacognosy (study of drugs from natural sources) at Purdue University, no herbs have been proven to help you lose weight except for Ma Huang, which contains the stimulant ephedrine. But Ma Huang can be dangerous—as you'll see in Chapter 8.

Pros: Let's see . . . if the herbs aren't dangerous, you may get a placebo effect?

Cons: There's no serious scientific backup to show that adding a bunch of herbs to your diet—that is, a bunch of expensive herbs—will make you any thinner any faster.

Examples: By way of example, here's an excerpt from an herbal system I picked up from HerbalLife's web-site: "Thermojetics Green & Beige Herbal Tablets— Discover how millions of people around the world are shaping up faster than ever! Thermojetics Green and Beige Tablets help you shed weight, look great, and feel better than ever without starving or over exercising. And they can also help you feel more in control, boost your confidence, give you the visible results you want." The ad goes on to explain that Green and Beige Tablets "work syner-gistically with each other," come from Chinese and Amazonian herbs, and "create a synergism that helps keep your body in favor of reducing fat."

The issues:

1. You've got to take something called "Green and Beige Tablets" seriously.

2. Just because something's an "ancient" herb or comes from the Amazon doesn't mean it works.

"Food Combining": These diets recommend certain food combinations and forbid other combinations, or they rotate foods so you don't eat them within a certain number of days. Among the rationales: improves digestion, enhances weight loss, and enables you to conquer food allergies.

Pros: None. Even if the diet is ultimately balanced, what a pain it would be to go around making sure you don't have meat and starch within a certain number of hours of each other!

Cons: It's quackery. Food-combining rules vary among the different diets, based on the author's whim, not science. And please, someone should get it through to these folks that a) there are no secret pockets in the body where food can sit and ferment, and b) we come equipped with enzymes and other substances that break down protein, carbohydrates, and fats. As long as you stay away from rocks and other non-food substances, your body can digest what you feed it.

Examples: This is the fad that won't die, one that reached super-stardom in the 1980s with a few runaway best-sellers that have been reissued, such as Harvey and Marilyn Diamond's wildly popular *Fit for Life* diet. Here's how they explain it: "Food combining is based on the discovery that certain combinations of food may be digested with greater ease and efficiency than others. Food combining teaches that THE HUMAN BODY IS NOT DESIGNED TO DIGEST MORE THAN ONE CONCENTRATED FOOD IN THE STOMACH AT THE SAME TIME" (their uppercase letters). A concentrated food, they go on to explain, is any food that is not a fruit or vegetable. In their book, putting milk on your cereal is a no-no, as is topping your cracker with cheese.

The *Beverly Hills Diet* (revised for the 1990s as *The New Beverly Hills Diet: The Latest Weight-Loss Research That Explains a Conscious Food-Combining Program for Lifelong Slimhood* by Judy Mazel and Michael Wyatt, Health Communications, 1996) has equally kooky rules: "When you go from fruit to fruit, wait one hour. When you go from one food group to another, wait two hours minimum (three hours would be better). Once you've eaten protein, eat at least 80 percent protein for the remainder of the day." Earth to Judy? But oh the reward: She tells you to expect a 10 to 15 pound weight loss in three to five days—that's over 2 pounds a day! With a weight loss rate that big, kooky is starting to sound dangerous. I guess you could lose that much on Mazel's diet though. After all, on Day 1 all you eat is pineapple, corn-on-the-cob (sorry, no salt or butter), and salad with her dressing recipe. For a change of pace, on Day 2 you get 8 ounces of prunes, strawberries, and baked potatoes. She's not too fussy about amounts of these foods, but after some harsh lessons on the toilet, you probably won't be overdoing it.

Then there's *Dr. Berger's Immune Power Diet* (by Stuart Berger, Signet, 1986). This is sort of a variation on the food-combination theme, where certain foods can't be eaten within three days of each other. (More on him in the next chapter.)

The Rotation Diet: This can mean two things. It's the title of another 1980s big seller by Martin Katahn, Ph.D. that's still slinking around bookstores. Katahn wants you to switch calorie levels every few days to prevent the drop in metabolic rate (the rate at which your body burns calories) that sets in when you go on a low-calorie diet. For the first three days, women take in 600 calories (men get 1,200); then 900 for women and 1,500 for men for the next four days; then a week on 1,200 for women and 1,800 for men. Katahn says you'll lose 10 to 20 pounds that way. After that you're supposed to stop dieting, then go through the cycle again. In case you haven't guessed, this isn't healthy. First of all, the rapid weight loss phase is sure to be dangerous and debilitating. And since he's simply switching you back and forth among low-calorie diets—especially low for women—it's hard to believe your metabolism wouldn't slow down. Save yourself some misery and skip this one.

The other rotation diet is a food faddish favorite. In this one, you rotate your foods so that you never

66

The Beverly Hills Diet, in other words, is a step-by-step outline of how to binge and purge, with natural laxatives." So says Laura Fraser in her book *Losing It* (Dutton, 1997), which basically skewers the diet industry. The "natural laxatives" are the mountains of fruit you have to eat on that diet.

99

eat the same food on consecutive days (sometimes you have to wait four days) in order to prevent "getting allergic" to any one food. There's no scientific basis for that one.

Fasting: When people talk of fasting they're usually referring to a juice fast, where you have nothing but fruit juice and water for a day or more.

Pros: Some people may experience a spiritual benefit. For instance, during Ramadan, Muslims fast from sunrise to sunset. But after sunset they eat, so it's not deprivation, just self-control.

Cons: Whether it's complete fasting—nothing but water for a day or two—or just juice, there's no known health benefit. Proponents claim that the quick weight loss from a day or two of fasting motivates you to go on the "real" diet. Just as likely you'll be so weak and discouraged that all you feel like doing is bingeing on Lorna Doones. Others claim that fasting "detoxifies" and "purifies" your body. Ask exactly which toxins are being released, and you never get a straight answer. Seriously, folks, if we were full of toxins we probably wouldn't be around for much longer. The whole toxin theory is quackery at its apex. In fact, fasting can actually produce the semi-toxic substances called ketones that we discussed earlier in the chapter. Processing ketones can damage your kidneys. Also, fasting can be really constipating because there's no bulk to stimulate the intestinal muscles.

Some useful "not-entirely-diet" books

These books are light on the food prescription, heavier on the life management. Their sound advice can help you in your weight loss effort.

- *Eating on the Run,* 2nd ed. by Evelyn Tribole, MS, RD (Leisure Press, 1991). One-minute meals and snacks, a critique of convenience foods and fast foods, time-saving strategies, and how to organize your kitchen for quicker meal-making make this a good resource for those in a hurry.

■ *Nancy Clark's Sports Nutrition Guidebook,* 2nd ed., by Nancy Clark, MS, RD (Human Kinetics, 1997). If you're serious about exercise, this is a great resource. Find out how much protein athletes really need, how to carb-load before the big event, the best ways to stay hydrated, and much more.

■ *The Complete Idiot's Guide to Eating Smart,* by Joy Bauer (Alpha Books, 1996). This is a great primer, covering all the important areas of nutrition. It's incredibly hands-on and practical, chock-full of tips and specific instructions on eating for health, weight loss, pregnancy, college, and athletics.

■ *The Complete Idiot's Guide to Losing Weight,* by Susan McQuillan with Edward Saltzman (Alpha Books, 1998). In a simple yet comprehensive fashion, this book goes through the basics of weight loss, with lots of practical tips for cutting back on fat and calories and increasing exercise.

■ *The 8-Week Cholesterol Cure,* by Robert E. Kowalski (HarperCollins, 1990). If you're trying to lower your cholesterol, this book does a good job of including all the dietary links. If his dietary recommendations—a low-fat diet, plenty of oat bran (yes, oat bran can help lower cholesterol), and other helpful foods such as fish—aren't enough to lower your cholesterol, Kowalski suggests taking high doses of the B vitamin niacin. This works for some people, although there are

Timesaver
It's easy to grab five minutes to plan five meals. Do it while waiting for a meeting to start, waiting in line, waiting for an appointment, waiting anywhere.
(Source: *Eating on the Run,* by Evelyn Tribole, MS, RD. Leisure Press, 1991.)

side effects and you must only do so under a doctor's supervision.

- *The Diet-free Solution,* by Laurel Mellin (HarperCollins, 1998). The book is an outgrowth of nearly two decades of research at the University of California at San Francisco. Mellin found learning and practicing six skills helps people lose weight and keep it off. They are: strong nurturing, effective limits, body pride, good health, balanced eating, and mastery living. This is heady, heavy stuff; you need to work at this one and do some real soul searching. It seems worth it because her published research results show that not only do people lose on her program, but they continue losing two years later. If the book seems like too much to tackle on your own, investigate the possibility of joining one of her "Solution" groups, described in Chapter 6.

The following table lists Laurel Mellin's bright ideas (also backed by years of research) on the causes and cures of a weight problem from *The Diet-free Solution* (HarperCollins, 1998):

THE CAUSES	THE CURES
Mind	
1. Weak nurturing	Strong nurturing
2. Ineffective limits	Effective limits
Body	
3. Body shame	Body pride
4. Poor vitality	Good health
Lifestyle	
5. Unbalanced eating	Balanced eating
6. Stalled living	Mastery living

- *Living Without Dieting,* by John P. Foreyt, Ph.D., and G. Ken Goodrick, Ph.D. (Warner Books, 1994). Although the authors do give advice on what to eat, emphasizing a low-fat, pyramid-style diet, the book is really about changing the way you think about food, about being overweight, about dieting, and about exercising. Both men are psychologists specializing in obesity, and it shows. Through quizzes and self-evaluations and an emphasis on social support, the book leads you into a way of coping that reduces reliance on food and opens your world to other positive opportunities.

- *Thin for Life,* by Anne M. Fletcher, MS, RD (Houghton Mifflin, 1994). Fletcher interviewed 160 "masters" at weight maintenance, who lost at least 20 pounds and kept if off for three years or more. The insights from the masters are invaluable (I've used some in this book) and inspiring. Fletcher synthesizes their advice down to 10 instructive "Keys to Success." Her follow-up book, *Eating Thin for Life* (Houghton Mifflin, 1997), shares advice from the same 160 masters on coping with food, including 122 low-fat recipes.

Why do we believe the bad ones?

If so many of these diets are not only ineffective, but potentially harmful, how come we're still buying into them? One reason is because they throw up the illusion that this time it will be easy. Painless. Chocolate-filled. Anyone who's been around the diet block a few times knows that losing weight and keeping it off is hard work, but diet book authors, infomercial hosts, and product manufacturers deftly lead us back into the fantasy we desperately want to believe. Says author Malcolm Gladwell in a February 1998 *New Yorker* magazine piece about obesity: "If you read a large number of popular diet books in succession, what is striking is that they all seem to be making things up in precisely the same way. It is as if the diet-book genre had an unspoken set of narrative rules and conventions, and all that matters is how skillfully those rules and conventions are adhered to."

First, Gladwell notes, authors discuss their pain over being fat kids, or disillusionment with other diets out there. Then, writes Gladwell, comes "the Eureka Moment, when the author explains how he stumbled on the radical truth that inspired his diet." Later, the "Eureka Moment is followed typically by the Patent Claim—the point at which the author shows why his Eureka Moment, which explains how weight can be lost without sacrifice, is different from the Eureka Moment of all those other diet books explaining how weight can be lost without sacrifice." For instance, the Patent Claim of Robert Atkins, author of the best-selling *Dr. Atkins' New Diet Revolution,* is that insulin is principally to blame for weight gain, and that "the metabolic defect involving insulin can be circumvented by carbohydrates." He still hasn't proved this claim.

Diet book authors play into your frustration over your weight problem and repeated failures, offering you hope that finally, this time, you've got the answer between the book covers. And it's still hard for some people to believe that a book written by an MD, Ph.D., or other credentialed person could be bogus. Also, when your friend just lost 10 pounds on the latest diet, it's irresistible, no matter how unlikely the plan seems. Unfortunately, a few months later, when you've gained back that 10 pounds, the diet won't seem so irresistible to either of you. And good diets, like *Choose to Lose,* take effort and habit change. The typical American eats about one, maybe two fruits and vegetables daily. Total. Often the vegetable is french fries. Switching to five or more unfried vegetables and fresh fruits is radical. Fad diets make things seem easier and they never tell you whether anyone does well on them long-term. So, when you're ready to roll up your sleeves and do the healthy diet and exercise thing, a good diet book can be an inspiration and a teacher. If your eating and exercise habits are really out of whack, you may need more than a diet book to get back on track. If that's true for you, go back to Chapter 6 to get clued in on the wide world of nutrition programs to choose from.

Just the facts

- Learn the buzzwords and avoid buying a diet book dud.

- Sane and healthy diets are usually either low-fat, high-carb, or based on the Mediterranean and Asian diets.

- Diet books without a specific diet prescription can be helpful.

- Don't let your frustration with the system lure you into buying a useless book.

"
There's one message that comes through really clear: If you want to lose weight and keep it off, you really have to have a commitment to permanent changes in your lifestyle.
—Mary Lou Klem, Ph.D., Senior Research Fellow, University of Pittsburgh School of Medicine and a researcher with the National Weight Registry study of nearly 1,000 people who've successfully maintained their weight loss.
"

GET THE SCOOP ON...
Weight loss drugs ▪ Weight loss herbal
supplements ▪ Scam alerts ▪ Phony clinics,
dubious credentials

Diet Drugs, Weight Loss Supplements, and Scams

Chapter 8

They know your pain, they know your magic weight loss pill fantasy, and they're making good money off it. With varying degrees of truthfulness and responsibility, manufacturers are churning out drugs, supplements, creams, and devices that claim to help you fight fat. As of press time, few of these things have been proven to work. Those that do won't make you thin, but they may modestly boost your weight loss.

Diet drugs

Should you take a drug to help you lose weight? At this point, given the drugs on the market and their side effects, most of you shouldn't. However, for a minority of you, drugs may be warranted if all the following apply:

- You've lost all the weight you can after doing your very best with a diet and exercise approach.

201

- You are still carrying an amount of weight that is dangerously raising your blood pressure, blood cholesterol, or blood sugar.

- A responsible, trustworthy physician sees the need (but you still might want to get a second opinion).

- You respond well to the drug: It truly enhances weight loss and side effects are minimal.

Unofficially . . .
Although patients are asking their doctors for diet drugs— over 380,000 prescriptions were written between April and September of 1996—about 75 percent of patients stop taking the pills. Probably because they are disappointed by the small weight loss or disturbed by side effects.

The reason I'm so negative is that the drugs only work as long as you take them, they all have side effects, and the extra weight you lose can be as little as 5 pounds (the range is 5 to 22 extra pounds over diet alone). And since studies of more than a single year's duration haven't been carried out for most of these drugs, it's hard to say whether the drug will continue working over time and what the side effects of long-term use will be.

The argument made by the drug companies, and by the university researchers testing the diet drugs, is that obesity is a disease, and like many other diseases, it needs to be treated with drugs. But those same experts admit that, given the side effects and unknown long-term effects of the currently available drugs, taking drugs over the long haul might be dangerous. Hence the conclusion of the National Task Force on the Prevention and Treatment of Obesity (which included many prominent scientists who consult for the drug companies) published in the *Journal of the American Medical Association:* "Because obesity is a disorder that cannot be expected to remit without continued treatment, short-term (weeks or months) treatment of obesity with drugs is generally not warranted. Treatment with medications will likely need to be continued for years, and perhaps for the lifetime of the patient, to sustain weight loss and improve health." With about a third of America meeting the definition of obese, the money-making potential of an obesity drug that works is staggering.

But there are arguments against drugs. Those who believe that obesity is usually a symptom of an unhealthy lifestyle worry that people will just take a pill, forget about exercise and eating right, and become unhealthy thinner people instead of unhealthy fatter people. This won't happen if you take the existing drugs, since they don't take off that much weight. Even with drugs, people who have lots of body fat to lose will still need to exercise and watch their calories. But more effective pills may come onto the market in the next decade. Another argument against diet drugs is put forward by the anti-dieting movement folks and those who argue that obesity is not as big a medical risk as it's made out to be. These people see diet drugs as just another risky way of exploiting obese people.

Yes, drugs do carry risks. That's why you *must* go over the risks and benefits thoroughly with your doctor, says Arthur Campfield, Ph.D., Distinguished Research Leader in the department of metabolic diseases at the Nutley, NJ–based drug company Hoffmann LaRoche, Inc. "Since obesity has different origins," says Campfield, "we need a variety of drugs that work in different ways to meet people's individual needs." Also, the drugs have different risk factors, so people who can't take one type may safely take another. He says that one of the reasons the now-banned diet drugs fenfluramine and dexfenfluramine became so dangerous was that doctors were indiscriminately prescribing them, partly because of high patient demand for them. It got to the point where one doctor was handing out

Watch Out!
Although doctors are allowed to prescribe amphetamines for weight loss, these drugs, and closely related compounds such as ben-zpheteramine are not recommended because you could get hooked.

prescriptions for a fee over the Internet, recounts Campfield. "If patients are more reasonable and physicians more careful, we'll figure out how to use the drugs safely," he says. So, if and when safer, more effective drugs come out on the market, the reasons for taking them may become more compelling. Especially if diet and exercise aren't thrown out the window. Who knows? If a pill can safely help you take off a substantial amount of weight, it might even make it *easier* for you to exercise.

The caveats

Here are the major issues to keep in mind when considering whether to use prescription (and some non-prescription) diet drugs:

- They are recommended for people who are obese, not those with just a few pounds to lose. The National Institutes of Health recommends using them only if the obesity has put you at medical risk. The experts I consulted advised not going on them unless your BMI is 30 or more; some went down to a BMI of 27 if there was evidence of obesity-related disease such as high blood pressure or diabetes. And, as I mentioned, all suggest that you first give the diet and exercise route a fair chance.

- Not all drugs work for everyone. The research suggests that if you don't lose at least four pounds over four weeks on a particular drug, then it's unlikely to ever help you.

- They only work as long as you take them. In most studies people gained back the weight after stopping the medication. According to the chronic disease model of obesity, many people may need to stay on this type of medication for life, just as they'd take high blood pressure medicine for life. But the long-term safety of diet drugs is unknown—most research studies end after a year or so.

- The longer you take them, the less effective they are, probably because you develop a tolerance to them. Most studies show that your weight levels off after you've been on them for four to six months. And at this point, the Food and Drug Administration (FDA) doesn't want anyone taking higher doses than those currently allowed.

- They don't work, or don't work nearly as well, if you don't also curb calories and/or increase physical activity. So if you take the drugs, definitely get into a program of some sort (see Chapter 6 for suggestions).

- The drugs are approved for use for only a few weeks, although doctors are allowed to prescribe them for longer. This is where the weird politics of the FDA come into play. The FDA regulates how a medicine can be advertised or promoted and what can go on the label. But once a drug's out there, doctors are allowed to use it in ways other than what's on the label. This practice is called off-label use. So, your doctor could continue prescribing these drugs for the rest of your life. Another example of off-label use is combining two diet drugs. Both types of off-label uses may be risky because, as mentioned, there are no long-term safety studies.

- There are side effects—some mild, some dangerous.

Watch Out!
People with high blood pressure, abnormal heart rhythms, clogged or diseased heart arteries, or angina (chest pain) should not take sibutramine (brand name Meridia), a relative new-omer on the diet drug scene. Clinical trials have shown that the drug can increase blood pressure and heart rate and cause abnormal heart rhythms.

Here's what's up, doc

Ultimately, you and your doctor together will decide whether it's appropriate for you to take diet drugs. Since these drugs do have side effects, there's some important information you've got to pass on to your doctor. Of course, the doctor should remember to ask, but you know much can be skipped in those rushed appointments, so be prepared to bring up some of these issues yourself. Here's what should be discussed:

▪ Your weight, especially where the weight is distributed (belly fat being the most risky). Remember, it's generally assumed that these drugs are appropriate only for BMIs of 30 or above with accompanying medical risks.

▪ Your weight history. If you haven't given it the good ol' diet-and-exercise try a few times, come back after you're sure nothing else works.

▪ Your medical history and the medical history of your family. You're a better drug candidate if you have diabetes, high blood pressure (except you can't take the diet drugs that raise blood pressure), high blood cholesterol, and any other medical conditions that will improve with weight loss. Your doctor might consider a family history of these diseases reason enough to prescribe. Still, before considering drugs you should at minimum take a blood pressure test, a blood test to measure cholesterol and triglycerides, and a test for diabetes.

In addition, be sure to tell the doctor if you have any of the following conditions:

1. History of drug or alcohol abuse (diet drugs may be addictive for this group).

2. History of an eating disorder, depression, or manic depression (other types of therapy or other drug treatments may be more appropriate for you).

3. Use of monoamine oxidase (MAO) inhibitors or antidepressant medication (diet drugs may interact negatively with these medications).

4. Migraine headaches requiring medication (again, to avoid drug interactions).

5. Glaucoma (diet drugs may worsen this condition).

6. Diabetes.

7. Heart disease or heart condition, such as irregular heart beat (the drugs may worsen these conditions).

8. High blood pressure (ditto).

9. You're planning on surgery that will require general anesthesia.

10. You're pregnant or breast-feeding (the drugs haven't been tested for safety in these cases, so even if your doctor gives you the OK, there'd better be a very good reason to take them).

What we're taking

After the 1997 drug scare that sent two diet drugs off the market, we're still left with a few other choices. The two drugs—fenfluramine and dexfenfluramine (the "fen" in fen/phen)—were voluntarily withdrawn from the market because they caused heart valve damage in an estimated 30 percent of people. The "phen" part of fen/phen, the drug phentermine, is still on the market because the Food and Drug Administration (FDA) hasn't found evidence that it causes heart damage when taken alone.

Bright Idea
If you ever took the now banned fen/phen combo of diet drugs, the U.S. Department of Health and Human Services recommends that you see your doctor to check for heart or lung damage. The heart-valve damage caused by this drug combo can also lead to lung problems. The government recommends getting an echocardiogram, an ultrasound reading of the heart, to make sure you're okay.

What's left in the prescription market are a few drugs that act by suppressing your appetite and/or slightly boosting your basal metabolic rate (which increases the number of calories you burn). The Food and Drug Administration has approved some of them for treatment of obesity, while others are approved for treating depression, but doctors are allowed to prescribe them for obesity.

It's not completely clear exactly how these drugs work, but they seem to increase one of two types of brain chemicals involved in appetite: serotonin or catecholamines. The result: When combined with diet and exercise the drugs may help you lose anywhere from $4^1/_2$ to 22 pounds more than you would with diet and exercise alone.

Three types of drugs are used to treat obesity. All have some appetite-suppressing effect, and they may also raise metabolism, so you expend more calories. Of the three, the antidepressant SSRIs (selective serotonin re-uptake inhibitors) are the most disappointing. Studies show that although people lose weight when they first go on the drugs, by about the fourth or fifth month on the medication, many have gained back all the weight they lost. So, at this point, most researchers agree that antidepressants aren't the way to go for weight loss unless there's depression involved.

Over-the-counter diet drugs

Even if you've never taken them, it's hard to miss the Dexatrim ads on TV—slender women in clingy clothing credit their great bodies to the diet pill. Dexatrim and Accutrim, are based on phenyl-propanolamine (PPA), an appetite suppressant with an M.O. similar to the catecholaminergic prescription drugs that affect the appetite centers in the brain. Besides PPA, the other approved over-the-counter anti-obesity drug is benzocaine, but manufacturers aren't currently adding it to their products. (It was in the Ayds appetite suppressant candies so popular in the 1970s.)

Future drugs

The current diet drugs work by suppressing appetite, but some of the drugs now in development will strike at other fat-promoting areas. Here's what could be coming down the pipeline:

■ **Orlistat,** brand name XENICAL™. Imagine if 7 of the 22 grams of fat in that large order of fries you scarfed down didn't count. Poof, they just exited your body. That's the promise behind Orlistat—to block 30 percent of the fat you eat before the body can absorb it. Although not yet approved by press time of this book, the industry buzz is that it will be on the market very soon. Its weight loss potential seems in line with the other drugs on the market, maybe a little higher. In research studies lasting one to two years, conducted by manufacturer Hoffmann LaRoche at several clinics in the U.S. and Europe, 4,000 people took either Orlistat or a placebo. They also stuck to a moderate dietary fat level of 30 percent of total calories. The average Orlistat taker lost 10 percent of his or her starting body weight—that's 22 pounds, since the average starting weight was 220 pounds. About three times as many Orlistat takers lost 10 percent of their body weight as those taking the placebo. For the more modest loss of 5 percent of body weight, Orlistat takers outnumbered placebo takers two to one. Those on Orlistat also lowered their blood cholesterol and blood

Unofficially . . .
PPA, used in over-the-counter diet drugs like Accutrim, is a danger to teens, according to Frances Berg, RN and LN, anti-dieting advocate, and author of *Afraid to Eat* (Healthy Weight Publishing Network, 1997). "One in three teenage girls has taken diet pills in some studies," she says, and some have died from overdosing. Although the label recommends that anyone under 18 consult a doctor, kids don't follow that advice, and they are allowed to buy the pills.

pressure in a more medically significant way than the placebo group. When Orlistat takers switched to the placebo (part of the study design) they started gaining the weight back, and when placebo takers switched to Orlistat, they started losing weight.

Orlistat works by interacting with fat globules from food in a way that prevents an enzyme called pancreatic lipase from attacking the fat. Normally, pancreatic lipase breaks down fat molecules into particles that can be absorbed by the intestine. At the recommended dose of Orlistat, 30 percent of the fat you eat becomes pancreatic lipase-proof and gets excreted with the feces. But here's where the side effects come in, caused by an unnatural situation—undigested fat—in the large intestine. Actually, according to the research reports, only 3 percent of clinical trial patients reported more than two adverse events (two episodes of any one adverse event), and very few dropped out of the study because of gastrointestinal problems. What helped is that they were counseled to keep their diets low in fat. According to Hoffmann LaRoche's Arthur Campfield, a high-fat meal could make things uncomfortable, especially in the beginning. But, he says, the intestines seem to adapt, and most of the discomfort happens when you first start the drug, not later on. Another potential side effect is lower levels of absorption of fat-soluble vitamins and other beneficial food compounds. Dr. Campfield recommends taking a multivitamin also. But there's still the question of all the other disease-fighting compounds not in a multi.

But a far more serious potential side effect—breast cancer—is what caused the Food and Drug Administration's (FDA) advisory committee to stop short of giving Orlistat their full seal of approval and issuing instead what is known as an "approvable letter." When the FDA is largely satisfied with the research and performance of a drug but wants additional scientific data or has yet to reach agreement with the manufacturer as to the wording of prescription or label information, it issues an approvable letter. This delays the decision for full approval until the FDA receives the requested additional information and agreements. The situation that caused the FDA to request further research involved nine cases of breast cancer among Orlistat takers—compared to two cases in those taking the placebo. On the basis of the available research, Dr. Campfield believes that Orlistat probably isn't the culprit. He said that a microscopic examination of the breast tumors indicated that those taking Orlistat had developed the cancer before the study. Also, the placebo group had a lower than normal rate of breast cancer, making the Orlistat group's rate look particularly high. Still, he recommends, "Until further studies clarify the issue, if you're at high risk for developing breast cancer, you might want to discuss the issue with your doctor." Hoffman LaRoche anticipates submission to the FDA of all additional requested data by late 1998, with potential FDA marketing approval to follow shortly thereafter.

■ **Leptin.** As explained in Chapter 3, leptin, also called Ob protein (Ob for obesity, leptin derived from "thin" in Greek) is a hormone that works to make you thinner. It is discharged from fat cells to signal the brain to put a lid on appetite and increase physical activity. In other words, it's a fat-fighter—and a potential dieting gold mine, more effective than anything we've seen yet, if a drug company could just figure out how to use it. So far, injecting overweight people with leptin hasn't panned out. It seems that large people produce even more leptin than thin people, so perhaps their brain isn't as sensitive to its signals, or they produce a defective form of the protein. In fact, cases of defective leptin have been found in a few families where many of the family members are obese. Drug companies are taking different research tacks: Hoffmann LaRoche is trying to develop a drug that would make the brain more responsive to leptin. Other companies are working on developing a leptin look-alike, which could be taken while losing weight to combat the natural dip in leptin that occurs while dieting. According to Campfield, we're still about a decade away from seeing a leptin-based drug.

- **Neuropeptide Y blocker.** This hormone does the opposite from leptin—it stimulates appetite, lowers the metabolic rate, and encourages fat storage. In fact one of leptin's functions is to decrease neuropeptide Y production. Pharmaceutical companies would like to create a drug that would block the production of neuropeptide Y.

- **Melanocortins.** A family of proteins that may promote weight loss. These proteins seem to be linked to leptin, doing their job when leptin levels are high (leptin levels increase with an increase in body fat).

- **UCP.** UCP stands for "uncoupling protein." The uncoupling refers to a chemical event inside cells such as muscle or fat which leads to energy release and calorie burning. Lab animal research shows that UCP becomes extra busy when mice are put on a high-fat diet and seemingly helps them burn off the excess calories. It could be that thinner people's UCP works better, or they have more.

Fringe fat fighters

Watching a late-night infomercial a few nights ago, I was transfixed by the bald-faced, shameless lies told about a product that supposedly traps fat from the diet. Go ahead, have that prime rib meal, the product hawker dared. "It's like you never ate it," he said solemnly. The product was a tablet based on *chitin*, a fiber-like substance derived from marine animal shells (described later). Can chitin or another supplement help you lose weight? As of mid-1998, nothing's been scientifically proven to, except for the risky ephedrine or Ma Huang described a little later. But that doesn't stop manufacturers from raising false hopes, as you can see from the seemingly endless supply of single supplements and multi-pill "systems" in drugstores and health food stores that make weight loss claims. And they're expensive; one "system" of various pills costs $80 for a few weeks' worth. According to the Federal Trade Commission, Americans spend about $6 billion a year on fraudulent diet products, many of them pills and powders.

Now, I'm not saying that *none* of the "natural" supplements work. It's just that very few of them

Bright Idea
Before going to a clinic that promises an unusual-sounding weight loss technique, contact state and local health authorities covering the region where the clinic is located to see if it's kosher. The Federal Trade Commission warns against going to healthcare clinics that require patients to travel away from home to receive treatment for untested, unapproved therapies; they may be ineffective or even dangerous.

have stood up to the rigors of scientific testing. That means that most of these substances haven't undergone the gold standard experiment, the "double-blind, placebo-control" trial. That's a study in which groups of people are divided into two groups, each group similar in terms of body weight, disease risk, and age. In the case of a weight loss substance, the two groups have to be on similar diet and exercise regimens. One group takes the substance, the other a placebo (dummy, inactive pill). It's called "double-blind" because neither the researchers nor the subjects know which pill they are taking. At the end of the trial, the researchers break the code and report on the results. In order for the results to be meaningful, the study must also use a minimum number of subjects (varies according to study design). And then, other researchers in other labs must be able to get similar results. Finally, the results should be published in what are called "peer review" journals—scientific journals that accept only papers that adhere to strict scientific research standards. Then the scientific community will feel comfortable that the substance works.

Manufacturers of weight loss supplements usually fail to follow the full scientific procedure outlined here and try to trick you with science claims that aren't really scientific. Some of their tricks include the following:

- Their "scientific study" was done on rats, not humans. Just because a rat loses weight doesn't mean you will.

- Yeah, the study was tested on humans but the results have little to do with the claims on the label. For example, in the research study, 100 mg daily of Substance X helped people lose weight. But for various reasons (safety, pill size, who knows?) the label instructs you to take 30 mg daily. It's not at all clear whether that amount will do anything.

■ The study was so poorly executed its results are meaningless.

■ They reference an "article" of theirs in a legitimate scientific journal, but it turns out that the "article" is only a letter to the editor.

So, before taking a pill or powder that claims to be "scientifically proven" see if the manufacturer can answer three simple questions:

1. Was the research done on humans?

2. How much did the research subjects take, and how much weight did they lose?

3. And, most importantly, where are the peer review journal articles of the research?

And even if a substance works, is it safe? Whereas drugs require long testing periods for side effects (and still, look what happened to fen/phen) there are no such rules for dietary supplements. Any of us could go down to the basement, put together a concoction of amino acids and vitamins, and market it as a weight loss miracle. The FDA will step in and recall it from the market only after people start getting sick or dying from your concoction. So, with many of these supplements, wait until better research comes out, or take them at your own risk.

The Federal Trade Commission (FTC), the government's consumer watchdog, offers the following advice on how to spot false claims:

■ If it sounds too good to be true, it probably is.

■ The promoters use key words such as "scientific breakthrough," "miraculous cure," "exclusive

> " Consumers should not assume that everything they buy in stores or in the mail has been approved by the government for safety or effectiveness. That's not the reality of the marketplace.
> —Leslie Fair, Division of Advertising Practices, Federal Trade Commission "

product," "secret ingredient," or "ancient remedy."

- The promoter claims the medical profession or research scientists have conspired to suppress the product.

- The advertisement includes undocumented case histories claiming amazing results.

- The product is advertised as available from only one source, and payment in advance is required.

If you're even a little plugged into the weight loss supplement scene you'll recognize at least one of the compounds in the following list. These nutrients or herbs regularly crop up in the ingredient lists of the so-called weight loss aides or muscle builders:

Chromium picolinate. A form of chromium, this is a vital mineral nutrient (for more on this mineral, check out the chart in Chapter 5).

Claim: Enhances fat loss and muscle gain. The theory is based on the fact that chromium is necessary for proper insulin functioning (insulin is a hormone involved in blood sugar and blood fat and protein regulation). Faulty insulin is linked to increased weight gain. But unless you're chromium deficient, taking extra chromium shouldn't affect insulin. And even if you are chromium deficient *and* have faulty insulin, there's no proof that taking chromium will help your lose weight.

Evidence: This is one of the few supplements with a number of decent research studies under its belt. Hope for this one was fueled by results of a USDA study years ago, indicating that chromium supplements slightly enhanced muscle and may have helped reduce fat in a group of young athletic men compared to a placebo. But since then, about four legitimate published research studies have failed to replicate the USDA findings, and the word is, that chromium does zip for weight loss.

Hydroxycitric acid. This is an acid derived from an Asian fruit called *garcinia cambogia.*

Claim: Helps prevent carbohydrates in the diet from turning into fat.

Evidence: Rat studies done 25 years ago indicated that this substance may help prevent the conversion of excess carbohydrates in the diet into rat body fat. But it seems that eating this stuff was an appetite turn-off, so the weight loss was probably the result of a lowered calorie intake. The few human studies using *garcinia* aren't considered scientifically valid. Until proven helpful and safe, I'd stay away from it.

Ma Huang. This Chinese herb is a natural source of the stimulant ephedrine and is often combined with another stimulant—caffeine—in so-called diet aides.

Claim: Raises metabolism, thereby helping burn more calories and causing greater weight loss.

Evidence: Research has shown that taking ephedrine and caffeine together can raise metabolism and slightly enhance weight loss. But at a high price: heart attack, stroke, and even a few deaths have been linked to the combo. Because of the health dangers the FDA has passed a law limiting the level of ephedrine in dietary supplements and requiring warning labels on the products. Bottom line: This is certainly one to avoid.

Herbal fen/phen. Trying to cash in on the prescription fen/phen pulled from the market, the supplement version, of course contains neither fenfluramine nor phentermine. It's usually based on the stimulant ephedrine (see Ma Huang, above) and St. John's Wort, an herb that may work as a mild

Unofficially . . .
Supplement manufacturers can get away with outrageous claims because the government doesn't have the staffing needed to police the market, and dietary supplements don't have to be tested for safety and effectiveness like drugs do. The FDA removes supplements from the market only after they've caused harm. And since the FTC deals on a case-by-case basis, it can fine one company for making false claims, but 10 others can continue doing the same thing, hoping they'll be overlooked.

antidepressant. The FDA has cracked down on these products, removing them from the market. The FDA's beef is that their name implies they do the same thing as the prescription drugs and that this combo may be unsafe. I've also seen the ephedrine/ St. John's Wort combo under the name "Diet Phen."

Claim: Promotes a "positive mental attitude" while dieting, speeds up metabolism, helps you lose more weight than diet and exercise alone.

Evidence: Although there's evidence that ephedrine can boost metabolism, it can also be dangerous (see Ma Huang). And there's no conclusive evidence that St. John's Wort promotes weight loss.

Fiber pills. Fiber from psyllium or other concentrated grains in pill form.

Claim: The pills will help you lose weight by suppressing appetite or trapping dietary fat, which gets excreted instead of absorbed.

Evidence: Research shows that taking 15 to 18 fiber pills daily (between 7 and 10 g of fiber) while dieting helped people lose an extra pound or two a month. That's a lot of pills for the amount of fiber you could easily get from a bowl of bran-based cereal. Also, there's some research indicating that lean people eat more fiber than obese people. Fiber's trimming power takes several tacks: It isn't digested or absorbed, so for all intents and purposes it's calorie free; but it expands in the stomach so you feel full. Insoluble fiber, the type in wheat bran, speeds intestinal transit time, meaning food moves through you more quickly so you probably absorb slightly fewer calories. (The intestines are where food is absorbed into the body.) Soluble fiber, the type in oats and beans, coats the intestines, partially blocking food absorption.

If all fiber's factors worked for you at once, you could be absorbing 5 percent fewer calories, which makes a slight difference over time. Bottom line: While they won't hurt you, you're better off skipping these and eating the type of diet outlined in Chapter 5. That'll give you plenty of fiber. If you really can't seem to eat high-fiber foods (or you're slowly developing a taste for them), try the fiber pills and see if they help. Remember, no supplements, including fiber pills, will do any good if you're taking in too many calories.

Chitin or chitosan. A few years ago this fiber-like pill came on the scene, based on a chitin, a fibrous material from the shells of marine animals.

Claim: Depending on the manufacturer's gall: That chitin will trap anywhere from a small percentage of the fat from your diet to "Prime rib dinner? It's like you never ate it."

Evidence: Neither I nor my experts could find any good scientific proof of these claims.

Cellulose-bile products. The way they are supposed to work is by creating a web in the intestines, trapping bile acids (the body's "detergent," which breaks up fat particles for better absorption), so fat is less easily absorbed.

Claim: Promote weight loss by reducing the amount of dietary fat your body absorbs from food. Some combine fiber with ox bile extract; fat is supposed to be caught up in the fiber and bile acid web and excreted with it. Possible side effects: diarrhea and stomach cramping.

Evidence: According to the FTC, scientific research does not demonstrate that these products prevent or significantly reduce the body's absorption of fat from consumed food. The FTC has gone after

Watch Out!
When you increase fiber, either through pills, cereal, or other foods, drink more water. Otherwise, fiber can actually be constipating; it needs water to expand in the gut and then move on through.

two manufacturers of these tablets, the makers of "Lipitrol" and "Sequester," fining them for unsubstantiated claims. Bottom line: Without enough good science behind these products it's hard to tell what they'll do. Take at your own risk.

Herbs and slimming teas. Since herbs work as either diuretics or laxatives, they may make you feel less bloated, but they won't burn fat, according to herb expert Varro E. Tyler, Ph.D., Emeritus Professor of Pharmacognosy at Purdue University.

Claim: Herbs and teas will slim you down, shed pounds, promote weight loss.

Evidence: Except for ephedrine (discussed earlier), none of the herbs will help you lose body fat. Yes, you might lose weight, but it's just temporary water-weight loss.

Herbs such as buchu, celery seed, dandelion, and Juniper act as diuretics, causing you to lose more body water through the urine. This might make your skirt fit a little better until your next glass of water. Since diuretics can cause potassium loss, you shouldn't take them unless your doctor prescribes them. Some of the "slimming teas" may contain senna, a stimulant laxative, which, like any other chemical laxative, has the potential for abuse. Other stimulant laxatives in teas include cascara, buckthorn, aloe, and rhubarb root. Reliance on herbal or pharmacologic laxatives causes the muscles in your intestines to weaken so that you'll be constipated unless you rely completely on laxatives. A fiber supplement, such as Metamucil, is a much safer alternative to chemical stimulant drug or herbal laxatives. Better yet, have a high-fiber diet that includes a high fiber cereal every morning.

Blue-green algae or spirulina. These are both types of algae, microscopic plants that grow in ponds and lakes.

Claim: In addition to purportedly boosting energy, and "detoxifying" (this meaningless word is always a tip-off to snake oil), this little plant is also supposed to suppress the appetite.

Evidence: The Food and Drug Administration concluded that there's no evidence that it's an appetite suppressant, and several companies have received court injunctions for misleading advertising.

DHEA. Reading the outpouring of hype on this hormone, you'd think it was the fountain of youth. DHEA is short for dehydroepiandrosterone, a hormone similar in structure to the sex hormones testosterone and estrogen.

Claim: In addition to claims that it increases sex drive, longevity, and energy, and prevents cancer, heart disease, and Alzheimer's, it's also marketed as a weight loss aid. Starting at about age six our bodies manufacture it; blood levels peak in our mid-20s, then start to decline so that by the time we hit 75 we have about 20 percent of the DHEA circulating in the blood that we had in our 20s. You can see the attraction: If it's something we had lots of in youth, then taking it might keep us young.

Evidence: Serious DHEA research is underway, but so far, there's not much to go on. First of all, no one knows what it really does in the body, except that it gets converted to other hormones, especially estrogen and testosterone. This could actually be potentially dangerous, since these hormones are associated with breast and prostate cancer later in life. And the preliminary research shows contradictory effects. For instance, a University of California

Bright Idea
Fiber from foods is better than fiber from pills. Here are some fiber heavy-hitters to fall back on when the rest of the food is fiber poor and the grams of fiber they contain.

apple or orange: 3 g

$1/2$ cup cooked Brussels sprouts: 3 g

1 ounce bran flake cereal: 4–8 g

$1/2$ cup canned or cooked dried beans (like lentils or black beans): 5–8 g

1 oz. high fiber cereal: 10–15 g

study gave DHEA to eight men and eight women
ages 50–65 for three months, then gave them a
placebo for three months. While DHEA seemed to
add on more lean body mass (muscle), it was also
associated with more body fat in women (less in
men). Another study tracking 2,000 men and
women for 12 to 14 years found that men with high
DHEA levels were 15 percent less likely to die from
heart disease, but DHEA levels made no difference
in women's risk. Bottom line: Don't take it until the
scientific research proves that it's safe and effective.
And beware! DHEA's side effects include increased
body and facial hair on women and cessation of
menstrual periods, probably because it's getting
converted to the male hormone testosterone. And
anything that increases testosterone production in
men could increase their risk for prostate cancer.

Growth hormone releasers. These are products that contain one or more amino acids (things we eat every
day; the building blocks of protein).

Claim: Ingesting them on an empty stomach stimulates the pituitary gland to produce growth hormone, which burns fat and causes weight loss.

Evidence: None. Although injecting large amounts of
the amino acid arginine can raise blood levels of
growth hormone, there's no scientifically valid
proof that taking it in pill form will do the trick.
Anyhow, elevated levels of growth hormone doesn't
cause weight loss, but chronically elevated growth
hormone can cause acromegaly, a deforming condition of enlarged hands, feet, and face. I'd stay away
from this stuff.

Pyruvate. This is a type of acid formed naturally in
the body as a by-product of the conversion of blood
glucose to energy.

Claim: Supplementation with pyruvate increases metabolism and accelerates fat loss. One ad says "27 years of extensive research and clinical studies with human subjects at the University of Pittsburgh Medical Center have shown that groups using the nutrient calcium pyruvate experience: 37% more weight loss, 48% more fat loss, and 20%–50% more endurance and physical performance." The ad goes on to explain that pyruvate accelerates fat loss by increasing cellular respiration, or the amount of energy the mitochondria—the cells' metabolic furnace—use. Pyruvate has even been shown to reduce fat without exercise.

Evidence: The research was done at the University of Pittsburgh Medical Center and one study showing enhanced weight loss in a small group of men and women was published in a respectable journal. Also, there's a little animal research showing that pyruvate lowered levels of body fat in pigs. However, the experts I spoke with who are familiar with the pyruvate research are pretty skeptical, saying that the experimental group was too small, and that they need to see the research results replicated by a scientist that doesn't hold patents to the form of pyruvate used in the experiments. Although the journal article didn't report any side effects (except sounder sleep!), as you now know, the Food and Drug Administration doesn't require safety tests for dietary supplements, so the long-term effects aren't known. At least this one has some research behind it, but I'd feel more comfortable about it when a few corroborating independent studies have appeared in the literature.

Ergogenic aids

Ergogenic refers to the use of nutritional, physical, mechanical, psychological, and pharmacological

Moneysaver
Don't waste your money on chromium supplements in hopes that they'll lower your blood cholesterol. In addition to ergogenic claims, recently cholesterol-lowering claims have been showing up on chromium picolinate supplement ads. The reliable research studies has found no effect on cholesterol.

techniques or aids to improve athletic or work performance. You've probably heard of anabolic steroid use disqualifying athletes from the Olympics or other competitions. Anabolic steroids are drugs that act similarly to the major male hormone testosterone; in some people they seem to increase muscle size. Steroids are drugs; on the nutrition front, supplements also make claims for increasing muscle, endurance, or performance. Some, like pyruvate (described earlier), also claim to increase weight loss. Here are a few popular ergogenic aid ingredients:

Creatine, in the form of creatine phosphate, is a major energy supplier for muscles. Our bodies make it, and we get it from meats and other foods.

Claim: Supplementing with creatine gives you bigger, stronger muscles and enhances performance.

Evidence: Research shows that indeed, supplementing with 5 to 10 g of creatine daily seems to make you slightly stronger. But only as long as you keep taking it, according to Steven Toler, Pharm.D., Ph.D., Senior Clinical Research Investigator, Pfizer, Inc., and a consultant toxicologist. Toler published a review on the supplement in a scientific journal. Supplementing with creatine means a larger store of energy for muscle cells so you have more energy stores for acute, short-term exercise like bench pressing or maybe the beginning of a short sprint. For instance, one study found that people taking creatine for 28 days could bench press a weight that was six percent heavier than what they could bench before taking creatine. But the 28 days is misleading, says Toler. Really, he says, creatine's effects max out in about five days; taking it for longer won't make you much stronger. And the reason your muscles look bigger on creatine is because it pulls more water into muscle cells, not because you've built up muscle mass. Stop taking the creatine and muscles deflate back to their original size in about a month. *Safety issue:* As with all these dietary supplements, the issue is safety. True, creatine is a natural substance that we normally get through food on the order of 1 to 2 grams daily. But supplementing with it may be harmful for people who have kidney problems, since the kidneys end up processing creatine for excretion into the urine. So if you've got kidney problems of any kind, don't take creatine; there's evidence that it can further damage kidneys. Without long-term safety research, you don't know what the recommended 5 to 10 grams levels will do to you. Also, at those levels, you'd better be taking a clean, pure product; if other impurities crept in you could be in trouble. It's nearly impossible to tell how pure the products are; you could start by asking the manufacturer for a copy of the contaminants report.

HMB (Beta hydroxy beta methyl butyrate). A chemical that is derived from the amino acid leucine. Amino acids are building blocks of protein.
Claim: Builds bigger, stronger muscles and causes faster fat loss. The theory is that it suppresses muscle breakdown (our bodies are always tearing muscle down and building it up), which favors a net gain in muscle.
Evidence: Okay, there is a teeny weeny bit of evidence that there might be something to this, but really not enough to go on yet. And, as always, it's best to wait until more evidence emerges that it's both effective and safe. Especially to the tune of $90 for a bottle of 360 pills (you're supposed to take four daily).

L–Carnitine. It's a substance in muscle that the body makes and that we get from eating meat and

Bright Idea
Studies show that although about a third of Americans use some sort of alternative therapy such as supplements, massage, acupuncture, and herbs, about 70 percent never tell their doctor. Be sure and mention any alternative therapies to your physician; they may interfere with the standard medical treatment.

other animal proteins. Among other things, it helps transport fat into muscle cells to be burned for energy—easy to see why it's being marketed as a weight loss aid.

Claim: Enhances muscle building and lowers body fat.

Evidence: The problem is, there's no proof that supplementing with carnitine will burn more fat or give you bigger muscles. Carnitine is just one part of a complex mechanism of burning fat. While research shows that supplementing with carnitine raises blood levels of carnitine, it doesn't show that this translates to weight loss.

Outrageous scams

Now I'm not suggesting that any of you would believe that (much less buy) an insole for your shoes burns fat. That is, I don't think any of you would under normal circumstances, but, as Jodie Bernstein, director of the Federal Trade Commis-sion's (FTC) Bureau of Consumer Protection puts it, ". . . consumers' anxiety about their weight and diet can easily overwhelm their better judgment. Real health consequences associated with obesity—such as heart disease, high blood pressure, and cancer—can make some consumers easy prey for diet fraud hucksters." Most of the products on the following list were targeted by the FTC, which, since 1927, has been slapping fines on manufacturers of fraudulent weight loss products. Here are a few companies and products in the doghouse with the FTC:

▪ Slimming Insoles, by Guildwood Direct Limited, or Slimming Soles, by Body Well, Inc. They purportedly make you lose weight through the principle of reflexology, where certain areas of the foot correspond to certain areas of the body. With each step you take, says the manufacturer, you massage reflex zones connected to the digestive system, stimulating this system to burn fat. Ads for Slimming Soles had the gall to say that the reflexology points would "force" your body to get rid of its surplus fat, and that you can lose "over 15 lbs. in just six weeks without dieting or doing any extra exercise!" The FTC has fined both companies for unsubstantiated claims.

- Fat Burners and Fast Burners, tablets and drinks that were sold under 11 different names as part of the "Fat Burners System" by AmeriFIT, Inc. Among other things, the FTC court settlement required the company to print the following on its label: "The dietary supplement in this system is for nutritional use only and does not contribute to weight loss or loss of body fat."

- "Svelt–PATCH." A transdermal patch (intended to penetrate the skin layer and deposit the effective substance into the bloodstream) that supposedly controls appetite and raises metabolism. The ads told us: "Amazing Skin Patch Melts Away Body Fat," and that scientific tests found that 56 percent of the participants lost at least 20 pounds in two months (between 20 and 71 pounds in only two months). (The company had to fork over $375,000 for that untruth.)

- Sauna suits and other nylon or rubber garments that make you sweat. Sure, you'll sweat and lose water weight, if you're lucky you won't get too dizzy and dehydrated, but you won't lose any more fat. And soon after you eat and drink that water weight will be right back. Several young male wrestlers died wearing sauna-type suits;

Watch Out!
Don't believe everything you read in the brochures and literature that accompanies supplements; that's where some of the real lies lie. Since manufacturers can be fined and forced to change labels that make false claims, they often save the really outrageous claims, for brochures that lie around on the shelves where supplements are sold.

they were losing weight rapidly to qualify for a weight category. Doctors believe the suits contributed to the deaths by causing dehydration.

Unofficially . . .
To do a background check on a doctor, call Medi-Net. For a charge of $15 you can verify the doc's educational background, residency, board specialty certifications, and licensing. You can also find out if disciplinary action was taken against him or her. To order the physician report, call (888) ASK-MEDI, or go to their website: www.askmedi.com. If you want to talk to an employee, call (800) 972-MEDI.

- Cellulite cures. Those whose job it is to terrorize women really did it right with cellulite (which isn't a real medical term). An entire industry feeds off our fear of dimpled thigh skin. Cellulite is plain old fat, like the fat anywhere else on the body. The waffling effect is caused by the way fat bulges between the bands of tissue that connect the subcutaneous (right below the skin) fat to the underlying tissues. Having cellulite appears to hereditary; the dimpling seems to worsen with age as skin gets thinner and less elastic, but you may be able to improve the appearance with weight loss. However, enzyme injections, vitamin and mineral supplements, and cremes have not been proven to reduce cellulite. In fact the FTC cracked down on one lotion, Ultima II proCollagen anti-cellulite body complex for reduction of cellulite, for making misleading claims.

- Food scents. These devices exude the odor of food. They're based on the questionable theory that simply inhaling the scent of a doughnut or a banana or chocolate is so satisfying you won't want to eat the real thing. There's no science behind this theory; in fact these scents could sent you on an emergency Krispy Kreme mission.

Exercise equipment

Home exercise equipment can be a very useful part of your weight loss and weight maintenance, but you've got to make sure you don't get sucked in by scams. For more on the benefits of these machines, see Chapter 14. When buying equipment, you've got to be wary of three possibilities:

1. You'll get a great product, but it'll collect dust in your basement because you never use it.

2. You'll get a good product that advertises unrealistic weight loss claims. For instance, cross-country ski exercise machines can give you a good aerobic workout. But the FTC says that the claims made by NordicTrack, Inc., a leading manufacturer of these machines, are unsubstantiated. NordicTrack claimed that 70 to 80 percent of consumers who purchased a NordicTrack cross-country ski machine to lose weight lost an average of 17 pounds; that 80 percent maintained all of their weight loss for at least one year; and that those who used the machine for 20 minutes daily, three times a week, lost an average of 18 pounds in 12 weeks. The company settled with the FTC, agreeing not to make these types of claims unless it has reliable evidence to back them up. The FTC also cracked down on Life Fitness, AbFlex, and Icon Health and Fitness, Inc., for making unsubstantiated weight loss claims. Again, it's not that the equipment is bad, it's just that they exaggerated the benefits.

3. You'll get a worthless product. "Passive" exercise machines such as vibrating belts and tables that you lie down on that vibrate or mechanically lift up your legs and arms will not "eliminate excess water and acid waste" (whatever that is) or loosen up fat so it's easier to shed. They won't help you lose weight. Sorry.

This quiz, developed by the Federal Trade Commission, will help you tell which exercise equipment claims to believe. Mark each question true or false:

Pump fiction. What's your exercise IQ?

1. Be wary of exercise devices that promise total fitness in just three minutes a day.

2. Even when they are relaxing, people who exercise regularly burn more calories than inactive people.

3. The total price of an exercise machine that's advertised at four easy payments of $50 is about $200.

4. Weight lifting has no health benefits.

5. Sit-ups and ab crunches are the best way to burn fat off the stomach.

6. Cross-training is the best route to overall fitness.

7. It's best to buy exercise equipment that comes with a money-back guarantee.

8. No exercise device can help you spot reduce.

9. Before and after claims in ads for exercise devices may be misleading.

Quiz answers

1. True. Real fitness requires regular activity, sensible eating, and a healthy lifestyle. Exercise need not be grueling, but there are no "three minutes a day" shortcuts to better flexibility, improved muscular strength, enhanced physical endur-ance, or improved cardiovascular or respiratory efficiency or weight loss.

2. True. Everyone burns calories while they're exercising. But one of the great benefits of an

active lifestyle is that it can boost your metabolism even when you're at rest.

3. False. Shipping charges, postage, handling, delivery, or other hidden fees can add on to the cost of exercise equipment. Whether you order by phone or buy at a retail store, find out the real cost before making a purchase.

4. False. Strength training isn't just for the "body beautiful" types. Lean muscle burns more calories than flab. Sensible weight training helps maintain muscle tone and endurance.

5. False. The most common cause of a "beer belly" is fat—not weak muscles. Sit-ups may help tone the abs, but only a sensible diet combined with regular exercise can turn a "beer belly" into a "six-pack stomach."

6. True. Cross-training—a regular program combining different types of activity—is your best route to fitness. A combination of your favorite activities—walking, swimming, biking, dancing—can help you shape up while avoiding the boredom and burnout of one kind of exercise.

7. True. But get the facts first. Not all money-back guarantees are the same. How long do you have to return the equipment? If you order through the mail, how much will it cost to return it? Who pays for repairs?

8. True. No exercise device can burn fat off a particular part of your body. The reason: Everything you eat has calories, and everything you do uses calories. Your weight depends on the number of calories you eat and use each day. Increasing your daily physical activity will burn extra calories.

9. True. Before-and-after pictures can be eye-catching, but they may not always tell the whole story. Regular exercise is an important ingredient in moving from plump to "pumped," but diet plays a key part, too.

Quack watch

Lets face it, the properly credentialed nutrition professionals, myself included, haven't been able to keep Americans from getting fatter. But, neither have the alternative practitioners. None of us have licked the war on the waistline, but some—both mainstream and alternative—aren't doing any harm, and others have helped lots of people lose weight and keep if off. Then there are those that prey on the overweight, selling false hope at a very high price. I remember getting a frantic call in the late 1980s from someone I hadn't heard from in ages. She'd spent $3,000 on three or four visits to a New York City clinic run by Stuart Berger, MD. At the time, Berger's brisk business was fueled by his popular diet book, *Dr. Berger's Immune Power Diet,* based on all sorts of hokey theories and recommending very high levels of vitamins and other supplements. It's still in bookstores. (Berger died at age 40, obese, with heart disease.) When my friend called she was megadosing on vitamins and minerals—some at 100 times the recommended levels—and eating a completely unbalanced diet. She could hardly drag herself to work. She was furious when I explained that the money she'd given Berger for phony tests and outrageously priced supplements was a complete waste.

Before wasting your time stepping foot into a clinic, call them up and see whether they meet the

criteria in the "Shoppers guide to weight loss programs" section in Chapter 6. And then, just in case
they were just telling you what you wanted to hear,
ask them whether they use any of the following
theories or techniques, surefire tip-offs to a quacky
program:

- **Hair analysis.** The only legitimate role for hair
  analysis is to test whether you're suffering from
  arsenic, chromium, or lead poisoning. Testing
  your nutritional health by taking a swatch of
  your hair is a classic hallmark of a quack; con-
  veniently, these people sell you supplements to
  "correct" your "deficiencies." Although hair
  analysis is not exclusive to obesity treatment, if
  the clinic does it, then it's probably doing a lot
  of other fishy things. Stephen Barrett, an MD
  who has devoted much of his career to "quack-
  busting," sent two identical hair samples from
  two healthy teenage girls to 13 commercial labs.
  He sent the samples three weeks apart under
  two different names. The lab reports were all
  over the map, differing on the level of minerals
  in the hair and on what was considered standard. The reason hair analysis is hokey is
  because:

1. Hair grows too slowly to determine what's
   going on right now.

2. Shampoos and other hair treatments interfere with analysis.

3. A single hair strand differs in composition
   up and down its length.

4. No standards have been set for normal,
   high, or low levels of nutrients in hair.

Unofficially . . .
Grapefruit pills
will not burn fat.
Somehow, grape-
fruit got embed-
ded in the food
faddist con-
sciousness, prob-
ably starting
with the grape-
fruit diet. The
claim: Grapefruit
contains fat-
burning enzymes.
It's utter
nonsense.

Moneysaver
Don't rely on
promises of a
money-back
guarantee for
weight loss
remedies. Many
fly-by-night
operators will
not be around to
respond to a
refund request!

▪ **Nutritional blood analysis.** This hokey "test" involves viewing a drop of your blood, highly magnified, on a video screen. Typically, you'll be told your blood shows too much clumping and other "abnormalities," which are usually caused by the fact that the blood's drying out. The scam continues when they sell you enzyme pills which supposedly get rid of that awful clumping. Even if you needed these enzymes (for reasons not yet known to science!) after your stomach acids do a number on them, they'd be unrecognizable as enzymes. Your bloodstream would never see them because enzymes are proteins and, like other proteins, your stomach acids digest them, rendering them into a completely unusable form. (Again, this test is not necessarily performed for obesity treatment, but is a warning sign that you've entered a quacky establishment.)

▪ **Selling vitamins.** Although there is a role for judicious use of supplements, a practitioner who sells you vitamin/mineral tablets or supplements such as the ones described in this chapter has overstepped the bounds of science. As you've seen, none of these things have been proven to enhance weight loss.

▪ **Rapid weight loss.** If they want you to lose over two pounds a week, hang up.

▪ **Restrictive diet plans.** You should be able to eat any food in moderation. High-protein diets that limit carbohydrates may make you lose weight a little faster, but they're unhealthy and are nearly impossible to stick with over the long haul. Likewise for diets that forbid combining certain foods. The exception: very low-fat diet programs for preventing heart disease, such as

Dean Ornish's diet, described in Chapters 6 and 7. The exclusion of high-fat foods on his very low-fat diet appears to be key in preventing and reversing heart disease in those at risk.

■ **Injections of vitamin B12 or other substances.** B12 injections may be necessary for those who have a hard time absorbing this vitamin— mainly the elderly. But otherwise, I can think of no good reason to get injected with anything, unless you're participating in a legitimate scientific study at a reputable university or clinic.

Just the facts

■ Diet drugs produce only modest results and have side effects, so try the diet and exercise approach first.

■ At best, most weight loss supplements haven't been proven to do a thing; at worst, they are outright frauds and even harmful.

■ The Federal Trade Commission is starting to crack down on exaggerated claims—make sure you don't believe any of them.

■ Finding out whether a weight loss clinic uses fraudulent tests can save you a lot of money.

Eating Habits Rx

PART IV

GET THE SCOOP ON...
How attitude helps ▪ Dealing with cravings ▪
Taking control at parties and restaurants

Chapter 9

The Weight Loss Head Trip

You know what to eat, you know you shouldn't be using the vending machine to cope with office stress, you know you should exercise—so how come you can't make yourself do it? Learning to cope with life in a nonfood way, and adopting the attitudes that promote good eating and exercise habits is by no means an overnight process. But it's what you've got to do if you really want to keep your weight down once and for all. That's the word from those ex-overweight people I keep telling you about. In research studies they consistently report that the key to their success—often after years of yo-yoing—was changing the attitudes and habits that were keeping them heavy. Sometimes it takes a while to make the necessary attitude shifts but that's okay—you can still work on new habits in the meantime.

Attitudes and feelings follow action. "Go ahead and change the behavior and start acting like you've

❝
When you want
to eat even
though you are
not physiologi-
cally hungry, it
means that
something is up.
You went to food
for comfort
because you did
not know what
was troubling
you, or because
you could not
comfort yourself
in another way,
or because you
felt compelled to
flee. (Source:
*When Women
Stop Hating Their
Bodies,* by Jane
R. Hirschmann
and Carol H.
Munter, Fawcett
Columbine,
1995.)

❞

changed, even if your major attitudes haven't yet. They will," assures New York City–based psychotherapist Dinnah Pladott, Ph.D., A.C.S.W. For example, even if you want to stick a cookie in your mouth because your boss yelled at you, go out and take a short walk instead. The attitude that food is the antidote to stress will change, says Pladott. This chapter will present both the pound-paring attitudes of successful "losers" and ways of changing food habits.

You may not be aware of many of your undermining habits; that's where the food record described in the next chapter comes into play. By filling out the food record for a few days you'll not only admit to yourself that, yes, you did go through an entire box of Wheat Thins in one day, but you may also find out why by looking at your mood and hunger ratings.

Watch your attitude

It's not that people who are fat all have the wrong attitudes and everyone who's thin has the right attitudes. It's just that thin people, if they're genetically thin, can get away with bad attitudes. (Weight-wise that is—don't worry, a problem like not accepting responsibility will trip up the thin person in other areas of life.)

I compiled a list of positive attitudes from conversations with psychologists, from reports on people who've successfully maintained weight loss, and from my own counseling experience. But before we get to it, here's a set of books I've drawn upon for this chapter—they can also be enormously helpful to you: *Living Without Dieting,* by John P. Foreyt, Ph.D., and G. Ken Goodrick, Ph.D. (Warner Books, 1994); *Thin for Life,* by Anne M. Fletcher, MS, RD, (Houghton Mifflin, 1994); *Emotional Eating: What*

You Need To Know Before Starting Another Diet, by Edward Abramson (Jossey-Bass, 1998); and *The Diet-free Solution,* by Laurel Mellin (HarperCollins, 1998). See Chapter 7 (under "Some useful 'not-entirely-diet' books") for a description of the topics these books cover.

If you're already equipped with one or more of the attitudes I set forth in the following sections, then you're that much ahead. As for the ones that you still need to work on—there's no set formula for adopting these attitudes. This is complex business, definitely not suited to one-size-fits-all advice. Ultimately, you may want to invest in a good psychotherapist.

Take care of yourself

That box of Oreos at your side may be your attempt to soothe and gratify yourself because you aren't taking care of your own needs. And it does—temporarily. But while eating is nurturing, especially when the foods are healthful, overeating is not: It destroys your body, and I don't have to tell you about the psychological ramifications. But if you could figure out what it is you really need and how to fulfill it, you wouldn't substitute "Band-Aid nurturing." As Laurel Mellin puts it in *The Diet-free Solution,* the nurturing process amounts to asking yourself three questions—"How do I feel?," "What do I need?," and "Do I need support?" If for years you've been out of touch with your wants and needs, stuffing down feelings, then learning to self-nurture will take some practice. Mellin's book gives an excellent step-by-step approach.

The peace and satisfaction that comes from getting your needs met, means you can finally focus your energies away from food and develop other

Unofficially . . .
What matters to your body is what you do—what concoction of food chemicals you pour into yourself. The message is that what you eat does matter, and as nurturing as it is to eat tasty food, it is not nurturing to overeat. So, as essential as it is to avoid a sense of deprivation, it is also essential to eat foods that provide our bodies with their full measure of health. (Source: *The Diet-free Solution,* Laurel Mellin, HarperCollins, 1998.)

parts of your life: closer relationships, work, and other interests such as theater. And, in turn, with more enriching facets in your life, body weight and eating become less central, less of a preoccupation.

Take responsibility

In a survey of 541 Weight Watchers group leaders who'd kept their weight off for about six years, 77 percent named "taking responsibility for one's own behavior" as one of the top three most important factors toward maintaining their weight loss. This is about accepting that it's not your husband or your job or other external factors that have made you fat, but your own eating habits. Of course a husband who's constantly waving ice cream cones and french fries at your face needs to change his ways, and if you work at Dunkin Donuts, you've got to find a new job immediately.

Taking responsibility means eliminating those fat-inducing situations. And it means learning about the fat and calorie content of foods, so you really know what you're getting into when you eat at Burger King. But what about a genetic propensity toward obesity? True, you can't change that, but you can take responsibility for the fact that your eating and exercise habits are simply feeding into those genes.

Do it for yourself

This means losing weight for yourself, not to please anyone else. One study of people in commercial weight loss programs found that those who were doing it for themselves—to improve their self-esteem or lower their health risks—were more likely to stay in the program long enough to reach their goal weight than those who were motivated by external, temporary reasons like fitting into a wedding dress. In *Thin For Life*, author Anne Fletcher asks the successful maintainers, "What was different that last time you lost weight? Why, at this one point in time, were you able to change your life forever?" It soon became clear that when they decided to take action for that final, successful time, there was one common theme: something happened that spurred them to "take the reins." They stopped looking to others for all the answers and decided to lose weight for no one but themselves. With that attitude, eating right and exercising becomes something you do to please yourself, something you really want to do.

Be realistic

If, after many attempts at getting thin, you realize that it's just not where your body wants to be, aim for a healthy weight that's not "thin" (see Chapter 1 for the healthy weight range). As explained in Chapter 3, most overweight people's set point isn't pointing at "thin." But it sure can point to something a lot thinner than obese. The authors of *Living Without Dieting* suggest people ". . . go through a grieving process to say good-bye to the thin self they will never attain. Otherwise they will be continually reverting back to their old dieting ways with yo-yo fluctuations and ultimate failure to make any significant changes."

Another example: After months of training, which included 18-mile runs, Oprah Winfrey was down to her goal weight of 150 when she ran a marathon. Her realistic attitude toward her weight comes through in her book, *Make the Connection*, where she admits that she's gained weight since the marathon. She's philosophical about it, saying that the amount of exercise she needs to stay that slim is impossible to keep up on her busy schedule, so she's

Bright Idea
Many of the attitudes and approaches that will help you keep your weight off are taught in "Solution" groups across the country. The Solution was developed by dietitian Laurel Mellin, an outgrowth of about two decades of research at the University of California at San Francisco. For more on this program, see Chapter 6.

accepted the fact that she'll be a little heavier. And she's got a personal trainer and cook! So, don't be so hard on yourself. Figure out a weight that's really achievable in the long run.

See failures as learning experiences

This applies to what happened today as well as what happened over the past decades. You stopped off and wolfed down a few doughnuts on your way to work this morning? Treat this as a great opportunity to analyze: Hmmm, could it be because you didn't eat breakfast? Or were you feeling particularly down on yourself? Why? Because you hate your boss and dread going to work? Okay, now how to avoid this happening again? You get the idea. Also, a scan through your weight loss history can be very helpful. First, because the fact that you ever lost any weight is heartening, you know it can be done. Second, because you can try to pinpoint why, in the past, you weren't able to stick with a lifestyle conducive to keeping the weight off. Was the eating plan you followed too restrictive, causing you to feel deprived, then binge? Had you not yet dealt with emotional eating? Those previous weight loss experiences are a gold mine from which to gather a wealth of knowledge for this go-around.

Rethink deprivation

Successful maintainers have turned the whole concept of dieting deprivation on its head. Instead of feeling impoverished because they can't dine at Outback every night or because they have to drag themselves out for a walk, they feel deprived if they can't make it to the gym or miss out on healthy meals. As Success Story Richard Drezen said in Chapter 1, he doesn't feel deprived "Unless I have to miss a workout, then I feel deprived." And Success Story Mandee deals with deprivation by making sure she works in a few higher-calorie treats—in moderation. When you've internalized the desire to do good things for your body—to eat healthily and exercise—then the bad old habits seem just that— bad old habits, not old ways that you yearn to go back to.

See shades of gray

Black-and-white, all-or-nothing thinking is the downfall of many an overweight person. As my friend said to me last week, "Since I had a quarter-pounder with cheese I figured I'd blown it, so I ordered another. With fries." Sometimes "blowing the diet" or gaining a few pounds just messes people up for a day, for others it throws them completely off course and ends the weight loss effort.

When you've overeaten, put it behind you. You haven't fallen into the black pit of your weight loss effort; you simply overate. And starting from the end of that splurge, you can pick up where you left off before the splurge. "Well, after overdoing it by 1,000 calories, what's another 1,000 calories?" the same friend asks.

Well, it's another 1,000 calories that you'll have to work off. Think of it this way: If you left your car too long in one spot and got a $50 ticket, and you knew that if you left it there for another few hours they'd ticket you again (which they do in Washington D.C., where I live) wouldn't you get in that car and drive it to a new, legal spot? You cut your losses and start afresh. Same thing when you stray off the good eating and exercise habits road. A slip is just a little detour—you can quickly get right back on the main road.

Watch Out!
The obsession with thinness is starting earlier. Fourth grade girls in rural Iowa were "very often worried about being fat," and 40 percent of fifth graders in a University of South Carolina study wanted to lose weight, although 80 percent weren't overweight. Help your kids develop a good body image before it leads to an eating disorder.

Unofficially . . .
Somewhere
between 22 and
25 percent body
fat is considered
"normal" for a
woman. However,
our body role
models—fashion
models and many
actresses—have
only 10 to 15
percent body fat.

Accept less-than-skinny

Learning to like your body, and—trite but true—
love yourself, fat or thin, will not only spare you a lot
of grief over your weight, but will *ultimately help you
lose weight.* This ties in with "Be realistic," but it goes
even further: seeing beauty in body shapes that
don't fit the slender ideal of the past 30 years.
Remember: It's only recently that thin was in; it's
been out for most of history. I'm sure you can come
up with lots of examples of sexy, attractive people
who aren't skinny or don't have fashion model bodies: Rosie O'Donnell, Bill Clinton (depending on
the month), Delta Burke, . . . and even some of your
own friends. It's just that we're not used to seeing
these bodies on TV, in movies, or in print ads. But
the few chances we get to see "nonconformist" bodies in the media can be heartening. For instance, I
remember how lovely actress Pauline Collins' body
looked when she stripped and jumped into the
Mediterranean Sea in the charming movie *Shirley
Valentine.* For me, it was the most memorable symbol
of liberation among many in this story of a middle-
aged English woman who leaves her humdrum exis-
tence for adventure on a Greek island.

Disliking your body, or certain parts of the body,
is connected to how you feel about your inner self,
notes Laurel Mellin: "Because body and self are
intertwined, unraveling them is very difficult. What
people don't like about themselves becomes pro-
jected onto some part of their body, which they
then disparage. And what people dislike about their
bodies becomes fodder for rejection of the self.
Rejection of the body and self add to the buildup of
emotional distress inside. We stop seeking comfort
from within ourselves and start seeking external
gratification" (*The Diet-free Solution*).

"Skinny is a relative concept," says psychotherapist Dinnah Pladott. Redefine for yourself the meaning of 'thin'; there are no absolute definitions." And, she reminds us, concepts of beauty are always changing. For instance, until the 1960s, there were no black beauty queens; white features were the standard of beauty. Then the "Black is Beautiful" concept exploded and afros became so stylish that Barbara Streisand got one!

And in other cultures, plump, not skinny, is the standard of beauty, as you can tell from this passage from the Egyptian writer Najib Mahfouz: "Without meaning to, he observed the lines demarcating the divisions of her voluminous body. He could not help but marvel when her hips came into view, for their crest almost reached the middle of her back, while their bottom flowed down over her thighs . . . Then she approached the table with her glorious body." (Source: *Palace of Desire,* Najib Mahfouz, Cairo: American University Press/Bantam Doubleday Dell, 1991.)

"Start moving the 'locus of value'—the place or source from which you derive the manner and the criteria for your values—from the outside to the inside," urges Pladott. "That means, stop measuring your value by how you stack up to a Calvin Klein billboard. Start defining what YOU consider beautiful, attractive, desirable. And in addition, start seeing what you've really got to offer inside the physical package."

Pladott recommends the classic exercise for learning to accept your body: Stand in front of the mirror naked, and say "I love my body." "In the beginning this feels contrived, but as you do it regularly, after a while it seeps in," assures Pladott. If

you're feeling very negative about your body,
acknowledge the feeling, likening it to the feelings
you have when your child misbehaves, she suggests.
"The anger you feel toward your child, just like the
negative feelings you have about your reflection in
the mirror, are both transient. What's permanent is
that you love your child and you love your body," she
says.

Accepting and loving your body will improve self-
esteem, which in turn will help you feel more confident about your weight loss efforts. But when you
hate your body, self-esteem plummets, making it
harder to succeed at anything, including weight loss.
So, paradoxically, accepting your body—and your
inner self—will fortify you for your weight loss effort
and make it all the more successful. And other wonderful opportunities may open up. "The moment we
accept the uniqueness of our bodies and stop trying
to put ourselves into a cookie cutter, we start accepting our other differences. It's what's different about
a person that leads to creativity, to great innovations
and pioneering," notes Pladott.

Some resources to support you in your "body
acceptance" effort include the magazines *Radiance*
and *Big, Beautiful Woman* and the National Association to Advance Fat Acceptance, which has local
chapters.

Enjoy yourself

Take a break from worrying about food and your
weight: Go to the movies, go shopping, set aside
time for a good novel, get artistic, see a ball game,
pamper yourself by getting a massage—whatever
floats your boat. "Many dieters figure that since they
haven't met their weight loss goals they don't
deserve to do anything nice for themselves; they see

pleasure as self-indulgent," says Edward Abramson, author of *Emotional Eating: What You Need To Know Before Starting Another Diet.* "They have the idea that in order to lose weight they have to be very hard on themselves, but that's counterproductive. Making the effort to change habits takes mental resources; if you go out and do things you enjoy, you'll have more psychological energy and enthusiasm for your weight loss effort," notes Abramson.

Habits of highly effective weight losers

As you've probably figured by this point in the book, there are no guaranteed formulas to maintaining weight loss except sticking with a level of diet and exercise that keeps you at your goal weight. In fact, it appears that finding your own path to weight loss, creating a unique way of dealing with food and exercise, increases your chances of success over simply trying to plug yourself into someone else's pre-scribed system. So, I'm throwing out a bunch of techniques that others have found helpful. See which ones address your biggest problems and try them out for size. If something doesn't seem right for you, skip it.

Graze responsibly or don't graze at all

Grazing—eating small meals and snacks throughout the day—works for some people—people who eat lots of carrots and seltzer. But for others it turns into a daylong vending machine fest with calories adding up alarmingly. Try these approaches:

1. Safest strategy: Don't graze; eat three meals and one or two snacks. Ways to keep from grazing:

   ▪ Have three satisfying meals of at minimum 350 calories each plus snacks (see Appendix C for examples).

66

I dream of white thighs; and I dream of a man in golden tights, who loves me. I wake up caught in a web of con-flicting impulses and desires. Exposure, and defense. Hiding, and revelation. I decide to go on a diet. In earnest. For real. Redoubling all past efforts. I mean it this time. I mean it every time. I float above my body, regarding myself from a great height; I regard this body with pity, amuse-ment, weariness, and love. (Source: *An Accidental Autobiography*, Barbara Grizzuti Harrison, Houghton Mifflin, 1996.)

Moneysaver
Conquer a junk food habit and you save money. Let's say you typically go through the equivalent of a big bag of chips and a half a box of Oreos daily— about $5 a day. Quit that habit and save $150 a month, $1,800 a year. Bet you can come up with a few nice ways to dispense with $1,800.

▪ Eat a real breakfast to tide you over until the next snack or lunch.

▪ Carry around a toothbrush and brush your teeth after eating; you may be less likely to put something in your mouth right away.

▪ Keep your environment graze-free by keeping food out of your office and car. At home, clear the kitchen of chips, cookies, and other nutrient-void foods, keeping around fruits and vegetables. It'll be interesting to see how much grazing you do with those foods. If you don't live alone, beg and plead with your family or housemates to minimize the junk food. Have them keep their snacks in a separate cupboard which is off-limits to you.

2. Interim strategy (before you give up grazing or get the grazing down to a decent calorie level): Don't buy in bulk. Want a cookie? Go to the bakery and get one, *just* one.

3. More risky strategy, but doable if you proceed with caution: Graze, but plan ahead, and try to include one "real" meal. It's really important to stick with low-calorie, low-fat foods.

Your splurges should be small, mini, little: three Hershey's kisses, $1/3$ cup frozen yogurt, a small order of fries (and give some away). Using the pyramid guidelines in Chapter 4 and the diet guidelines in Chapter 10, figure out how much you should eat total. Divide the food up into small snack-size portions and don't stray. If you work outside the house, bring as much as you can from home, and carefully plan the carry-out or restaurant food. For instance, cut up the red pepper and carrot strips the night before and put appropriate portions of foods in baggies. When the food runs out, stop eating. When you get home, decide what you'll have that evening and don't have anything else.

Eat aware

We've all done it—eaten without really being aware what just happened. As my friend, after eating a huge bakery cookie while flagging down a taxi and getting in the cab aptly put it, "Suddenly, it was gone, and I hardly remember eating it, much less what it tasted like." "Unconscious" eating is dangerous because, hey, if you forgot you ate it, you've still got plenty of calories to spare, right? And the eating goes on. Another reason that it leads to more eating is because you've missed out on sensory pleasure and satisfaction that comes with appreciating food. So you seek that out again. Here are some solutions to the problem:

1. When you eat, stop what you're doing and really focus on the food. Turn away from the computer; get off the phone. If you're eating while walking, slow down and think about each bite. Enjoy it.

2. If you're eating in front of the TV, wait for the commercial break, turn the TV off or the sound down, turn away from the tube and focus on your food. Finish the meal at the next commercial break. Typically, nutritionists advise never eat while watching TV, but I don't like one-size-fits-all advice. However, if you find you usually overeat when watching TV, better listen to those nutritionists.

3. Make a mental note when you have a big cookie, a soft drink, or another high-cal, low-nutrition

Timesaver
Healthy grazing can be time-consuming with all the cut-up vegetables and preparation of mini-meals. Wash and cut vegetables up to three days in advance, and store them in the fridge in plastic containers. Instead of making little sandwiches each time, make one whole one, cutting it into quarters and storing the uneaten part for later. This also helps you get a handle on how much food you're eating.

Watch Out!
Women are more
likely to binge
when they
are lonely or
depressed, men
when they're in
social situations
making them feel
happy, excited or
encouraged to
eat. That's what
turned up in a
study of 1,184
obese patients
enrolled in
Structure House,
a residential
weight loss pro-
gram described
in Chapter 6.

food: "Today I've had one calorie splurge so I'll wait until tomorrow to have another."

GRAZE IN NUTRITIOUS PASTURES

If you're going to graze, do it right; little nib-bles at a time, not the whole pasture! Here are some good grazing foods:

Morning snacks (80 to 150 calories)

- 1 cup of skim milk, plain, or as a latté or cappuccino

- 1 cup plain or $3/4$ cup lemon or coffee low-fat or non-fat yogurt (these are lower in calories than fruit yogurts)

- half a $3^1/_2$-inch (2.3-oz.) bagel

- small ($2^1/_2 \times 3^1/_2$ inch) bran muffin

- half a regular muffin

- slice of whole wheat bread with jam or $1/_2$ tsp. butter or margarine

- 3 whole wheat graham crackers

- 2 40-cal rice cakes

- 6 oz. fruit juice

Afternoon snacks (100 to 150 calories)

- 3 to 4 cups ($3/_4$ to 1 full oz.) of air-popped or reduced-fat popcorn—no more than 120 calories and 5 g fat

- 1 oz. pretzels, preferably whole wheat

- 1 oz. baked tortilla chips dipped in salsa or bean dip (make your own by mashing canned black beans with a little cumin or check out those made by Guiltless

Gourmet or Hain, or any other brand with no more than 40 calories per 2 Tbsp.)

- 1 cup of skim milk, plain, or as a latté or cappuccino

- 3 whole grain low-fat crackers topped with 1 tsp. of peanut butter or 1 oz. of low-fat cheese (no more than 5 g of fat per oz.)

- 1 cup sliced carrot, cauliflower, cucumber, or any other vegetables except avocados, which are loaded with fat and calories. Dip in reduced-fat salad dressing or other low-fat dip

- 1 apple, pear, peach, orange, or 1 cup chopped fresh fruit

- 1- to 2-oz. slices of lean turkey or chicken breast with mustard or a little chutney

Evening snacks (100 to 160 calories)

- $1/2$ cup flaky bran or whole grain cereal with nonfat milk

- 1 cup hot chocolate made with nonfat milk and a teaspoon of thin chocolate syrup or from cocoa

- $1/2$ cup non-fat plain yogurt with 1 tsp. of honey and half a banana

- 1 cup non-fat milk with a graham cracker or small cookie or biscotti

4. As much as possible, make a routine out of eating, having breakfast, lunch, dinner, and snacks

at roughly the same time each day. That way, anything extra will seem out of the ordinary; you'll notice it.

5. Plan your snacks. Anticipate the times and places when you usually snack and bring healthier foods with you or have them available at home.

6. Keep a food diary (described in Chapter 10).

GRAZING DAY

A day of mainly grazing, with one "real" meal can be a healthy proposition when done in moderation. Here's what that looks like (actual calories per item may vary slightly):

8:30 am: latté with non-fat milk (90 cal)

10 am: small bran muffin (90 cal)

11 am: an orange (80 cal)

1 pm: cup of sliced vegetables with $1/3$ cup black bean dip (180 cal)

2 pm: 1 oz. of baked tortilla chips; about 15 (110 cal)

3 pm: cappuccino with non-fat milk and a biscotti (180 cal)

4:30 pm: slice low-fat cheese with a couple of Finn Crisp crackers (130 cal)

6:30 pm after work: 4 oz. wine (80 cal)

7:30 pm "real" meal: $1^{1}/_{2}$ cups cooked pasta with shrimp marinara sauce and a tablespoon of parmesan with a 2-cup salad and 2 tsp. dressing (480 cal)

9 pm snack: ¹/₃ cup vanilla frozen yogurt
(check label for no more than 120 cal
per half cup or 4 oz.) with strawberries
(120 cal)

Daily total: 1,550 calories

Pyramid group tally: four starches (bran muffin, chips, crackers, pasta); three vegetables (sliced vegetables, salad), two fruits (orange, strawberries) two dairies (latté, cappuccino), two proteins (bean dip, slice of cheese, shrimp); one fat (salad dressing); low-cal extras: biscotti, frozen yogurt, wine.

Curb cravings

Mine's chocolate, typical female that I am. I've worked it out: I get a little every day, and chocolate leaves me alone. Chocolate ranks highest as the most craved food for about half of women and about 15 percent of men. Cravings—an intense desire for a particular food—strike most of us, 97 percent of women and 69 percent of men according to one Canadian study. Women's cravings lean toward the sweet side: cookies, chocolate, ice cream, while men's are more on the salty/savory side: meat, pizza, chips. The causes are a complex mix of psychological and physiological factors, seemingly a response to hormones, stress, dieting, and a variety of other things. The hormone connection comes into play in the sharp rise in cravings premenstrually. Interestingly, there's not much evidence that pregnancy increases cravings; it seems that women simply give into them more because they feel they can eat more while pregnant. Stress,

Unofficially . . .
How come
chocolate is the
most craved
food? It could be
the stimulants it
contains such as
caffeine and a
compound called
theobromine. It
could also be
any number or
combination of
the 400+ com-
pounds in this
extremely com-
plex food.
Another theory:
The amino acids
tyramine and
phenylethylamine
may be slightly
arousing (the
latter spikes in
the brain when
we fall in love).

well, you know if you've ever headed straight for food in response to a deadline, or a fight, or a huge task ahead.

In extreme cases, cravings may be an addiction; there's evidence that these foods may be acting like drugs. Some people may use food to self-medicate, according to Adam Drewnowski, Ph.D., professor of psychology and director of the Program in Human Nutrition at the University of Michigan. In his fascinating series of studies, he gave women who regularly binged on high-sugar/high-fat sweets such as ice cream a drug called naloxone, which blocks receptors on a pleasure center of the brain. Suddenly the foods no longer produced the same pleasure, and the women's cravings—and bingeing—stopped. "These studies support lab animal research indicating that foods high in sugar and fat release endorphins in the brain," says Drewnowski. Endorphins are mood-elevating brain chemicals such as those produced during a "runner's high." He suggests that there's a craving continuum: At one end, a small subgroup of the population who are truly addicted, perhaps because of depression or other disorders caused by faulty brain chemistry that produces too few "feel good" chemicals. At the other end are amazing people who have no cravings. The rest of us fall somewhere in between. But whatever the causes, caving into cravings too often can foil your weight loss and weight maintenance efforts. Here's how to deal with them:

1. **Investigate causes.** Figure out why they strike. Do they often hit when the baby cries or when lots of demands come at once? Cravings can fall into a pattern: You crave peanuts when you go to that bar with your buddies after work, or you

have a hankering for cookies when you step into the kitchen? The food/mood record in the next chapter will clue you in.

2. **De-stress.** If cravings are stress related, then work on eliminating or reducing the stress.

3. **Pleasurable nonfood substitutes.** Find appealing substitutes you can swap for eating such as a catch-up phone call to a friend (don't use the kitchen phone!) or an inexpensive purchase such as a magazine. This gives a sense of reward without adding pounds.

4. **Take a walk.** I know it seems like walking couldn't begin to replace chocolate, but often a few minutes into the walk the craving goes away. Could be that exercise helps boost levels of mood-elevating chemicals.

5. **Give in to them.** Not with binges, but with reasonable portions. "The mistake people make is to try to banish certain foods altogether," says Ted Weltzin, MD, an eating disorders specialist and director of Weltzin and Associates, a psychiatric group in Madison, Wisconsin. "And that just sets you up for a binge later on." You tell yourself you can't have cookies, you start craving them, dreaming of cookies, and pretty soon you go out and eat a whole box of Pepperidge Farm Milanos. Then you feel guilty, deprive yourself for another week or so, and have another binge. Weltzin recommends including the food in moderation. Start by slowly reducing the number of times you give in and the amount you consume each time. For example, if you've been eating two scoops of ice cream nightly, try one scoop. As your resolve

> **"**
> I would not be happy in a world without chocolate, so I have developed a Häagen-Dazs meditation. When I eat the teaspoon of ice cream, I close my eyes and meditate— on the rich flavor, the cold rush, the wonderful sensations as the ice cream melts on my tongue. I would prefer to have a small spoonful of Deep Chocolate Fudge Häagen-Dazs than a pint of fake-fat frozen dessert.
> —Dean Ornish, MD, in *Eat More, Weigh Less* (HarperCollins, 1993).
> **"**

builds, try skipping a day here and there. And don't kid yourself: A carrot stick isn't going to cut it when you feel like Godiva, so have a little piece of chocolate.

6. **Seek help.** If you think your cravings are a response to depression, an eating disorder, or severe PMS, a good psychotherapist can do wonders.

Diffuse emotional eating

Intense have-to-have-it-now cravings are one type of emotional eating, but eating nonchalantly out of boredom, loneliness, depression, anger, or anxiety is another. It's become a sitcom classic, the 20- or 30-something single female, dateless, in front of the television, spoon in a pint of Ben and Jerry's or Häagen-Dazs. But that person could be a mother, a guy living with housemates, a sibling in the middle of a big house with a big family. The house may be crawling with people, but you're feeling unimportant, unconnected or there's a lack of intimacy in your life. So food becomes the companion, a temporary filling of the chasm. Much of this springs from the lack of self-nurturing described at the beginning of this chapter.

The most extreme form of emotional eating is binge eating, described in Chapter 12. Some researchers speculate that some emotional eating springs from biochemical imbalances in the brain. For instance, some people may not produce enough of a calming brain chemical called serotonin. Or, they may experience serotonin dips at certain times of the day. Carbohydrate-rich foods, such as cakes, cookies, and ice cream, may temporarily boost serotonin. But other researchers point out that it's not any old carbohydrates; we're not going for whole grain bread and rice cakes, but high-fat, sugary carbs. So it's hard to say whether it's really the carbohydrates that we need or the comfort and taste stimulation from the sweets.

Here's how to get a grip on emotional eating:

1. Fill out the food/mood record described in the next chapter. In addition to writing down everything you eat, you'll also write down your mood before eating, providing valuable clues to what's triggering all this. You'll start seeing patterns: For instance, your emotional eating is under control during the day but crops up at night. Sometimes, notes Abramson, it's hard to pinpoint the feelings that triggered the eating, other than a vague feeling, such as anxiety or being upset. "In that case," says Abramson, "right then as you're standing in front of the fridge nibbling on something, stop and recall what you were thinking about before eating. Often after recognizing the thought you can identify the feeling. For example, if you are thinking that your boss treated you unfairly, you are probably feeling anger." Get it down in your food/mood record.

2. Make a plan. "Once you know your patterns, take a few moments during a low-stress time to make a plan. Figure out how to make food less available during the times when you're prone to emotional eating," suggest Abramson. For instance, if you know that you tend to eat when you do tedious, boring tasks like ironing or paying the bills, do them on the day before you go food shopping, when there's nothing good to eat in the kitchen.

Bright Idea
Lunch and dinner foods can also make great snack foods. For instance, Brandy Whiteside, a ninth grader, snacks on canned corn when she gets home from school (she got her nutrition education in fifth grade with CATCH, a National Institute of Health–sponsored nutrition education program). So rethink "snack": Open it up to any healthful favorite.

3. Recognize that emotional eating may be a consequence of dieting. If you've been restricting calories to the point of hunger and irritability, it's no wonder you're overeating—your body is demanding it! In that case, stop the diet, or if it's basically a healthy diet but just too low in calories, increase the calories to the point where you're not hungry. Or try eating more filling, but low-calorie foods such as vegetables, low-fat or air-popped popcorn, and fruit.

4. Go out and do something fun. "Fun," of course, is in the eye of the beholder. Go take a walk with a friend, set aside an hour a day to so some non-food-related activity you enjoy—plan a trip, hit some golf balls. As I mentioned above under "Enjoy yourself," this can only help your weight loss efforts.

5. If the emotional eating seems related to a serious depression, get help. Shop around for a good psychotherapist. If the emotional eating seems linked to stress and anxiety, think about how to reduce the stress. Get a baby-sitter once or twice a week, delegate tasks to your employees, or take a yoga class or a stress management class.

Slow it down

If your meals go into your mouth as if they've been vacuumed off your plate, you could be doubling or tripling the calories you'd have eaten if you just slowed down. The physiological signals that tell our brains "I'm full" have a delayed reaction time, kicking in about 15 or 20 minutes after eating. That's why you can down a double cheeseburger, fries, milk shake, and a big hunk of cheesecake and feel like there's room for more, but a half hour later you're heading for the medicine cabinet. See if these techniques will help slow things down:

1. At home, serve yourself one reasonable portion, leaving the rest of the food in the kitchen. Tell yourself you won't go back for seconds until a half hour after eating. If you're still hungry, then go back for half portions.

2. Chew well and slowly.

3. Put your knife and fork down between bites.

4. Focus on eating; don't get too distracted by TV or conversation.

5. When eating with others, get into the mealtime conversation. Since you don't want to talk with your mouth full (now do you?), talking draws out the meal.

6. Eat bulky foods such as vegetables, baked beans, and whole grain breads; you have to chew them longer, and once they go down, they expand in the stomach, making you feel fuller sooner.

7. Eat lower-fat foods. Before you tame your speed-eating problem, at least make the go-down-easy foods as low in calories as possible, such as low-fat cheeses, skim milk, and reduced-fat ice cream.

Home in on hunger

Hunger is a great thing, signaling us to eat when we need to, making eating all that more enjoyable. But hunger can mess us up in two ways:

First, we get so hungry that we overeat. Avoiding excessive hunger is simply a matter of better planning. Spread those calories evenly throughout the day, and you won't get hungry. Oh yeah, and

Watch Out!
Nuts are
dangerous for
speed-eaters.
Inhale a cup of
addictive dry-
roasted mixed
nuts and there's
814 calories
down the hatch.
Pistachios are
a better bet
because you
have to take the
time to open
them, eating
them one at a
time. A reason-
able portion:
a quarter cup
(with shells) will
amount to about
100 calories.

something else: get enough calories. Those 1,000-calorie diet plans are never going to be enough. Time to revisit breakfast, lunch, and dinner interspersed with a snack or two. One of the reasons people skip breakfast is because they're not hungry because they overate the night before. Well, the reason they overate the night before is because they skipped breakfast, and by evening the body was demanding it's daily calorie rights. As I explain elsewhere in this book, the foods we tend to snack on at 10 or 11 pm are usually not healthful breakfast foods like skim milk, high-fiber cereal, and fruit. More likely you'll reach for chips, pizza, ice cream, and the like, and lots of it because you're hungry.

Second, we lose our hunger reflex from weird eating patterns and overeating. Ideally, we should eat when we're hungry, but not starving, and stop eating when we're satisfied, not stuffed. "However," as Laurel Mellin puts it, in *The Diet-free Solution* "in some situations your body's hunger signals may *not* be accurate. For instance, if you chronically overeat, have been gaining weight or carry your weight in the middle, your levels of insulin and the various gut peptides that regulate appetite may be turned up so high that you *think* you're hungry when you're *not*. Moreover, if you're preoccupied with thoughts of food, you'll stimulate changes in some of these levels, again mimicking hunger when your body does not need food." Here are things you can do to recalibrate your hunger reflex:

- Stop dieting, advises Frances Berg, LN, author of *Afraid to Eat* (Healthy Weight Publishing Network, 1997). "When you're counting calories you're responding to external controls. So it's impossible to listen to your body signals and eat when hungry and stop when full; instead you stop at an artificial calorie level. You want to move into internal control of hunger," says Berg.

Timesaver
An eat-in dinner in no time flat: Stop at the supermarket, grab pre-washed and cut salad either from the salad bar or the produce section, some rotisserie chicken (remove the skin), and you're set.

■ Do the same thing recommended to prevent extreme hunger: Eat three meals a day, interspersed with small snacks if needed. At first you may not be hungry at regular meal times. Build up to it by eating something at the meal, even if it's very small. For instance, have a quarter of a bagel for breakfast. Then don't eat a thing until lunchtime unless you truly feel hungry. Make that in-between snack also small, just enough to quell extreme hunger. Hopefully, you'll be hungry by lunch. Have a real lunch. If you're hungry between lunch and dinner, make sure it's real hunger by waiting for 15 or 20 minutes. If it doesn't go away, have a piece of fruit or something equally low-cal. Then, enjoy dinner. Stick with this structure and you'll soon be able to trust your hunger cues again.

■ Along with this structure, make sure to get some exercise. Do what you're capable of—say, a 10- to 30-minute walk at least once a day. Exercise has an appetite-balancing effect, perhaps because it helps regulate blood insulin, a hormone involved in appetite.

■ Learn to recognize your own hunger signals, which may be different from other people's. For instance, usually I have the classic gnawing stomach sensation, but occasionally that doesn't happen and instead I feel a little lightheaded and can't think clearly. I have a meal, and I'm fine. So the fuzzy lightheadedness is one of my hunger signals. Other people's hunger makes

Bright Idea!
Getting a good night's sleep may help keep your weight down. Studies show that when people are sleep-deprived, they eat 10 to 15 percent more calories. The extra intake attempts to increase energy and may be the body's way of fighting the lowering of its core temperature that results from lack of sleep. And being "Z-deficient" means being too tired to exercise.

them weak, crabby, tired, or they develop cold hands and feet.

- Also, learn to recognize the sensation of being satisfied, not stuffed. (See the discussion of speed-eating earlier in the chapter.)

Derail deprivation

Have something you love to eat every day. Not a big something but a little one, like two mini Reese's chocolates. Do as diet guru Dean Ornish does: Stop everything and really savor the food. Don't guiltily gulp it down as you tap on the keyboard, or paint the room, or run for the bus. Savoring is so much more satisfying; you may actually not crave more. All-out splurges take some planning; make them count. For instance, I love the pecan sticky buns at the Uptown Baker near my home. Fortunately, they make them only on Saturdays. So, one or two Saturdays a month I have one. I try to make the rest of the day a little lighter in fat and sugar to make up.

Eating out

The four-grams-of-fat Classico spaghetti sauce topping a little pasta and a side of salad with just enough dressing coming out of your kitchen is all fine and well. But your aunt's holiday fest, the land mines of T.G.I.Friday's and Burger King, and the temptations at your favorite pricey restaurant are another. Here are ways of coping.

Civilized social eating

You do fine at home, but you tend to overdo it when you go out to a dinner party or, the ultimate temptation, a holiday buffet. An occasional splurge is fine, but if social eating is messing up your weight loss eating, it's time to take action.

- Don't go starving. Don't worry, you'll still have room to enjoy the goodies there, but you'll be less likely to eat too much. Eat a little something before going out to dinner or to a party, especially if the event happens past your normal dinner time and you're getting hungry. For example, have a piece of fruit or a slice of toast with a little low-fat cheese or jam.

- Keep a cap on the booze. Alcohol loosens your control of overeating just as it loosens your tongue and your inhibitions. Have something in your stomach before your first drink. Each of you has a different tolerance level: Stop before you get to the point of "Hell, I think I'll eat the rest of that pie."

- Divide and conquer. When there are more than a few dishes, mentally divide the spread into foods you really want and foods you can do without. Leave the "do withouts" alone for the rest of the meal. Now that you've narrowed it down, take reasonable portions. Try not to go back for seconds unless you're still hungry 20 to 30 minutes after eating.

- Make one, maybe two items your splurge. Eat less of everything else on your divide-and-conquer list to save room for the foods you're really excited about.

- If you're full, but you really want dessert, share it with someone.

- Remember how you'll feel later: You never regret NOT overeating, you only regret stuffing yourself.

Unofficially . . .
Americans eat
out, on average,
4.1 times a
week; the aver-
age annual
household
expenditure for
food away from
home was $1,702
in 1995, the
latest year this
statistic is avail-
able. The most
popular restau-
rant meal is
lunch. (Source:
The National
Restau-rant
Association, a
Washington,
D.C.–based
association
representing
the restaurant
industry.)

Assert your restaurant rights

An occasional restaurant splurge isn't a big deal, but with the frequency most of us eat out, restaurant splurges can quickly send you into calorie overload. All the recommendations made under "social eating" apply to restaurants; in addition, here are a few more suggestions for eating well while eating out:

- Avoid restaurants where the only low-fat item on the menu is a green salad. That's too boring for a whole meal; you'll wind up eating something high in fat.

- As often as possible, pick the restaurant yourself. Your friends will be relieved; people are always stymied when trying to decide where to go.

- Unless you've really got the buffet willpower thing down, avoid them. Even going in with my strongest resolve, I've always come out of a buffet groaning.

- Don't fill up on the bread basket or on the tortilla chips in Mexican restaurants. When eating alone, ask the server not to bring it, or have him or her hover for a few seconds while you take what you want and return the rest to the kitchen. Unless you've factored buttered bread into your day, ask in advance for unbuttered. When you're with a bunch of people you may have to forego these tactics; if so, keep the plate at the other end of the table from you.

- If you're unsure how a dish is prepared or want it prepared more healthfully, ask the waiter. This doesn't have to turn into a *When Harry Met Sally* shtick ending with a murderous waiter. Just politely ask whether you can get the fish grilled

instead of fried, whether you can get the burrito with just a little cheese and no sour cream,
or whether they can poach the eggs instead of
scramble them. I've gone even further, getting
chefs in Chinese restaurants to cut back on the
oil in stir-frying, my local wrap restaurant substitutes salsa for an oily pesto sauce, and I can
usually convince the waiter to bring me the vegetable special in place of french fries.

- Order half portions of main dishes plus a salad
  or low-cal soup. Restaurants are starting to serve
  half portions, and even if they're not on the
  menu, it doesn't hurt to ask.

- If the portion is large, ask the server to doggy-
  bag a portion of it immediately, before you take
  a bite.

- At pancake houses, get buckwheat or other
  whole grain pancakes. Ask for a fresh fruit topping or a pureed fruit topping; you probably
  won't need to add syrup or butter.

- Show your appreciation by returning to the
  restaurant. Waiters are happier to accommo-
  date you when they know you (and you tip
  decently).

- Don't assume that items marked "lean" or
  "heart-healthy" or "diet" are. The old hamburger and cottage cheese plate with a slice of
  melon "diet plate" is still on menus from the
  days when starch was considered fattening.
  And truly low-fat dishes may be served in such
  large portions they're no longer low-calorie.
  Definitely look over those items; they may truly
  be the best bets, but be critical.

Bright Idea
Before going to a
restaurant, a
good way to size
up the diet con-
sciousness of the
meals is to read
about the restau-
rant in a newspa-
per review or
guidebook and to
go to its website,
suggests Judy
Dausch, Ph.D.,
RD, LN, and a
nutritionist with
the National
Restaurant
Association.
"Many restau-
rants now have
Internet sites
which give infor-
mation on how
the food is pre-
pared, and, in
some cases, a
nutrition analysis
of foods," says
Dausch.

Support system

Your dad helped move you off of training wheels; thanks to that really great high school teacher you finally understood algebra; you don't know how you could have gotten through your divorce without your friend to lean on. You know it, a helping hand can bolster your success in so many areas of life. And the research shows the same to be true for weight loss. As John Foreyt and Ken Goodrick, renowned psychologists specializing in weight loss put it in their book *Living Without Dieting*, "When you falter, support people are there to comfort and encourage you to keep going. When you succeed, they will be there to give praise. This will help to prevent the damage to self-esteem from failures and will boost self-esteem with every success." This, they say, will help break up destructive thinking patterns dieters fall into, like beating themselves up for going "off" the diet, which causes self-esteem to plunge, and, in turn, saps enthusiasm for the weight loss process.

People who are truly supportive aren't those who scold you for that second piece of pie. Supportive people empathize with your weight loss struggle, usually because they've been there themselves. Ideally, you should find a person or a support group of people who have lost the weight and kept it off because, in addition to empathy and support, they're an inspiration. "The most important help a support person can give is to *lend emotional support and a clear-thinking brain* when you are having a temptation crisis," write Foreyt and Goodrick. That crisis could be the urge to binge, or go on a restrictive diet, or to cancel your gym membership— anything that knocks you off your course.

Some people have found it helpful to pick a "buddy," a specific support person. If you do this, you've got to be clear with that person about how you want to be supported, stresses Kelly Brownell in *The LEARN Program for Weight Control* (American Health Publishing, 1997). "A common and critical mistake is to expect your partner to read your mind," says Brownell. He advises making very specific suggestions such as eating sweets in another room, or going to exercise with you, or not scolding you when you slip up. And Brownell reminds you to reward your partner for helping you and to see how you can help him or her, so it's not a one-way relationship.

If you're a socially isolated person, you may be thinking "When I lose weight, I'll get back in touch with people; when I'm thinner I'll make new friends." Sorry, you've got it backward: Now's the time you need the friends and support the most to help you deal with the lifestyle changes you're making. If you have no one appropriate to turn to, try a support group—not only will you meet people in the same boat, but you may perhaps strike up a real friendship.

Chapter 6 describes the two most well-known support groups, TOPS and OA. Chapter 12 describes eating disorder support groups. Some of the people I interviewed, and many of the 160 "masters" of weight loss interviewed in *Thin for Life*, used support groups as needed, as occasional boosters, even after they'd lost the weight. A good support group makes you feel inspired and enthusiastic about losing weight, not bad about it. Get out if any of the following things happen:

> **"** It is not the perfect but the imperfect, who have need of love. It is when we are wounded by our own hands, or by the hands of others, that love should come to cure us—else what use is love at all?" (Source: *An Ideal Husband*, by Oscar Wilde.) **"**

- The group gets competitive about who loses the most weight.

- Group get-togethers lead to overeating.

- Your weight loss efforts have faltered since joining the group.

The attitudes and habit changes sprinkled throughout this chapter may take a while to set. And I've just given you the barest details; the books

---

Success Story: Peggy Newman

"I was really skinny at age 17, then I gained steadily until I was 180 at age 19, about 200 in my early 20s." But for the past 20 years Peggy Newman, a singer-songwriter-mom in Nashville, Tennessee, has been about 140 pounds (except for the occasional 10 pounds she gains and loses around the holidays), which look great on her 5'9" frame. Peggy says her overeating was her rebellion against a repressively religious upbringing where "everything was a sin, including gluttony." Add in some self-loathing, fueled by her obsession with fashion magazines and models, and you get a pretty potent psychologically triggered obesity brewing. "I tried every diet in those magazines, would lose 5 or 10 pounds, then gain it back. It was the magazines that taught me about bulimia—tried that for a few months but didn't like it."

Things started to turn around for her when she left home, started singing and performing, and met a guy who thought she was beautiful, even at 200 pounds. "He didn't try to control my weight, and that's when I started shedding the pounds. And I started to realize that God didn't hate me, I wasn't going to burn in hell, and I started feeling better about myself." One morning she woke up and had an epiphany: "I had a conversation with God, told him that if being an overweight person was my part in the scheme of things, I can accept that. I just want to be healthy. So I'll eat healthily and see what emerges—a thinner person or a fat person." Right then she canceled all her subscriptions to fashion magazines and concentrated on eating a low-fat diet with a generous amount of fruits and vegetables. "I never deprive myself; if I want bread and butter I have it but now I eat half-size portions of the more caloric foods." She also exercises 20 minutes, five days a week— "No more, because I hate to exercise." The scale went out with the fashion magazines— Peggy gauges her weight by how her clothes fit. The only thing left to work on is her body image: "I'm still not satisfied with my body; I still see a fat person even though part of me realizes I'm not."

quoted here are much better at actually helping you make the changes. They lead you step by step through new ways of thinking and coping. Most of you know that a grilled chicken breast is lower in calories and fat than a double cheeseburger. But going ahead and making that choice involves the concepts outlined here. Once you start making the "head" changes, the food changes described in the next chapter will come more easily.

Just the facts

- Getting the psychic energy up to lose weight and keep it off may involve changing some fundamental beliefs about yourself.

- Coping with cravings, overeating, emotional eating, and other fattening habits involves real strategizing.

- Yes, parties and restaurants can be fat traps, but come prepared and you won't fall in.

- Research and common sense tell you that emotional support helps you stick to your weight loss guns.

- Don't try to go it alone.

GET THE SCOOP ON...
Dieting derailments ▪ Good food choices
you can live with ▪ Carefree calories ▪
Fat and sugar substitutes

Chapter 10

What to Eat

"Betcha can't eat just one," the ads taunt, and they're right. It's as if those Midwestern food labs are taking a page from the tobacco industry manual on how to addict us, with the perfect blends of sodium, sugar, and fat. Addictive junk food, huge, supersized fast food and restaurant food, and cookies, bagels, and muffins that have tripled in size over the last 15 years are making us fat. So's overeating the other stuff, pouring on too much dressing, eating big portions of decent food, and eating too little of the good stuff like fruits and vegetables. All of this wouldn't be such a big deal if we were out there exercising. But let's tackle the food part in this chapter and save the exercise part for Chapters 13 and 14.

Ideally, according to everything nutrition science has been able to glean from the research so far, we should be eating according to that USDA pyramid sitting in Chapter 4. Actually, the low-fat, high-fiber version of the pyramid is outlined in Table 4.3. Eat pyramid-style, and you don't have to get so hung up on calories. It's almost as if weight loss is simply a

Bright Idea
While focusing on lowering fat and calories we sometimes lose sight of sodium, which for some people can raise blood pressure. Most of our sodium comes from processed foods, not the salt shaker. Compare food labels, buying the lower sodium choices. A rule of thumb: limit processed foods that contain more than 480 mg of sodium to one a day. Ideally, we should get no more than 2,500 mg daily.

side effect when you keep a lid on high-fat and low-fat/high-sugar foods.

You'll learn what to eat in this chapter. The previous chapter, equally important, gives you insight on how to eat, how to change your eating patterns, and how to stop using food to cope with life issues.

The state-of-the-art, healthiest, most fat-shedding way of eating advice in this chapter is only useful when you're ready to take it. If, after reading this, you still find yourself reaching for the cookies and ignoring the fruit, still overeating high-fat foods, then go back to Chapter 2, take the readiness tests, and see where you're stuck. If you haven't read Chapter 9, go there; you may recognize yourself in the some of those weight gaining attitudes and see some solutions.

Making the eating changes I'm suggesting here is a big deal if you've been living the high-fat life. If you think you're ready enough, but it seems overwhelming, get some help: Hire a nutritionist for a few sessions or join a weight loss group. Chapter 6 will point you in the right direction. Or try one of the responsible diet books or workbooks I recommend in Chapters 6 and 7; they give you a more prescriptive, step-by-step approach than I do in this chapter.

I've focused much of the chapter on fat because studies of people who have successfully maintained their weight loss show eating low-fat is a key element to their success. Lowering the fat content of your diet automatically drops the calorie content, unless you're scarfing down entire boxes of fat-free Entenmann's and the like. Also, there's some evidence that a low-fat diet slightly revs up metabolism, meaning you burn more calories. The other main factor is regular exercise.

Pinpointing the problem

Since this is a guidebook, not a diet book with a specific eating plan, I'm letting *you* mastermind your diet change strategy. Besides, I don't know your individual tastes, particular eating habits, and problem areas. (The closest I come to a prescribed eating plan is Appendix C, which lets you create low-fat, high-nutrient days drawing from 10 breakfasts, 10 lunches, 10 dinners and 10 snacks.)

Here's the deal: Using your food record, *you* figure out what you've got to work on to get your diet to look more like the body-fat shedding, low-fat/high-nutrition pyramid in Chapter 4. I'll give you ways of working on it. For instance: eating too many sweets? For solutions, go to "How sweet it still can be" further on in this chapter. Or, are meatball subs, fries, and the like your Achilles heel? The "Grease-ball cures" section of this chapter should help you out. And so on. But first, you've got to figure out where to begin. The food record and fat and fiber quizzes are your starting points.

The food record

Where is your diet going wrong? I mean beyond "I eat too much," or "I eat too much fat." Let's get specific, so you can really tackle your own individual diet foibles. That's what keeping a food record will do for you. It's a fantastic tool for building a better diet, and later, it may be the thing that keeps you on track. The food record (also called diet diary or food diary) is simply a complete, honest list of everything you eat for a few days, a week, or however long it's kept. An even better food record is one that also records when and where you ate, your hunger level, and your mood. Then you've got the information to figure out what, exactly, is undermining your diet.

Unofficially . . .
As you change to healthier, lower-fat foods, one thing shouldn't change: the pleasure of eating. Try not to suffer it out with rice cakes and dry toast. Go for tasty grilled fish and chicken with a sparkling salsa and savor that little piece of chocolate; make eating light even better than eating heavy.

Food record basics! You know those "before" and "after" shots of overweight people who become slender? The food record can be your "before" and "after" snapshot of your diet. It's the most valuable instrument we've got for figuring out where you're at now, and where you need to make changes. See the box here to learn how to use it.

Food Record Basics

■ For one week, or three days, write down every last morsel you eat, plus the when/where/hunger/mood part. A week is ideal; at minimum go with three days: two weekdays and one weekend day.

■ Eat the way you normally eat and try not to change your diet so you can see where you're overdoing it and, hopefully, why.

■ After the week (or three days) take some time to review the records. You'll start making the connections.

■ A good way to rate your diet is to compare it with the USDA's Food Guide Pyramid in Chapter 4 and the low-fat pyramid suggestions in Table 4.3. For instance, does your average daily fruit and vegetable tally come close to the pyramid's? Your meat consumption? Are you eating low-fat, high-fiber breads, cereals, and other grains?

■ Work on just one or two problems at a time.

■ In a week or two, when you feel that you're starting to eat better, fill out the food record again, and see how you've improved or what you're still doing wrong.

■ Fill out food records as needed throughout your weight loss and maintenance. For instance, if you start gaining back some weight, just the act of filling out a food record can be enough to get you back on track.

> ▪ Don't become obsessive. The food record
> is a tool to help assess your current diet
> and point out areas you need to work on.
> Try not to let it feed into obsessions
> with eating or with dieting and guilt.
> Although some people find it helpful to
> pretty much always record their food, I per-
> sonally find that obsessive. My hope is that
> through this book and the programs I rec-
> ommend, you can develop normal eating
> patterns that free you from food and
> weight obsessions.

Let's get back to the "complete and honest" part
for a sec. Meaning, you don't skip a thing: That was
four Reese's peanut butter cups? Put four, not three.
Eyeball that pasta with clam sauce dish—it's big,
maybe four cups. You finished it all. Write down
four cups pasta with clam sauce. "Starbucks latté"
isn't good enough: a tall (12 oz.) made with 2 percent milk, no sugar—that really tells you something.

If you've never done this before, it's going to be
enlightening. And even if you have, it's critical that
you do it again because diet patterns shift. Also, our
ability to be honest with ourselves changes. Study
after study shows that people tend to underreport
what they eat. Instead of being embarrassed—even
to yourself—about what you really eat, you should
feel relieved if you're overeating. If that's how you
got fat, then there's something you can do about it.
If you truly were eating like a bird, then it's either a
bad case of genetic obesity or some other serious
issue.

"JOE'S" SAMPLE FOOD RECORD
DATE: SEPTEMBER 5

How Much of What Food	Food Group Guesstimate*	Time of Day	Where	Hungry? (not, a little, very)	Mood (before/after)
8 oz. cup coffee with 2 Tbsp. 2% milk and 2 packets sugar	1/8 dairy	8:45 am	Kiosk	not	good/good
Subway meatball sub with cheese (foot-long, about 6 meatballs, asked for no mayo), 3/4 oz. bag of Ruffles, 20 oz. coke	4 carbs, 4 proteins, 1 dairy, 1 high-fat food, 1 high-sugar food	12:30 pm	Subway	very	irritable/good
1 12 oz. Coke, 4 Oreos	2 high sugar, high sugar	3 pm	office (meeting a deadline)	a little	stressed/stressed
1 Nestles Crunch	1 high fat/sugar	3:45 pm	ditto	not	stressed/guilty
8 handfuls peanuts, 2 beers	1 high fat, 2 alcohol	6 pm	bar (happy hour)	a little	trying to relax/ guilty
Spaghetti with white clam sauce (about 4 cups), small side salad with 2 Tbsp. Italian dressing, 8 oz. wine, 2 medium slices garlic bread, 1 cannolli, 1 espresso w/1 tsp. sugar	9 carbs, 6 fats, 1 protein, 1 vegetable, 2 alcohol, 1 high fat/sugar	8 pm to 11 pm	Italian restaurant (with clients)	not	tired/guilty

Here's a sample food record. Get your blank food record from Appendix F and make lots of photocopies of it before using.

*Based on Joe's data in the preceeding table, here's how Joe guesstimated the food groups from this meal:

9 carbs: 4 cups spaghetti equals 8 complex carbs, 1 slice Italian bread equals 1 complex carb

6 fats: approximately 4 tsp. oil in the clam sauce equals 4 fats, 2 Tbsp. salad dressing equals 2 fats

1 protein: about 2 oz. clams equals 1 protein

2 alcohol: 4 oz. wine equals 1 alcohol, Joe had two 4 oz. servings or 2 alcohol

1 high fat/high sugar: the cannoli

Joe's day's tally (check Chapter 4 for serving sizes for each of these groups):

Dairy:	1¹/₈
Carbs:	13
Fruit:	0
Vegetables:	1
Protein:	5
Fat:	6
High sugar and/or high fat:	6
Alcohol:	4

This is the food record for a day in the life of "Joe," a guy who's eating in reaction to stress and, as is typical with men, overeating in a social situation. And it looks like he's feeling too guilty about the overeating to enjoy it much. The "Food Group Guesstimate" column may be a little tough to figure out sometimes, but do your best because it's pretty revealing stuff. Those are the numbers you plug into your "day's tally." Look how telling Joe's tally is! It's pretty clear that high-sugar/high-fat foods are his downfall, at least on this day. And he's running really low on fruits, vegetables, and dairy. He's got his work cut out for him.

An honest food record will show you how your diet is making you fat and, just as importantly, why. Take it a step further and strategize ways to solve the issue. Look at Table 10.1 to see how this works.

TABLE 10.1   LET YOUR FOOD RECORD BE YOUR GUIDE

Food Record Said You Ate	Lightbulb Goes Off	Strategy
Danish or doughnut at 11 am 3 days this week	"Oh, that seems to happen on the days I skip breakfast."	Eat a healthy breakfast.
Eight fistfuls of peanuts, 7 chicken wings, and 3 beers at happy hour w/friends	"Drinking alcohol definitely makes me eat things I normally wouldn't."	Have 1 beer, keep peanuts at *their* end of the bar. Or eat a real meal during happy hour.
Two chocolate bars and 4 Oreos in the office at 4:15 while under a deadline	"Whoops, I know I head for chocolate when I'm stressed, but I didn't realize it was *that* much chocolate."	Cut down to 1 (or no) chocolate bar and bring in lower-fat food (air-popped popcorn or 3 to 5 Hershey's kisses.
Half an 8-oz. brick of cheese and a half box of Triscuits over a three-hour period	"Grazing all day when I'm home is dangerous."	Keep lower-fat grazing foods around like cut-up vegetables, seltzer, and fruit.

Do it slowly and permanently

Don't make it hard on yourself; make the diet changes gradually. Yes, you'll lose the weight more slowly this way, but why not? Why not boost your chances for real success this time? When you get impatient at not losing 30 pounds in 30 days, remind yourself of all the other times. How you went on drastically different low-calorie diets only to go right back to your old habits—and your old body weight. Each of you will approach diet changes differently according to where you're coming from. Here are some ways to tackle it:

- Pinpoint problem areas. Using your food diary, make a list of problem areas.

Watch Out!
Studies show that overweight and obese people systematically underreport their calorie intake by 30 to 40 percent. They especially tend to under-report foods high in fat and sugar.

- Take your time. Tackle one at a time; it doesn't matter whether it takes one week or one month, go at it until you're comfortable with the change. Sometimes a seemingly small change has major repercussions. For instance, if skipping breakfast is your normal pattern, deciding to eat a healthy breakfast may involve shifting all your mealtimes around. One of the reasons people skip breakfast is because they aren't hungry because they eat a lot late at night. Why do they eat so much late at night? Because they skip breakfast. So you can see how it could easily take a month to make this "little" change.

- Take on an entire food category. For instance, are fast foods your downfall? Next time, go into a fast-food restaurant knowing just what to order to keep fat and calories in check. The "Greaseball cures" section of this chapter and Appendix D, "Restaurant Foods," will clue you in. Or is dairy doing you in? Work on training your taste buds to go from whole milk or 2 percent to 1 percent, to skim, and try a few low-fat cheeses until you find something palatable.

- If you have access to the Internet, there's a great website that helps you analyze your diet, developed by a prominent nutrition researcher, Gladys Block. Her quizzes have been scientifically evaluated to do a good job of estimating intake. Versions of these screening tests are being used in the Mir Space Station to estimate the astronaut's diets. The website address is www.nutrionguest.com.

Eating more of the good stuff

If you've missed the National Cancer Institute's "Five-a-Day" slogan, you've been in nutrition denial. It's on airport billboards, plastic produce bags, and food labels, urging us to eat a total of five vegetables and fruits daily. Originally this advice was borne out of 200-plus studies linking generous fruit and vegetable consumption to lower incidence of cancer and heart disease in populations worldwide. Now there's even better proof: Research trials where subjects receive nutrition counseling, including advice to eat more than five a day (and lower fat), result in weight loss, and sometimes eliminate the need for diabetes and blood pressure medications.

This may sound insultingly obvious, but it's got to be said: You can't eat more fruits and vegetables and whole grain foods if you don't have them in your kitchen. However, for those of you who haven't gone to the grocery store in ages, whose meals come prepared and "to go," keeping stocked with healthy staples is a bit of a change. Here's what it takes:

Turn up the vegetable volume

If you haven't had a vegetable lately, join the masses, who as a rule avoid vegetables, reporting only a strong showing in the french fries category, which really doesn't count as a vegetable in this context. See if you can live with any of these strategies:

- Buy fresh produce twice a week for best taste.

- Make fresh salsas to liven up grilled chicken, fish, or lean meat; as a dip for vegetables (see, a double hitter); to add to homemade wraps; to accompany Mexican-style beans; and any other way that appeals to you. Be inventive; the tomato base can become tomatillos, carrots, cucumber, zucchini, and so on.

- Chop up a carrot and add it to soup, tuna salad, beans of any kind, or pasta or rice salads.

- Grate a carrot and cook it into spaghetti sauce, rice (with parsley), a savory pancake (along with some scallions), or in a tortilla with beans and salsa.

- Don't overlook frozen vegetables; they're often more nutritious than "fresh," which aren't so fresh after their long truck journey from far-away states. There are so many frozen vegetable combos to choose from, many without added butter or any sort of sauce. Some vegetables take to being frozen better than others: Personally, I prefer tiny peas, spinach, cauliflower, corn, Brussels sprouts, broccoli, and pureed squash, and I haven't had the best experiences with frozen asparagus, green beans, and potatoes. The trick is to cook them until they are just done, otherwise they can become a little rubbery. A semi-thaw and they're ready to be stir-fried, lightly sautéed, or steamed.

- Even canned is okay, depending on the vegetable. For my tastes, canned vacuum-packed corn is a winner, canned beans are fine if you rinse them in tap water to remove sodium, and canned spinach has its moments.

- Stuff them in sandwiches. If you're carrying the sandwich to work, tomatoes and lettuce can make things soggy, so slice 'em up and wrap them in plastic wrap. C'mon, it just takes a second. Add them to your sandwich just before eating.

Timesaver
For best taste, you've really got to buy fresh produce twice a week. Once with the rest of the groceries. Next time avoid waiting in supermarket lines by making a quick stop at a farmer's roadside stand during the season, or at a local health food store in the winter months. Not only will you save time, but you'll get better-tasting produce.

- If a green salad seems like too much of a fuss, do the Middle Eastern thing: chopped tomatoes and cucumbers with mint or parsley, a touch of lemon and olive oil. It's very portable.

- Bite the bullet and spend a half hour washing and peeling carrots, red peppers, cauliflower, or any other vegetables that you enjoy munching on raw or with a little low-fat dip. Make yourself a three-day supply, stick it in plastic containers, and you'll be grateful for it when it's saved you from a fattier snack.

- Two words: pasta primavera. For every cup of cooked ziti, rigatoni, linguini, or your other favorites, add one to two cups of fresh, steamed, or lightly sautéed vegetables. If you like tomatoes, use them with abandon; juicy tomatoes become, in essence, your sauce, so you can cut way back on the olive oil or other fatty sauces. Mix in generous amounts of fresh basil or other herbs, and you've taken care of at least two of the "five a day."

- Make meals based on salads. The classic: spinach salad with a hard-boiled egg, and, okay, bacon (but keep it to about a tablespoon crumbled). Another good choice that's becoming ubiquitous on restaurant menus: grilled chicken salad. I love bean salads; combine any beans (lentils, white beans, or garbanzos work well) with fresh herbs, lemon zest, and some chopped carrots and herbs and a tiny bit of olive oil, served on top of greens.

Figuring in fruit

The problem isn't that we don't like fruit—everyone likes some types—it's just that we forget to buy it. Or, that the stuff in the supermarket isn't the greatest quality. Try these ways of getting more fruit into your life:

- If it's at all convenient, go to a roadside farmer's stand or to farmer's markets. You'll remember what a joy bursting-with-flavor fruit can be, and it's usually cheaper at the stands than at the supermarket.

- In the warmer months, keep washed fruits in a mini-cooler in the back of your car for a rush-hour pick-me-up. This could thwart a trip to the fast food drive-thru.

- Roll up your sleeves and spend the half hour it takes to make a big fruit salad. It'll stay good in the fridge for about three days. To make it more dessert-like, add the following syrup to about four cups of fruit: $1/4$ cup fresh orange juice, one to two teaspoons honey, the peel of one orange or lemon, and even throw in a table-spoon of liqueur (Triple Sec and Grand Marnier work well).

- Make fruit salsas; they're great with grilled fish and chicken. Mango, cranberries, pear, papaya, orange, and grapefruit are all good candidates. Browse through some cookbooks for propor-tions, but basically you mix one or more of these fruits with diced onion, cilantro, or pars-ley, a little minced garlic, and, for spice, minced jalapeño peppers and/or minced fresh ginger. They last about two days.

- Top cereals and whole grain toaster waffles with sliced apples, pears, strawberries, blueberries, and of course the classic: banana.

- Blend fruit into a smoothie. Here's one of the zillions of combinations: $1/2$ cup nonfat milk,

$1/2$ cup nonfat plain yogurt, one ripe banana, $1/4$ to $1/2$ cup strawberries, one teaspoon honey, and a little ice.

- Bring grapes to work; the original melt-in-your-mouth-not-in-your-hands tidy snack.

- I've noticed that organically grown fruit is often tastier.

Gaining grains

Fiber can help you lose weight, and whole grains are a really good way to get fiber. Fiber expands in the stomach, making you feel fuller on fewer calories, and it may trap some of the fat in your meal sending it out of the body before it gets absorbed. Besides weight loss, fiber is linked to decreased risk of heart disease and colon cancer, and it may help reduce breast cancer risk. As opposed to foods made with low-fiber processed grains (a few examples: white bread, Cream of Wheat, corn flakes, most snack crackers), foods made with whole grains are richer in vitamins and minerals and contain disease-fighting compounds called phytochemicals. Convinced? Go to it:

- Buy breads with at least 2 g of fiber per slice. Freeze sliced whole wheat bread and toast slices as needed. Freezing keeps bread tastier; in the fridge the starch begins to disintegrate, which isn't a safety problem but a texture problem.

- Eat bran cereals or, at minimum, whole grain cereals with at least 4 g of fiber per ounce.

- Hot cereals are not all high in fiber (see Table 10.2).

We're supposed to get somewhere between 20 and 35 g of fiber daily. Fruits, vegetables, and beans will make a big dent in that number, and the rest should come from whole grains. See how much more fiber you get by making the following substitutions:

TABLE 10.2 WHOLER GRAINS

Processed Grain Food	g Fiber	Whole Grain Food	g Fiber
1 cup cooked Cream of Wheat	1	1 cup cooked oatmeal	4
1 cup (1 oz.) Corn Flakes	1	$3/4$ cup/1 oz. Kellogg's Nutri-Grain Golden Wheat	4
Healthy Choice Golden Multi-grain flakes	3	$1/2$ cup Kellogg's All-Bran Cereal	10
1 slice white bread or wheat bread	1	1 slice 100% whole wheat bread	2
$6^1/_2$-in. white pita	1	$6^1/_2$-in. whole wheat pita	5
large (4 oz.) plain bagel	3	Large (4 oz.) oatbran bagel	7
Thomas's regular English muffin	1	Thomas's Honey Wheat English muffin	3
8 reduced-fat Ritz crackers	0	8 reduced-fat Triscuits	4

Controlling "healthy" carbs

Although it is a lot easier for your body to turn food fat into body fat than to convert carbohydrates and protein from meals into body fat, overdo anything and you'll start putting on the pounds. So, even these healthy whole grain foods I've just pushed have to be eaten in moderation. Meaning, eat reasonable portions and give your body 15 to 20 minutes to register that it's full. If you're still hungry, get more. The point is to feel satisfied, not full. Some people feel a little out of control around carbs, piling their plates with pasta and eating the entire baguette. The problem isn't so much the carb calories, but the fat calories that go with. You're not eating mounds of plain, unadorned pasta; the sauce

Bright Idea
If your diet has been fairly low in fiber, then increase fiber gradually. Otherwise, you could be making hasty trips to the toilet all day. For instance, start out by using no more than $1/4$ cup of a high-fiber bran cereal and filling the rest of your cereal bowl with a lower-fiber cereal. Have no more than $1/2$ cup of beans to begin with. Your digestive tract adapts fairly quickly— within weeks. As you increase fiber, increase your water intake too—fiber *can* be constipating.

usually has some fat and so does the parmesan. These tips will help make a healthy high-carb diet more manageable.

Moneysaver
Dig into those bulk food bins for healthy cereals such as oatmeal, bran flakes, and unsweetened meusli. You'll pay a fraction of the price when you're not paying for packaging.

- Keep portions of starchy foods under control. Remember, just $1/2$ cup of cooked pasta, $1/3$ cup cooked rice, about $3/4$ cup of flaky cereal, and one slice of bread are each considered a serving, containing 80 to 90 calories. So if you're estimating six to eight complex carb servings on a food pyramid–based plan, you've used up three servings in a typical bowl of pasta.

- Switch to the high-fiber equivalent of a starch; it's harder to scarf down and easier to control portions. That includes whole wheat pasta, brown rice, and 100 percent whole wheat bread.

- Cut pasta, rice, and other grains with vegetables: about two cups vegetables per each cup of cooked starch.

- Still having a hard time with a particular starchy food, like bread? Leave that starch alone for a while and switch to another high-volume starch like air-popped popcorn (3 cups = 1 slice of bread) and vegetables.

- Eat some protein-rich foods at each meal; there's a little evidence that it has a hunger-quelling effect and may help keep appetite under control in general.

How much water should you drink?

No one quite knows where the standard eight-glasses-a-day recommendation came from, but turns out, it's right on target. First of all, it's the amount we naturally drink, according to a recent study of seven men at Brooks Air Force Base in Texas. When the healthy volunteers were confined to bed for

16 days, they drank, on average, eight glasses of water, more during the days they exercised. Study leader Victor Convertino, Ph.D., a research physiologist at the base, also just co-wrote a paper for the American College of Sports Medicine on exercise and fluid replacement. His rule of thumb: Drink 17 ounces of water two hours before exercising to keep body temperature and heart rate down. During heavy exercise, such as marathon running, follow it up with 5 to 12 ounces every 15 to 20 minutes. And don't trust thirst.

"Humans don't have a very sensitive system for detecting dehydration—they must consciously make themselves drink, especially when they exercise," Convertino advises. Eight glasses a day also sits well with American Dental Association spokesperson for fluoride, Michael Easley, DDS, MPH. That's enough to ensure that you get enough fluoride, which, he stresses, is as important for adults as it is for children. "As we age, our gums recede, exposing the roots of the teeth, which are not protected by enamel," he explains. Fluoride protects the exposed parts from root decay. Also, fluoride, along with calcium and vitamin D, may help prevent the bone-thinning disease osteoporosis. If you're drinking water low in fluoride (bottled or live in a low-fluoride area) Easley recommends a daily 1 mg fluoride supplement, available by prescription only.

While Susan Yanovski, an MD at the National Institute for Diabetes and Diseases of the Kidney, says there's "no magic number," she goes along with the eight glasses. She says you may need less if your diet is high in watery foods like fruits and vegetables and more if your diet is high in fiber, especially with fiber supplements that can actually be constipating without enough water.

Eating less of the bad stuff

Most nutritionists would slam me for calling any food "bad." One of the mottoes of the American Dietetic Association is that "there are no good or bad foods, only good and bad diets." Okay, true; in moderation, any food is okay, and I advise against yanking any food out of your diet. That's the food you're going to start getting a hankering for, and the food you may wind up bingeing on. But, c'mon, take a look at your food record, and you'll see that there are certain foods that are sending you into calorie overdrive. And it couldn't be purely coincidence that rates of obesity, heart disease, and nutrition-related cancers in Japan started rising at the same time we imported our fast-food restaurants to that country. So, here are some tips on decreasing the greasy, creamy, and sugary.

Putting the microscope on fat

Slather on butter, or suck the fat off a rack of ribs, and you know you're deep into fat. But the fat in some foods isn't so obvious.

FOOD	FAT CONTENT IN TEASPOONS
Obvious Fats	
Oil, 1 Tablespoon (Tbsp.)	3
Butter, 1 Tbsp.	3
Margarine, 1 Tbsp.	3
Vegetable shortening, 1 Tbsp.	3
Mayonnaise, 1 Tbsp.	2
Built–In Fat	
Olives, 7 large	1
Bacon, 3 slices	3
Nuts, 1/4 cup	4
Seeds, 1 oz.	2
Cream cheese, 2 Tbsp.	2
Sour cream, 2 Tbsp.	1

FOOD	FAT CONTENT IN TEASPOONS
Half-and-half, 2 Tbsp.	1
Table cream, 2 Tbsp.	1
Whipped cream, $1/4$ cup	2
Avocado, $1/3$ medium	2
Salad dressing, 2 Tbsp.	3
Cheese (most types), 1 oz.	2
Frankfurter, 1	3
Bologna, 1 oz.	2
Sausage, 1 oz.	2
Egg, 1 medium	1
Whole milk, 1 cup	2
Ice cream, regular supermarket, 1 cup	3
Ice cream, gourmet, 1 cup	8
Hamburger patty, cooked, 4 oz.	5
Cheeseburger patty, cooked, 4 oz.	6
Sirloin steak, 6 oz.	6
T–Bone steak, 6 oz.	8
Cooked–In Fat	
Potato chips, 1 oz. (about 15 chips)	2
French fries, 1 cup	2
Popcorn, microwave/movie theater, 4 cups	2
Fried fish, 3 oz.	2
Fried chicken, 3 oz.	3
Muffin, 1 oversized	4
Croissant, 1 medium	2
Doughnut, glazed, 1 medium	2
Danish, apple, 1 medium	2
Cheese sauce, $1/4$ cup	1
White sauce, thick, $1/4$ cup	2
Biscuit, 1 medium	2
Mayonnaise-based salads (potato, macaroni, coleslaw, $1/2$ cup)	2
Crackers, buttery snack-type, 5	1
Chocolate-chip cookies, 4 medium	2
Oatmeal cookies, 4 medium	2
Quiche Lorraine, 1 slice of an 8-inch diameter pie	10
Pizza, 1 slice of a 15-in. pie	2
Cheese enchilada, 1	3

Bright Idea
Your low-fat cheese options usually boil down to part-skim mozzarella (which doesn't even make the cut for no more than 5 g/oz.) or those grim fat-free cheeses. Take matters into your own hands and ask your grocer to start stocking more low-fat cheeses. Cabot makes some decent low-fat cheeses (Light Cheddar and Jalapeno Light Vitalait) and Tine Norway's Jarlsberg Lite is also convincing.

Slimmer snacks

Sometimes low-fat does equal boring; you have to go through a little trial and error before landing a tasty substitute. Here are some brands I like or that have gotten good reviews by friends:

Crackers (values per half ounce)

In comparison, high-fat crackers have about 75 calories and 8 g fat per half ounce.

Finn Crisp	60 calories	0 g fat
Ak-Mak Stone Ground Whole Wheat	58	4.5
Wasa Light Rye	37	0
Zaidy's Pletzel	50	0.5

Munchies (values per one ounce)

In comparison, chips, cheese balls, etc. can run as high as 160 calories and 13 g fat per ounce. And at 30 calories and no fat for two tablespoons, Guiltless Gourmet's Spicy Black Bean Dip makes a good partner for these snacks.

No Fries Cheese Puffs	120 calories	2 g fat
Snyders of Hanover Hard Sourdough pretzels	111	0
Smart Temptations Tortilla Chips	110	1
Newman's Own Organic Salted Stick pretzels	110	1.5
Baked Lays low-fat sour cream and onion potato chips	110	1.5

How sweet it still can be

I understand your sweet tooth; I rarely go a day without chocolate in some form. If you've got it bad, here are the basic ground rules and choices:

- Desserts shouldn't replace healthy foods. To work them in, make sure the rest of the day is filled with high-nutrient, low-fat foods (such as vegetables and whole grains).

- You eat full-fledged desserts (like a piece of pie, a slice of rich cake or pastry, a few scoops of Häagen-Dazs, or another high-fat ice cream) to your heart's content, and exercise like crazy.

- You eat reduced-fat or reduced-calorie desserts frequently and exercise almost like crazy. You've got to do some label comparisons in order to get a truly reduced-cal dessert. Just because it's lower in fat doesn't mean it's lower in calories.

- You save up and have a full-fledged dessert once, maybe twice a week. Or a reduced-calorie dessert three times a week. The rest of the week you satisfy your sweet tooth with tiny treats, such as those listed in the following box. And you get regular aerobic exercise three or more times a week.

- You get to the point where you can be satisfied by a very small portion, such as two or three Hershey's kisses or other treats in the Tiny Treats box.

Is sugar bad for you?

If you practice good oral hygiene, your biggest concern with sugar is weight gain, especially if you're eating high-calorie sweets and too many of them. And, if these constitute a large part of your diet, you

Unofficially . . .
Passing the
Cinnabon stalls
in malls is sure
to set your
brain's calorie
counter a-
whirring, but did
you figure on
670 calaories
and the equiva-
lent of 7 tea-
spoons of fat per
bun? That's what
the Center for
Science in the
Public Interest, a
consumer watch-
dog organiza-
tion, discovered
when they had
them analyzed.

Tiny Treats

These amount to about 50 calories each; a daily amount that you should be able to get away with if the rest of your diet is along the pyramid lines and you are getting some exercise.

2 Hershey's kisses	4 small gumdrops
1/2 oz. hard candy	12 jellybeans
5 peanut M&M's	15 regular M&M's
12 chocolate-covered raisins	5 small sesame crunch candies (total 1/3 oz.)
1 Fig Newton	1 Oreo
1 mini Reese's Peanut Butter cup	1 tablespoon Hershey's chocolate syrup
1 tablespoon jam	1 cup Swiss Miss fat- and sugar-free hot cocoa

---

may be skimping on vitamins and minerals by replacing these foods for fruits, vegetables, and other nutritious foods. But the other charges leveled against sugar—hyperactivity, yeast infections, diabetes and depression—have not been borne out by the research. Although there's no consensus on the ideal level of sugar in the diet, some of the experts I spoke to suggested no more than 20 percent of calories. That's 75 g on a 1,500 calorie-a-day diet; 90 g for 1,800 calories. Factor in about 40 g that naturally occur in two to three servings of fruit and two to three servings of dairy, and you're left with about 30 to 50 g (8 to 12 teaspoons) to play with—hardly enough for a can of soda.

Others told me it really doesn't matter how much sugar you eat as long as your diet is balanced and you're at a healthy weight. In other words, you can eat as much sugar as you want as long as it's on top of a great diet, not instead of. Problem is, most of us can't get away with that; we'd gain weight, especially since sugary foods are usually also high in fat. Dennis Bier, MD, a professor of pediatrics at Baylor College of Medicine and director of the USDA/Baylor children's nutrition research center in Houston puts it this way: "Within the context of an otherwise nutritionally adequate, balanced diet, there is no evidence that the amount of refined sugar consumed is detrimental in itself. In other words, there is nothing specifically biologically negative about sugar per se. On the other hand, if sugar intake is such a high proportion of one's diet that an individual's intake of other essential nutrients is compromised, or is causing the individual to gain weight inappropriately because of excessive calorie consumption, the intake of sugars should be moderated."

Greaseball cures

Addicted to burgers, fries, gyros, "ranch-style" breakfasts, and the like? You can recover; when people reduce the fat content of their diet, they lose their taste for these foods. In fact, many people report that just a nostalgic bite makes them queasy. As I've been saying, you can work any food into your diet, even a triple-decker cheeseburger if you get enough exercise and keep the rest of your day nutrient-rich and low-fat (or *several* days, in the case of the triple-decker cheeseburger).

Bright Idea
Extra-lean ground beef sounds low-fat, but a broiled 3-oz. burger will stick you with 14 g of fat; about 3 teaspoons. My father makes a mean burger with a lower-fat cut, top sirloin. At 6 g fat per 3-oz. burger, it's got enough fat to keep it juicy. Ask your butcher to grind top sirloin, trimmed of all fat.

Sugar By Other Names: The quickest way to spot sugar is to look at the "Nutrition Facts" section of the label under "sugar." The ingredient list on the label may not mention sugar, but it's probably in there under an alias. Here are some common sweeteners; all of them are just as caloric and nutritionally empty as sugar (except for sorbitol and mannitol, which are about half as caloric).

TABLE 10.3 SUGAR BY OTHER NAMES

Sugar	Description
brown sugar	crystals formed from molasses
confectioner's sugar	powdered sugar—white sugar more finely ground
sweeteners	sweeteners made from corn
corn syrup and high fructose corn syrup	a syrup made from corn starch
dextrose	glucose, sometimes mixed with water
fructose	a sugar found naturally in fruit and processed into a syrup or crystals
fruit juice sweetener	a syrup or crystal mixture of glucose and fructose obtained by boiling fruit juices into a syrup
glucose	the basic sugar that fuels our cells, sometimes added to foods, but usually combined with another sugar
honey	a mixture of fructose and glucose made by bees
invert sugar	liquid glucose and fructose
lactose	naturally occurring milk sugar
maltose	a combination of two glucose molecules
mannitol	a sugar alcohol
maple syrup	a combination of sucrose, glucose, and fructose from the sap of maple trees
molasses	residue from processing sugar cane or beet sugar into white sugar
raw sugar	crystals formed by evaporating the moisture from sugar cane juice
sorbitol	a sugar alcohol found naturally in some fruits—used in some dietary foods since it's absorbed more slowly than sugar
sucrose	a combination of glucose and fructose derived from sugarcane or sugar beets including granulated white sugar, raw sugar, brown sugar, turbinado sugar, and confectioner's sugar.
turbinado sugar	slightly refined sugarcane crystals

Fast Food Fake-Outs

Thought you were better off with chicken and fish? Not if they're prepared at fast-food joints. There are exceptions, but as you can see from the following list, in most cases, you're better off ordering the smallest burger on the menu than the fish or chicken offerings. Why? Because they either fry the chicken or fish or they include the chicken skin in the patty.

	Calories	Fat
McDonald's		
Hamburger	260	9
Grilled Chicken Deluxe	440	20
Crispy Chicken Deluxe	500	25
Fish Filet Deluxe	560	28
Wendy's		
Jr. Hamburger	270	10
Grilled Chicken Sandwich	310	8
Spicy Chicken Sandwich	410	15
Breaded Chicken Sandwich	440	18
Chicken Club Sandwich	470	20
Burger King		
Hamburger	330	15
Broiler Chicken Sandwich	530	26
BK Big Fish Sandwich	700	43
Chicken Sandwich	710	43

Unofficially . . .
Morningstar Farms Chik Nuggets are a clever vegetable protein knockoff of greasy chicken nuggets. Could be the power of suggestion, but they really do taste chicken–y. In addition to the high quality soy protein and fiber, they've got the nutritional pluses of chicken thanks to the addition of B vitamins and iron. Four chick nuggets come to 160 calories and 4 g of fat, compared to about 200 calories and 11 g of fat in the regular versions.

That said, it's still important to make these foods a very occasional part of your life. Unless you're a skilled juggler, these greasy foods set you up for a fall. And it's a good idea to wean your tastes away from these foods so you're truly satisfied with—even prefer—the healthier alternatives. For examples, check out the "Greaseball Reforms" box.

Greaseball Reforms

What a fat and calorie savings a simple switch can make! Hopefully, these switches keep the spirit of the food, just tone down the fat and calories. You'll find nutrition info on more of restaurant foods in Appendix D.

Instead of . . .	Have . . .	Approximate Savings*
Scrambled eggs plus 1/2 cup hash browns, 4 strips bacon, and a biscuit with 2 pats margarine (844 calories, 58 g fat)	Two boiled or poached eggs, 2 slices plain toast, and 2 oz. ham (380 cal, 15 g fat)	464 cal, 43 g fat
Quarter-pound burger with cheese (530 cal, 30 g fat)	Small cheese-burger (320 cal, 13 g fat)	210 cal, 17 g fat
8-oz. (large) beef burrito (usually some cheese and sour cream involved) (524 cal, 21 g fat)	8-oz. bean-only burrito w/2 Tbsp. grated cheese and no sour cream (341 cal, 9 g fat)	183 cal, 12 g fat
BBQ baby back ribs (14 ribs, 16 oz.) (770 cal, 54 g fat)	Sirloin steak, trimed of fat, 5 oz. (294 cal, 12 g fat)	476 cal, 42 g fat
Large order of fries (6 oz., about 3 cups) (550 cal, 27 g fat)	Small order of fries (small order is a little over 2 oz., about 1 cup). Better yet, split it with your meal companion. (200 cal, 9 g fat)	350 cal, 18 g fat

Instead of . . .	Have . . .	Approximate Savings*
Chinese Kung Pao chicken (with cashews, 1$^1/_2$ cups) (612 cal, 42 g fat)	Moo Shu Pork, 4 pancakes (432 cal, 16 g fat)	180 cal, 26 g fat
4 fried meat dumplings (243 cal, 16 g fat)	4 steamed vegetable dumplings (130 cal, 2 g fat)	113 cal, 14 g fat
Gyro sandwich (assuming they use about 5 oz. of meat and wrap it in a dense pita with a little yogurt sauce) (583 cal, 37 g fat)	Chicken kabob (souvlaki) sandwich (assuming they used about 4 oz. chicken, a little yogurt sauce, all wrapped in a dense pita) (369 cal, 14 g fat)	214 cal, 23 g fat
Subway foot-long meatball sub with cheese (920 cal, 38 g fat)	Subway 6 inch steak and cheese (398 cal, 10 g fat) or, even better, Subway turkey breast (289 cal, 4 g fat)	631 cal, 34 g fat

* To visualize your fat savings, remember that 5 g of fat is a teaspoon.

How critical are calories?

I'm de-emphasizing calories and focusing much more on reducing fat. While you still have to keep portions of even low-fat, healthy foods moderate, you don't have to count calories if you follow a low-fat, high-fiber version of the USDA's food pyramid in Chapter 4. And, of course, you should be getting regular, moderate exercise (see Chapters 13 and 14 for what that means). Calories will stay low enough, even if it seems as though you're eating a lot of food. And you'll be eating mainly complex carbohydrates, which seem to have their own safety

---

Salad Bar Barracudas

You can walk away from a salad bar with as much fat and calories on your plate as you would at a fast food restaurant and greasy spoon. While all unadorned vegetables, beans, and fruits are carte blanche, the items that follow should be avoided or limited. Decide which one or two of these items you need to liven up the salad, take a little portion, and leave the others alone:

Bacon bits, cheese, croutons, egg yolks (egg whites are fine), fried Chinese noodles, marinated Chinese noodles, macaroni salad, egg salad, tuna salad, potato salad, coleslaw, marinated mushrooms and other marinated salads, sunflower and other seeds, olives, any fried items such as egg rolls, and salad dressing. (A typical ladle holds 4 tablespoons of dressing. You definitely don't need more than 2 tablespoons of diet or regular.)

---

net: your body doesn't readily turn them into body fat. But as Table 10.4 shows, it's so easy to tip the balance on a high-fat diet because it seems as though you hardly ate anything. Here are the general guidelines for calories:

- Don't make yourself crazy counting calories. If you eat along the lines of a low-fat, high-fiber USDA food pyramid described in Chapter 4, sticking to portion sizes recommended in that chapter and get some exercise, you're golden.

- Go easy on low-fat or reduced-fat sweets. They're still loaded with sugar—not to mention calories—and can finally force the body to turn carbohydrate (from the sugar in these foods) into body fat.

- If you've had a high-fat day, leave it alone. Don't pile on healthy foods out of guilt; you're just adding even more calories. Just eat a littler lower fat than usual the next day, and try to get in an extra walk.

- Try to spread calories out as evenly as possible over the course of the day. Otherwise, hunger will get the better of you. There's no weight loss magic in eating before 7 pm or in eating many mini-meals as opposed to three squares, or in any of the other meal timing myths floating around.

For instance, when you skip breakfast, your body catches up with you eventually and demands calories later in the day. This wouldn't be a big deal if you were eating healthfully all day, but it's hard to get in the uniquely healthful foods we tend to eat at breakfast: fruit, fruit juices, high-fiber cereals, skim milk. Instead, you might end up satisfying those afternoon and late evening hunger pangs with junky foods. Same principle with skipping other meals; what's lying around for snacks may not be so good for you as what you'd get in a real lunch or dinner. If you know you get a hankering for late-night snacks, plan ahead and work one in.

As for six or more mini-meals throughout the day, that's a great way to go if you do it right: Don't overeat, and keep the meals nutritious (see Chapter 9 for how-to).

Moneysaver
Heavy-bottom saucepans and skillets are a must for low-fat cooking because you can use less oil without worrying about burning the food. But they can be expensive. Before spending upwards of $100 for a skillet, go to the hardware store and buy a cast-iron skillet—often under $10—and see how you like it.

As I've said,
it's a waste of
time to try and
count calories.
Modeling your
diet after the
pyramid will
keep you busy
enough. But in
case you want to
get an idea of
what a low-fat
day's worth (16
to 20 percent of
calories from fat)
of various calorie
levels looks like,
feast your eyes:

TABLE 10.4   WHAT LOW-FAT CALORIES LOOK LIKE

	1,200	1,550	1,700
Breakfast			
small bran muffin (about 2 in. by 1³/₄ in.)			
skim milk	1 cup (8 oz.)	1 cup	1 cup
1 cup small cantaloupe	¹/₂	¹/₂	¹/₂
calcium-fortified orange juice	¹/₂ cup	1 cup	1 cup
Lunch			
Lean roast beef sandwich with fancy horseradish cream (2 slices whole grain bread spread with mixture of 2 tsp. horseradish and 1 tsp. sour cream. Stuff with 2 oz. roast beef and sliced tomatoes)	1	1	1
sliced carrot and celery sticks	1 cup	1 cup	1 cup
seltzer	unlimited	unlimited	unlimited
apple or pear	1	1	1
Snack			
decaf skim milk latté	8 oz.	12 oz.	12 oz.
biscotti	none	1	1
Dinner			
cooked spaghetti	1¹/₂ cups	2 cups	2¹/₂ cups
your favorite red sauce (check labels: no more than 3 g fat per 1/2 cup or 4 oz.)	¹/₄ cup	¹/₃ cup	¹/₂ cup
grated parmesan	none	1 Tbsp.	1¹/₂ Tbsp.
3 cups mixed green salad with diet dressing	1 Tbsp.	1 Tbsp.	2 Tbsp.
Italian bread	none	1 slice	1 slice
vanilla frozen yogurt (check label: no more than 110 cal per ¹/₂ cup)	¹/₃ cup	¹/₃ cup	¹/₂ cup
topped with strawberries	¹/₄ cup	¹/₄ cup	¹/₄ cup

TABLE 10.5   WHAT HIGH-FAT CALORIES LOOK LIKE

	1,200	1,550	1,700
Breakfast			
apple danish	1 medium	1 medium	1 medium
2% milk	1/2 cup	3/4 cup	1 cup
orange juice	1/2 cup	3/4 cup	3/4 cup
Lunch			
McDonald's Quarter-Pounder with Cheese	1	1	1
order of small fries	1	1	1
Dinner			
lasagna	none	1	1
plain salad	none	none	2 cups
blue cheese salad dressing	none	none	1 Tbsp.

Cooking light

If you cook, you're ahead of the weight loss game. Making your own meals is a surefire way to control the amount of fat in your diet. There's still so much guesswork involved in restaurant and carry-out food if you get anything more involved than a turkey sandwich (no mayo) and a fruit salad. How much oil went into that grilled vegetable sandwich? This spaghetti with marinara sauce seems a little oily, wonder how bad? And pasta salads, tuna salads, and the like: Forget it! It's almost not worth ordering these things because the fat levels can shoot up so high.

When I say cook, I don't mean spending hours in the kitchen and learning a bunch of complicated techniques. I mean something as simple as boiling pasta, heating a low-fat spaghetti sauce, washing a carrot and some celery sticks in the meantime. Or,

← This day is similar to the low-fat day presented in Table 10.4—I've just substituted high-fat foods to reach about 45 percent of calories from fat. Notice how much less you can eat when foods are packed with fat and calories? On 1,200 calories, there aren't any calories left for dinner! And forget about fruits and vegetables. High-fat diets make it seem as though you didn't eat much, so the temptation to eat more is pretty strong.

Bright Idea
If you want something close to a diet plan to get you started, go to Appendix C where you'll find 10 breakfasts, 10 lunches, 10 dinners, and 10 snacks that you can mix and match to get nutritionally balanced 1,500-calorie days.

bringing home low-fat cold cuts, reduced-fat cheeses, and some whole wheat bread and bringing your own sandwich into work. Here are tips to make food preparation as painless and quick as possible. You know, you may even start enjoying it; cooking can be a creative outlet, especially pleasurable if someone else cleans up.

Get it right from the start

Just having the right ingredients in your kitchen is half the feat. Here are ways to make that happen:

- Stock staples. The following foods ensure that you can always put together a healthful meal, even on days when you were too busy to stop by the grocery store: canned water-pack tuna, can of beans (garbanzo and white beans are good in salads), sliced whole wheat bread in the freezer; carrots one can of soup (lentil, pasta and bean, tomato, or minestrone soup are good lower-fat, higher-fiber choices), bananas balsamic vinegar (a little drizzle makes most things taste good), a good mustard (ditto), spices depending on your tastes (I tend to reach for basil, oregano, curry, and cumin most often), and pasta.

- Buy lean cuts of meat, chicken, and fish. Beef: Lean cuts include top sirloin, round, bottom round, tip round, short loin/top loin, wedge bone sirloin, brisket, and skirt steak. Get cuts trimmed of all visible fat. Chicken: If you're not into skinning your own chicken, get the skinless, boneless breasts. They're a little more expensive, but very easy to work with. Turkey: Again, skinless is key. And remember, regular ground turkey is about as fatty as beef, with 11 g of fat per 3-ounce burger. But ground turkey breast is

Watch Out!
With little fat, lean cuts of beef and poultry and most fish get tough if cooked over high heat for more than a few minutes. Stir-fry or broil for one to four minutes (depending on the heat) just until the flesh is opaque and juices run clear.

very low in fat, at only about 1 g per 3-ounce burger. It is, however, a bit dry; best to use it in spaghetti sauce, meatloaf, and other foods that have other sources of moisture. Fish: Most fish is very lean and even the fattier fish, like blue-fish and mackerel, have only 5 g of fat in a 3-ounce cooked piece. However, some breeds of salmon are exceptionally fatty, such as farm-raised Atlantic salmon with 11 g of fat per 3-ounce piece; but since the type of fat in fish—omega-3—is so healthy, it's worth the splurge; just cut back somewhere else.

■ Have fresh, flavorful vegetables or decent frozen or canned (see tips earlier in the chapter in "Turn up the vegetable volume").

Give your cooking a makeover

My father, much more than my mother, is the chef. He learned to make over recipes he'd been cooking for 30+ years. Chicken broth now moistens and fla-vors his stews instead of oil, eggs are scrambled in a minimum of olive oil instead of butter, burgers are made with ground top sirloin, and everything that possibly can goes on the grill (corn on the outdoor grill is so good you rarely think of adding butter to it). Here are ways to cut the fat when you cook:

■ Use a heavy-bottomed skillet, such as cast iron. It will prevent food from burning, so you can sauté and stir-fry with a minimum of oil.

■ Cut oil/add broth. When stir-frying or sautée-ing, barely coat the pan with oil. Pam, or another vegetable oil spray, will keep you from overdoing the oil. When it seems as though the vegetables or meats are starting to get dry, add water, vegetable broth (available in some supermarkets and in health food stores), or chicken broth.

■ Add a splash of wine to sauces and stews to enhance flavor.

■ Splurge on fresh herbs; a tried and true way to distract your taste buds from the missing fat. Lighter herbs such as basil, parsley, and dill should be added at the very end of the cooking process—in the last minute or two—otherwise their flavor fades. Stronger herbs such as rosemary and thyme can be mixed in at the beginning or in the middle.

■ Bake or grill instead of frying or sautéeing. For instance, chicken dredged in flour and spices and baked works beautifully, so does, believe it or not, baked french toast (for recipe, see Appendix C). Grilled vegetables are better brushed in an oil-based marinade, but go light and remember that some of the marinade will be burned off.

■ In baked goods, such as muffins, pancakes, cookies, banana bread, and even some cakes, cut back on oil by substituting mashed fruit (applesauce and mashed banana work well, and pureed prunes mesh best with chocolate).

■ Try balsamic vinegar in salad dressings, marinades, and even sautéeing. Its musky sweetness adds interesting flavor to food, once again decreasing the reliance on fat for flavor.

■ Try low-fat or nonfat yogurt in place of mayonnaise or cream sauce. For instance, you can get a decently creamy pasta sauce going by mixing low-fat yogurt right into the cooked noodles.

Bright Idea
Need a break from low-fat spaghetti sauce? Make "everything but the kitchen sink" pasta, where you throw in steamed, lightly sautéed, or grilled vegetables and lean chicken or shrimp. Keep things moist by adding in very ripe, juicy, diced tomatoes. Chopped fresh basil makes it extra interesting.

And tuna, potato, and other mayonnaise-based salads work well with a three-to-one yogurt-to-mayo ratio.

Fat and sugar substitutes

I believe diet soft drinks, frozen yogurts, Swiss Miss cocoa, and all the other foods made with fake sugar and/or fat can play a useful role in a weight loss and weight maintenance diet. Especially if the high-calorie versions have traditionally played a big role in your diet. Switch from two regular cans of soda per day to diet and knock off 300 calories. This frees you up to use those 300 calories in a way that actually buys you some nutrition instead of wasting it on 20 teaspoons of sugar.

So, if foods made with sugar and fat substitutes help you switch from high-calorie to much lower-calorie versions of your favorites, fine. I'm not so sure it's a good idea to introduce these foods into your diet just because they're "diet." For instance, I don't see any good in starting up a diet soda habit when you never drank soda or eating potato chips made with Olestra (a fake fat) when you never were a chip eater. You're better off spending your money, time, and calories (some of these things still have calories) on the truly healthful foods. And there's always the danger that once you develop a taste for these foods, they might lead you into the junky real things.

Fat replacers

Too bad you can't just remove fat from food and wind up with a tasty burger or cookie or ice cream. And it's not even that fat has such an important taste—it's critical to what food technologists called

Timesaver
Cook up several soups (double or triple the recipe) over the week-end. Freeze them in small containers (enough for one meal) to reheat and eat all through the week. (Source: *Choose to Lose,* by Ron Goor and Nancy Goor, Houghton Mifflin, 1995.)

"mouthfeel." It's what makes ice cream smooth and rich instead of brittle and icy or makes a cake moist and tender instead of rough and dry. Here's what's out there:

- **Carbohydrate-based.** These are gums and other substances made from carbohydrates, such as pectin (a type of fiber that gives jelly it's jelliness) and starch. That's what "carrageenan" is doing on so many labels; it's a seaweed derivative, approved for use as an emulsifier, stabilizer, and thickener in food in 1961. They trick your taste buds into feeling a smooth, fat-like feel. These types of fat replacements have calories, but much less than fat. They get used a lot in low-fat ice creams and salad dressings.

- **Low-calorie fats.** Fats that have been chemically altered to be lower in calories, such as Salatrim, made by Nabisco. They've messed with the chemical structure of these fats, so that you only partially absorb them, amounting to about 5 calories per gram instead of 9.

- **Low- or no-calorie inventions.** Simplesse was the first one approved by the Food and Drug Administration. They cooked up this one by heating together a blend of egg white and milk protein in a process called microparticulation, in which the protein is shaped into microscopic round particles. Like a scaled-down version of jelly-like fish eggs, the microparticles roll easily over one another, creating a creamy feel. Simplesse can't be used for frying or baking in high heat because it breaks down and gets rubbery.

  However, the newest fat substitute on the block (as of press time), Olestra, can be fried, and they've gone straight for the potato and corn chips market. (Tasted the chips the other day, amazingly greasy feeling.) Olestra was approved by the Food and Drug Administration in 1996, but has really just started showing up in products recently. It's a chemical hybrid; a molecule of sugar replacing the glycerine core of regular fat, connected to eight fatty acids instead of the customary three. This structure, which looks and feels like fat, confounds our small intestine; our fat-busting enzymes can't break it up so it passes through unabsorbed. This one has stirred up a lot of controversy for two reasons. Studies show that in excess, it causes diarrhea and, even more repulsive, something called "anal leakage." I'll leave it to your imagination on that one. That's why you'll see the mandatory "This product contains Olestra. Olestra may cause abdominal cramping and loose stools" on labels of Olestra-containing foods. Also, Olestra opponents are worried that replacing fat with Olestra means missing out on types of vitamins called "fat soluble." These vitamins—A, D, E, and K—are present in dietary fat and are better absorbed in our intestinal tract in the presence of fat. But Olestra sweeps them out as it makes its own exit. To counter this, the manufacturer, Proctor and Gamble, has added these vitamins to its product (brand name, Olean). But there are other fat-soluble goodies such as beta-carotene and probably a bunch of yet-undiscovered ones that may be affected. Despite all these dire-sounding effects, a little Olestra probably won't hurt you, based on what we know so far. If you've got a healthy GI tract and eat only a small bag of

Bright Idea
Love linguini with white clam sauce? Make your own and cut fat by at least half (it usually has about 10 g fat per half cup, because of all the olive oil they throw in). Sautée a little garlic in a teaspoon of olive oil, add canned clam juice and fresh (let them steam until they open) or canned clams, and some chopped parsley and voilà! And done in under 10 minutes.

Olestra-fried chips a few times a week, it appears that you'll be okay. But in large quantities, you may be taking a risk.

Sugar substitutes

It's amazing how sweet these things are. The stuff you get in the packets has been mixed with corn starch to give it some volume, otherwise you'd end up flicking on a few tiny specks. Here's what you're eating:

66
Use by small children, especially those under two years of age, may not be compatible with their high energy needs. (Source: Position Statement by the American Dietetic Association: Fat Replacers, *Journal of the American Dietetic Association*, April, 1998.)
99

- **Saccharin** (Sweet 'n Low), an indigestible, calorie-free, petroleum-based product is 350 times sweeter than sugar. Used since the turn of the century, it was nearly banned in 1977, after studies linked it to bladder cancer in rats. But a public outcry kept saccharin on the market. Still, there are hints in the research that saccharin may be linked to bladder cancer. Recently, the National Toxicology Program's advisory panel on the government's *Report on Carcinogens* (cancer-causing agents) recommended keeping saccharin on the list of "anticipated" human carcinogens. This is better than getting on the list of *known* carcinogens, but still . . . Some organizations such as the consumer watchdog group Center for Science in the Public Interest do not recommend it.

- **Aspartame** (Equal or NutraSweet) is the combination of two amino acids, building blocks of protein. Technically, it has calories, 4 calories per gram just like any other protein and just like sugar. But since it's 200 times sweeter than sugar, the tiny levels used make it virtually noncaloric. Just after it got approved for use in dry foods and sodas in the 1980s, there was a scare when users reported dizziness, headaches, and other side effects. However, research studies didn't find these side effects. A recent report linked it to brain cancer, but that research was said to be so flawed that it was meaningless. Basically, experts I spoke with believe aspartame is safe for most people, but that it's possible that some will react badly. The FDA seems pretty confident about it, saying that the equivalent of 97 packets of aspartame per day could be safely eaten over a lifetime. There is a group for whom aspartame is absolutely off limits: those with phenylketonuria, an inherited inability to metabolize phenylalanine, one of the amino acids in the sweetener.

▪ **Acesulfame-K** (acesulfame potassium or Sweet One) is chemically close to saccharin, calorie free, and 200 times sweeter than sugar. This sweetener is used alone or in combination with others in dry beverage mixes, instant coffee and tea, gelatin, pudding, and chewing gum. Because laboratory rats developed tumors during testing, some consumer groups question its safety. The FDA, which approved acesulfame-K in 1988, claims that the tumors were unrelated to the sweetener.

▪ **Sucralose.** Though recently approved for use in the U.S. in 1998, people in other countries have been using it since 1991, and it was discovered in 1976. Sucralose starts out as table sugar, and through a chemical process loses some atoms and gains some others. This creates a molecular structure that the body doesn't recognize, doesn't absorb, and passes right out. It's approximately 600 times sweeter than sugar; you'll be seeing it in a variety of foods including baked goods, soft drinks, and as a table sugar substitute. So far, so good in terms of safety tests. Even normally suspicious groups such as the Center for Science in the Public Interest seem to be giving this one the nod.

Are sugar and fat substitutes worth it?

The burning question in the sugar and fat substitute research is: Does the body realize that you've tricked it and demand those calories later? So far, the research indicates that working sugar and fat

---

Success Story: Tom Kiely

You can be successful going it alone—no personal trainer, no commercial weight loss program, not even a diet book, as my 30-pounds-lighter friend Tom Kiely has proven. Well, I take that back, he didn't really do it alone, in fact getting in shape was his wife Joan's idea. "We mutually support each other; we're each other's big motivator." Picturing his father, overweight and diabetic, is another strong motivator.

Tom was athletic as a kid and weighed "165 forever" as an adult, until the weight started creeping up in his mid-30s. He stopped exercising when he became chairman of the religion department in a prestigious Catholic high school. "That and two kids at home left me too wiped out to exercise." So he thought. But when he hit 200 pounds (at 5'11") and he and Joan began their health kick, he found time to exercise. And the energy came back in droves. His exercise mainstay is jogging—three times weekly—and when the weather's bad he gets on the treadmill. A recent pulled tendon didn't set him back, he just switched to swimming.

The other part of the health kick (that's now become incorporated in their lives) is that the couple makes healthy meals together. It doesn't hurt that Tom was a professional cook before becoming a teacher. "I start preparing dinner when I get home. The cooking becomes a challenge, not a drag. I think: How can I do this differently to reduce the fat." He says, "You don't have to get maniacal to lose weight; my lifestyle didn't really change much. It's just that now I'm conscious of what I'm eating. I don't just grab. And I make sure to exercise. Yes, I still yen for the fat sometimes, but I've shifted my focus to so many other things that I don't obsess about what I'm going to eat next."

Unofficially . . .
A teaspoon of sugar is only 14 calories. Don't think you're doing yourself any favors by substituting it for a packet of artificial sweetener. That only starts to make a difference if you tend to have more than three teaspoons of sugar in your coffee or tea.

substitutes into your diet either does nothing or slightly lowers total calories. Seems like fake fats are more promising weight loss tools than the fake sugars, but that's probably because fat is a bigger weight gain culprit. Studies show that using fat replacers to move fat down from 40 percent of calories to 30 percent, lowers the total calorie level of the diet (people don't compensate by eating more calories). But those are studies that tightly control fat intake. Outside of a research study, it's hard to predict how people will react.

For instance, a University of Pennsylvania study indicated that some people take reduced-fat foods as a license to overeat. Women in the study were given the same type of yogurt labeled either "high-fat" or "low-fat," then fed lunch. Those who thought they'd had low-fat yogurt (even though it was high-fat) ate more at lunch than those who thought they'd had the high-fat stuff. It doesn't appear that sugar substitutes have done much good at keeping people slim: While their consumption has tripled over the past decade, there's been no reduction in the consumption of real, caloric sweeteners. Meanwhile, over this same period, the proportion of overweight people has gone up 8 percent; these trends may not be related, but it makes you wonder.

Ultimately, you want to be getting the bulk of your calories from naturally low-fat foods such as fruits, vegetables, and lean meats or beans. And, if you're exercising regularly, you can afford to eat a bag of real chips or a few scoops of Breyers. So perhaps these sugar and fat substitutes make useful crutches, weaning you off, but not completely off, foods you've come to enjoy in large quantities. And if you want to continue drinking diet sodas and eating Olestra chips forever, that's your decision. It's hard to gauge their safety. Many of the sweeteners and fat substitutes have been around for decades with no apparent adverse effects. Advice is mixed. Talk to the employees at the Food and Drug Administration, and you feel like going out and guzzling some Diet Coke just for the hell of it. Talk to the consumer advocates working at the Center for Science in the Public Interest and you feel like screaming "don't do it" when you watch people in

restaurants opening their pink and blue packets or
buying bags of Wow! chips made with Olestra.

Just the facts

- A food record is your most valuable tool for figuring out how to change your diet.

- With a little creativity and foresight, you can get
  more fruits, vegetables, and grains in your diet
  without much hassle.

- Give your greasy spoon and dessert habit a
  makeover by making substitutes you can live
  with and splurging in moderation.

- Eat à la the low-fat, high-fiber pyramid, get
  some exercise, and you don't have to worry
  about calories.

- Control fat by making it yourself; you don't have
  to be a chef to cook light.

- Fake fats and sugars may help you keep the
  weight off, but they aren't necessary and still
  have safety issues.

GET THE SCOOP ON...
Diet lessons ▪ Exercise lessons ▪ Psychological
lessons ▪ Outwitting maintenance saboteurs

Chapter 11

Staying Psyched

You're in luck. For the first time, we've got some scientifically supported advice on how to make that hard-earned weight loss stick. Up until now, it was pretty much anyone's guess. After decades of obsessing over the best ways to lose weight, obesity experts are finally shining the research spotlight on what helps people maintain their weight loss for two, three, and even five years. But don't get too excited—this research is still in its infancy. But there's certainly enough to go on, and the news is encouraging. That research is going to be the basis for much of the advice in this chapter.

People lose weight, lots of weight—50, 100, 200 pounds—all the time, sometimes many times throughout their life. But what percent maintain their weight loss? Up until recently, the answer was a grim 5 percent. However, that statistic may be way off, since it mainly came from research based on very obese people who lost weight through hospital-based programs, including physician-supervised liquid diets like Optifast. The outcomes were discouraging; when they caught up with these people

317

Unofficially . . .
Most people in the National Weight Control Registry, a large study of successful maintainers, reported that their weight loss "greatly improved their quality of life, health, and well-being, mood, mobility, and level of energy." However, a minority said that they had become more preoccupied with thinking about food and weight.

two or three years later, most had gained back the weight.

But the news coming out of other types of weight loss programs and from surveys of successful maintainers looks brighter. For instance, on Laurel Mellin's "Solution" program people kept losing weight years after they got out of the program (that program is described in Chapter 6). And studies of successful maintainers show that people can maintain big weight losses, even if they've been fat since childhood. I'll be referring a lot to the most exciting and comprehensive of these studies, The National Weight Control Registry, an ongoing examination of hundreds of people who've kept off at least 30 pounds for a minimum of a year. On average, the participants have lost 66 pounds and maintained at least 30 pounds of the weight loss for an average of five years.

The exercise advantage

I'm discussing this first because it seems to be the most important factor in keeping the weight off. Study after study shows that people who exercise maintain weight loss more successfully than those who try to do it with diet alone. Over 90 percent in the National Weight Control Registry regularly exercise, and, as you can see from Table 11.1, they're doing a lot of exercise, on average burning 2,830 calories weekly. That averages to 404 calories daily: an hour or more of brisk walking, an intense exercise class, or an intense bout on the treadmill, bike, or other aerobic equipment.

And the majority of the 160 "masters" of weight maintenance interviewed for Anne Fletcher's *Thin for Life* (Houghton Mifflin, 1994) cited exercise as one of the most important factors in their success.

Most masters exercised from three to seven times weekly—a third of them five or six times a week, and 16 percent exercised daily.

How much do you need?

The more weight you lose, the more exercise you need, says Thomas Wadden, Ph.D., director of the Weight and Eating Disorders Program at the University of Pennsylvania School of Medicine. He is one of the foremost weight loss experts; his latest research compares the effects of various types of weight loss programs on maintenance. He tells us: "Caloric needs probably drop about 10 calories for every pound lost. That means if you lost 40 pounds, you could be burning 400 fewer calories than before you lost the weight." So instead of having to shave off 400 calories from an already not-so-generous maintenance diet, exercise takes over that calorie burning, allowing you to eat more normally. Really, your exercise prescription is individual. But in general, the research points to three hours of heart-rate-increasing, aerobic exercise per week to really help keep your weight down. Doesn't matter what form the exercise takes—brisk walking (don't worry, you can start slowly and work up to "brisk," stationary or touring biking, an exercise class, tread-mill, stair-climbing machine, dancing—anything that gets your heart rate up for a sustained period of time will do the trick. Chapters 13 and 14 describe the ins and outs of various forms of exercise and why exercise works. In brief, exercise helps keep body fat in check long term because:

Bright Idea
Think of all the shopping and errands you could do in a "walking friendly" environment such as downtown or in a huge mall. Make an "errands" date with a friend and walk your way through the tasks instead of taking the car.

- You're building muscle when you exercise, whether it's aerobic exercise or strength training (weight lifting). The more muscle mass on that body, the higher your engine runs. In other

words, you're constantly expending more calories, even while you're asleep.

- Depending on how vigorously you exercise, you
  can knock off between 100 and 1,000 calories
  daily (more if you're a competing athlete).

- Exercise has an appetite-suppressing effect and
  may even dampen your taste for fat.

- Exercise may improve your mood, giving you
  more enthusiasm for sticking to good weight-
  maintaining habits.

Best maintenance diet

In all the major studies of people who've maintained their weight loss for at least two years, the
majority of people say that they stick to a low-fat
diet. And the other diet strategies are equally unsur-
prising: eating less overall, eating fewer high-sugar
foods, and eating less red meat. The 438 successful
maintainers tracked in the National Weight Control
Registry reported getting, on average, 24 percent of
calories from fat and 56 percent from carbohydrates. Men took in an average of 1,685 calories,
women only 1,306 calories. So, these people are eating a quarter to a third less than the average American—that is, if we can believe the U.S. Department
of Agriculture surveys on what Americans typically
eat. Many believe these surveys underreport intake
of calories.

This low-calorie intake may be necessary for
people who've been obese; research indicates that
formerly obese people run at a 15 percent lower
metabolic rate than those who've never been obese.
But fewer calories doesn't have to mean fewer nutrients. Even though the maintainers in the National
Weight Registry ate fewer calories than the average

TABLE 11.1   EATING AND EXERCISE HABITS OF WEIGHT LOSS MAINTAINERS IN THE NATIONAL WEIGHT CONTROL REGISTRY*

Habits	Average of 629 Women	Average of 155 Men	Average of All Participants
Calories per day**	1,297	1,725	1,381
Percent of total calories from fat	24	23	24
Percent of total calories from protein	19	18	19
Percent of total calories from carbohydrates	55	56	56
Eating episodes per day	5	5	5
Fast-food meals per week	<1	<1	<1
Restaurant meals per week (excluding fast-food meals)	2	3	3
Total restaurant meals per week (fast-food and other)	3	4	3
Total calories burned through exercise per week***	2,670	3,490	2,830
Calories burned doing:			
Stair climbing	186	202	189
Walking	1,058	1,241	1,092
Light-intensity activity (such as stretching or yoga)	234	170	221
Medium-intensity activity (such as cycling, aerobics, or treadmill)	501	637	527
High-intensity activity (such as weight lifting, running, step aerobics, stair-climbing machine)	690	1,239	797

*Adapted with permission from "A descriptive study of individuals successful at long-term maintenance of substantial weight loss," by Mary L. Klem, Rena R. Wing, Maureen T. McGuire, Helen M. Seagle, and James O. Hill, in *The American Journal of Clinical Nutrition*, Volume 66, 1997. ©1997 American Society for Clinical Nutrition.

**Keep in mind that people generally underestimate the amount of calories they take in.

***Keep in mind that people generally overestimate the amount of exercise they get.

American, their diets were richer in the five nutrients selected for examination by the researchers:
calcium, iron, vitamin A, vitamin C, and vitamin E.
The men got less iron, but that's okay since the
average American man exceeds his iron requirement, probably from eating so much red meat.
Although the research didn't go so far as to examine why the maintainers' diets were more nutrient-
rich, it's almost certainly a function of eating more
fruits, vegetables, and low-fat dairy. Still, on anything less than 1,500 calories, I'd take a standard
multivitamin/mineral tablet (Chapter 5 will help
you pick one).

"There's no question that a low-fat diet is best for
maintenance," affirms Thomas Wadden. Low-fat
diets work because:

- Your body converts fewer calories to fat. It's easier for your body to turn fat from the diet into
  body fat than it is to turn protein and carbohydrates. So, even if the two diets were the same
  calorie level, you body would burn more and
  store less as fat on the low-fat diet.

- Slip-ups aren't so bad. I've never heard of anyone gaining weight by overeating fruit. If the
  low-fat diet is also low-sugar (most of the sweets
  come from fruit), then it's hard to make a big
  calorie mistake even if you do overeat one day.
  Eating an extra cup of rice or pasta isn't going to
  do nearly the kind of damage as an extra cheeseburger. But be warned: Overeating low-fat/
  high-sugar foods such as reduced-fat cookies
  and ice cream can also put on the pounds.

- Low-fat diets train your tastes away from high-fat,
  calorie-rich foods. For instance, once people get
  used to skim milk, they typically can't stand to go

back to 2 percent or whole; these milks now taste oily. And those who have been on low-fat diets for a while report feeling queasy when they eat very fatty foods such as burgers or gyros.

▪ Low-fat diets are less addictive. "While your low-fat diet should be appetizing and tasty, one reason it works is because it doesn't excite your appetite in the same way as addictive high-fat foods such as snack foods and fast foods," explains Wadden.

Unofficially . . .
In a survey of Weight Watchers group leaders who've maintained their weight loss, the two most frequently cited challenges were "not going back to old eating habits" and "accepting that it's a lifelong commitment."

So, until the research hits on a better way, I'd stick with the low-fat version of the USDA's food pyramid that keeps cropping up in this book. Chapter 4 outlines the diet, and Chapter 10 gives you tips for incorporating it into your life. In addition to eating lower-fat levels, successful maintainers also eat less overall, which reduces calories and sets you up for less overeating down the road. That's because your stomach really does shrink, according to research from St. Luke's/Roosevelt Hospital in New York City that compared 14 dieters to nine people not on a diet. And "a smaller stomach is a good thing if you're trying to lose weight; you get uncomfortable before you overdo it," says the lead researcher of the study, Allen Geliebter, Ph.D., a research psychologist at the hospital's Obesity Research Center. After four weeks of a 600-calorie-a-day liquid diet, dieters lost an average of 20 pounds and shrunk their stomachs by an average of 27 to 36 percent, depending on which way it was measured (I won't go into the hard-to-explain measuring devices). But would this happen on a 1,200- or 1,500-calorie real food diet? Probably, if you had been eating a lot more before, speculates Geliebter. "Our research shows it works in reverse with bulimics; they've got stretched-out stomachs from eating massive amounts of food at one sitting," he says.

What helps you stay the course?

Okay, so a low-fat diet and getting regular exercise is what keeps people trim long-term. So how do you get the enthusiasm to choose marinara sauce over alfredo time after time and get yourself in that gym or out walking day after day instead of watching *Seinfeld* reruns, pint of ice cream in hand? A lot of it has to do with the attitudes mentioned in Chapter 9, which I'll bring into play again here. It all amounts to internalizing your motivation; you value being healthy much more than doing the things that make you gain the weight back. And even people who feel internally motivated can fall back into the bad old patterns, but they've learned to nip such slips in the bud and get the drive back. Here are some of the key factors that have helped people stick with it:

- *Admitting and accepting that you're in this for life.* That sounds overwhelming, and it's probably not helpful to remind yourself of this daily—the "one day at a time" motto is more manageable. But on some level, you've got to accept this. "When people go on a diet they have this fantasy that they can go back to their old ways at some point," says *Thin for Life* author Anne Fletcher. "But eventually, they stop seeing it as a quick fix. Instead of thinking 'poor me, what a horrible way to live' they see their new lifestyle as one that enables them to have what they want: to feel good." You reach this point when the price for bad habits is just too high to pay; it's not worth the agony you get in return.

Motivators

Here are ways of helping you stay on course, collected from interviews with researchers and maintainers.

- Recall the pain of being heavy.

- Keep a picture in your mind, or a photo somewhere in view, of your overweight self.

- Congratulate yourself often on how well you're doing.

- Focus on how much better you feel.

- Take the responsibility of becoming a role model to others.

- Try on your favorite outfit in front of the mirror.

- Touch the newly toned muscle in your arm.

- Don't say "never," "always," or "every day"—as in "I can never have pecan pie again," or "I will always eat low-fat," or "I will exercise every day." That way, if you break these impossible vows you'll feel like a failure. Replace them with "I will do my best to" or "I will try harder next time."

- Find a partner to exercise with.

- Take a low-fat cooking class.

- Forgive yourself when you slip up.

- Train for an event, whether it's a 5K race or an AIDS ride.

- Be patient; it's okay if the scale doesn't move down quickly.

"Making a lifelong commitment to weight control" was ranked the second most important factor to successful weight maintenance in a survey of 541 Weight Watcher's group leaders who had maintained an average 50-pound loss for six years. ("Taking responsibility for one's own behavior" was first.)

■ *Understanding that history doesn't necessarily repeat itself.* Just because you've lost and gained a number of times before, it doesn't mean you will inevitably gain the weight back. Nearly 60 percent of the "masters" in *Thin For Life* had gone through that cycle about five times before finally keeping it off. And 91 percent of those in the National Weight Control Registry had tried to lose weight before their final success; the average person had gained and lost 270 pounds. This same study confirms that just because you've always been fat doesn't mean you always will be. These people were pretty heavy—an average BMI of 35—before their weight loss (see the BMI table in Chapter 1). But now, they're maintaining at an average BMI of 24 for women, 26 for men. And their obesity set in early: 46 percent before age 11 and 25 percent between the ages of 12 and 18. In fact, your previous yo-yoing offers you rich insights on what *not* to do this time around. For instance, you may decide that *this time* "I'll never drop calories so low as to get really hungry," or "I'll let myself have an ice-cream sundae once a week instead of swearing off them and then bingeing."

■ *Finding your own way.* If you hate step aerobics, you don't have to do it just because your friend swears by it. Likewise, you don't have to follow the latest, hottest diet that forbids pasta, just because other people are losing weight on it (check back with them in a year and see how much they've kept off). Be creative, trust your instincts, and you'll fashion a system that works for you.

- *Developing attitudes that make it easier.* In Chapter 9 I describe ways of thinking and coping that are linked with successful weight loss and maintenance. To sum up they were:

  - **Take care of yourself.** As Laurel Mellin puts it in *The Diet-free Solution* (HarperCollins, 1998), the nurturing process ". . . amounts to asking yourself three questions: 'How do I feel?' 'What do I need?' and 'Do I need support?'"

  - **Take responsibility.** This means fighting the-dog-ate-my-homework syndrome. While, of course, you're not responsible for the genetic portion of your weight, you are responsible for your eating and exercise habits. "Taking responsibility for one's own behavior" was considered the most important key to success in a survey of 541 Weight Watchers "leaders" (those who conduct the Weight Watchers classes) who had, on average maintained a 50-pound weight loss.

  - **Do it for yourself.** This means losing weight for yourself, not to please anyone else.

  - **Be realistic.** If, after many attempts at getting thin, you realize that it's just not where your body wants to be, aim for a weight that's not *thin,* but healthy (the BMI chart in the first chapter gives approximations for healthy

Moneysaver
Before joining a weight loss program ask if it's got a maintenance plan. Often you get a discount if you buy into both the weight loss and maintenance plans at the beginning instead of paying for them separately.

weights). Twenty-one percent of successful maintainers in a survey of Weight Watcher's group leaders said that "setting a realistic goal weight" was one of the top three most important factors toward maintenance.

■ **See failures as learning experiences.** This applies to what happened today as well as what happened over the past decades.

■ **Rethink deprivation.** Instead of feeling deprived because they can't fill their days with cookies and fries, people who get really into a healthy lifestyle feel deprived when they have to miss a workout or a healthy meal.

■ **See shades of gray.** Black-and-white and all-or-none thinking gets you in trouble: You're either "on" or "off" your diet, you're either fat or skinny. When you can see grays, that chicken-fried steak and a shake lunch simply means you eat lighter and get more exercise tomorrow. So you're never going to be thin? Something in between fat and thin is just fine.

■ **Accepting your body.** This means seeing beauty in body shapes that don't fit the slender ideal and accepting your own body. Paradoxically, when you stop hating your body you free up all sorts of positive energy and develop self-esteem that goes a long way toward helping you lose weight.

■ **Not letting slip-ups turn into major relapses.** "A *lapse* is a slight error or slip, the first instance of backsliding," writes Kelly Brownell in *The LEARN® Program for Weight Control* (American Health Publishing, 1997—see Chapter 6 for more on the LEARN program). It is a single event like overeating, or gaining a few pounds. "*Relapse* occurs when lapses string together and the person returns to his or her former state. When relapse is complete and there is little hope of reversing the negative trend, *collapse* has occurred," states Brownell. So how do you make sure things don't reach the relapse/collapse point?

- **Believe that you can reverse the trend.** This ties in with the capability to see shades of gray so you're not "on" or "off" your weight maintenance plan. You simply overate or didn't exercise all week. While your slip may be cause for concern, and you may have gained a pound or two, just realize it's temporary, and go back to the ways you were maintaining. "It's an interesting paradox that patients of mine lose 40 to 50 pounds, but when they start to gain back four or five pounds they don't think they can lose them" notes Thomas Wadden. Wadden urges us to realize that, of course, we can lose these small amounts of regained weight. "Just as you have vicissitudes in moods and in the quality of your relationships, you will have ups and downs in your weight maintenance. Just because your weight's going up doesn't mean it can't come down," he assures.

- **Riding out the urge.** As Brownell explains in the LEARN manual, urges to overeat disappear if you wait it out. Think of urges as waves: They build, crest, break, then subside. Brownell instructs us to "urge surf": Identify the urges early in their development, then ready your skills

Timesaver
Instead of eating your way through the airport as you wait for your plane, take advantage of airport services. For instance: Get your shoes shined, get a manicure, write postcards, or catch up on phone calls. The plane will arrive before you have time to investigate the calorie-laden airport food.

and ride out the wave. "If the wave is upon you at full strength before you recognize it, you may wipe out no matter how well you surf. If you recognize the wave early, but cannot surf, you will also wipe out. Therefore both parts are important—early recognition and skills to cope with the urges." To cope in a nonfood way with the urges, look back at the suggestions made in Chapter 9 under "Curb cravings." Brownell suggests making your own list of activities you enjoy that can replace eating; his LEARN manual offers a list with room to write in your own additions.

- **Nip weight gains in the bud.** Here's the tricky part: staying vigilant enough to nip weight gains in the bud without becoming neurotic and obsessed about your weight. No easy task. It helps if you land on a weight that you can comfortably stick with, not one so low down the scale that you have to fight a hungry and exercise-obsessive fight to maintain. In *Thin for Life,* Fletcher says that nearly all the "masters" have a maximum upper limit—usually no more than 5 to 10 pounds above their goal—and they are adamant about not exceeding it. Fletcher describes many strategies they use when they cross that line including, of course, exercising more and eating less, but also not allowing themselves to feel guilty (so they don't get into self-destructive thinking). The success stories I interviewed in researching this book also had an upper limit, and when they hit it, increased exercise was the main way of dealing with it. Calories may be cut a little, but not much.

One obvious way of monitoring your weight is with the scale. "While you're losing the weight you shouldn't weigh yourself more than once a week because you'll get frustrated when you don't see the scale going down quickly enough," says Wadden. But once you've lost the weight, Wadden believes that frequent weighing is helpful. "Many successful maintainers weigh themselves daily or at least several times a week. These people are vigilant. If they gain some pounds that aren't due to pre-menstrual water weight, then they act quickly by increasing activity and eating less," says Wadden. Nineteen percent of maintainers in the Weight Watcher's survey weighed themselves once a week, probably because weekly weighings were part of their Weight Watcher's training.

However, others, especially those in the anti-dieting movement, see the scale as a ball-and-chain, imprisoning people in their weight obsessions. Some successful maintainers don't use the scale; for instance Peggy Newman, profiled in Chapter 9, threw out the scale with the diets; she can figure out when she's gained by the way her clothes feel and what looks back at her in the mirror. But Wadden, (and a number of his colleagues) begs to differ. "I can't support the philosophy of 'don't weight yourself at all, just see where your weight ends.' For formerly obese people, it will end up high," he states flatly.

Getting support from family, friends, and support groups is one tactic that appears on all the top ten lists of successful maintenance. The same

Watch Out!
TV-watching strikes again! In a huge ongoing Harvard study tracking 19,478 male health professionals, middle-aged men who increased exercise, cut down on TV-watching, and stopped eating between meals lost an average of three pounds while the rest of the group gained three pounds over a four-year period. (Note: None of these men were necessarily trying to lose weight.)

Unofficially . . .
A University of
Minnesota study
of 89 men who
had lost weight
on a weight
loss program
found that
successful main-
tainers were men
who believed
they could do
it, faithfully
attended the
weight loss pro-
gram, had social
support, and
improved their
diet and exercise
patterns.

reasons I gave in Chapter 9 for the importance of support during weight loss apply to weight mainte-nance: for comfort and encouragement, to bolster self-esteem, and to give you the psychic energy to keep it up. And the same characteristics of a sup-portive person described in that chapter apply: empathy and inspiration. You don't want a police-man or someone who makes you feel like a failure.

In *The Diet-free Solution*, a program that's had great maintenance results (see Chapter 6) author/researcher Laurel Mellin urges her readers to seek out support. It's an integral part to one of her six "cures"—strong nurturing. By asking for help, you are fulfilling a need, and when your needs are met, you have less tendency to turn to food for comfort. "Getting support from family and friends" was also cited as important in a Weight Watcher's survey of successful maintainers.

Not everyone needs a lot of support. The more you internalize your new exercise and eating habits, the less support you need, says Wadden. "Many maintainers feel a sense of autonomy; their changes are coming from inside rather than outside, so they don't need much help," he says. But until you reach that point, if you're struggling, then support can be the glue that holds your maintenance effort together. You may need something more structured than friends and family. Chapter 6 describes the sup-port groups such as TOPS or OA. Also, if you lost your weight on a commercial weight loss program, many of these have maintenance programs you can buy into. According to Wadden, the research indi-cates that you should go at least every other week for the group to be truly helpful.

Diet drugs

Do diet drugs help you keep the weight off? Maybe, but at a risk, since their long-term safety is unknown. Some of the researchers I spoke with said they'd be willing to give diet drugs indefinitely as long as the patient understood it may be risky and gave informed consent. "Medications make you less vulnerable to a high-fat environment; you're less responsive to Cinnabons and ice cream as you walk throughout the mall," says University of Pennsylvania's Thomas Wadden. But so far, drugs aren't a factor in studies of successful maintainers. It's not clear if this is because the drugs don't work, because the side effects are too bothersome, or because drugs still haven't caught on with the majority of maintainers. Only 4.3 percent of the National Weight Control Registry registrants reported using diet pills. Many of the 160 "masters" interviewed for Anne Fletcher's *Thin for Life* had tried diet pills, but none of them were using them to maintain their weight loss.

Outmaneuvering saboteurs

How come Richard Drezen, profiled in Chapter 1, did so well, kept his weight off for a year, then gained it all back in a matter of months? Stress. He moved from New York City to Washington, D.C., changed jobs, changed environments, and it threw him off. (As it turns out, he jumped right back into a weight loss program, lost the weight again, and has been holding steady for over a year now.) Trauma, change, stress, and people and situations that bring you down are all threats to your maintenance. Here's what to guard against:

"
It appears . . . that stressful interpersonal relationships can hinder and that supportive relationships can help. This emerges from the literature despite inconsistent methods of measuring support. From "Understanding and Preventing Relapse" by Kelly Brownell and others, in *American Psychologist*, July 1986.

Stress and negative emotions

Stress, depression, anxiety, and other upsetting emotional states of mind are risk factors for relapses of all sorts: smoking, drinking, and weight gain. One study found that 30 percent of relapses are in reaction to negative emotional states. This is not about taking a happy pill; stress, anger, sorrow, and other negative feelings are normal and inevitable. Interestingly, it's not necessarily the obvious using-food-to-cope-with-stress syndrome. You may be beyond that by the time you've been maintaining for a while; that's a habit you "fixed." It could be that you're feeling so overwhelmed, you've got so much to deal with ("multi-tasking" is Wadden's term) that something's got to go, and that something is exercise, or cooking light, or all the other ways you've been maintaining your weight loss. "It's hard to maintain that level of vigilance when other things are going wrong," says Wadden. If possible, the ideal solution is to work on reducing the cause of the stress or pain or anger or whatever else is overwhelming you. If you can't do much to change the situation, in the meantime keep up your exercise and healthy eating as best you can, even if you're not as rigorous as before. Better to gain back 10 pounds than 20 pounds.

Sabotaging spouses

Funny things happen on the way to a slimmer body, including contradictory behavior from your spouse or partner. Yup, that same wife or husband or partner that's been urging you to lose weight is now bringing home cookies and stopping off at Baskin Robbins when you take your walks together. As you lose weight and become more self-confident and attractive, your spouse—male or female—may feel

threatened or jealous. Studies on the topic found
that, sorry guys, husbands are worse saboteurs than
wives. Two-thirds of dieting women contend with
sabotaging husbands, whereas wives are generally
supportive, according to a study conducted by
George Blackburn, MD, an associate professor of
medicine at Harvard Medical School and chief of
the nutrition and medicine clinic at Beth Israel
Deaconess Medical Center at Harvard. "Husbands
frequently have mixed feelings about weight loss,"
says Edward Abramson, Ph.D., a psychologist specializing in weight issues whose book *Is Your
Marriage Making You Fat?* (Kensington Publishing) is
due to hit the stands in late 1998. While they want
their wives to lose weight, they're afraid of the consequences. Reasons for keeping their wives fat, says
Abramson, include:

- **Sexual jealousy.** "Now she'll be more attractive
  to other men and I'll lose her." Abramson suggests reassuring your husband by becoming
  more sexual with him. And that may be something you haven't been before because the
  shame of being fat can inhibit sexuality.

- **Spotlights his deficiencies.** "As long as she's
  overweight I can get away with my smoking/
  drinking/overweight/gambling because who's
  she to talk?"

- **Removes his line for "winning" arguments.** If
  she complains that he's inconsiderate, he counters that she isn't perfect either, "Look, you had
  two pieces of pie when you said you weren't
  going to have any." Most overweight women feel
  so guilty, they succumb to this emotional black-
  mail, says Abramson. His advice: divorce weight
  from other issues. "If the two of you are having

Success Story: Mohammed Yasseen

Growing up, I remember "Mr. Yasseen," a good family friend, as handsome, soft, and chubby (never obese). Now, at age 74, he's handsome, lean, and fit-looking. "I lost 20 pounds in 40 days over the stress of my first wife's death. That was 10 years ago, and I remember my doctor assured me I'd never keep the weight off. But I was determined to do it, so I went out and bought a scale and weighed myself every morning. If I gained a pound, I'd eat a little less for a day or so. That went on for six months: daily weighings, with my weight fluctuating by a pound or so. Then it seemed as though my stomach shrank, and I no longer wanted to eat big meals." The weight stabilized; he's had 155 pounds on his 5'8" frame for 10 years. Besides keeping portions moderate, Mohammed Yasseen walks three miles at least five times a week (in bad weather he uses a treadmill). He's one of those people happy with virtually the same lunch every day: a medium-size Syrian bread (pita), two in-season fruits, and a slice of cheese. He hasn't given up his favorite—steak—he just makes sure it's completely trimmed of fat. "I still use the scale, check it a few times a week to make sure I'm not gaining. But I'm not anymore."

a debate about the household budget and he brings up your weight, say 'That may be true, but if you want to talk about my weight we can do that as soon as we finish talking about the budget.' As you lose weight and your spouse can no longer hide behind your weight and eating issues, he'll have to deal with his own problems." Meanwhile, what to do when he brings home a gallon of Breyers? Abramson suggests telling him, "I'm confused. On one hand you say you want me to lose weight, on the other you're bringing home ice cream. What should I do?" Throwing it back to him will force him to confront his own feelings about your weight loss and, hopefully, curb the sabotaging.

Just the facts

- So far, nothing beats a low-fat diet for maintenance.

- People who exercise keep their weight off; on average, you need three hours a week.

- Adopting new attitudes, new ways of coping with urges to overeat, and developing good social support will improve your success at maintaining your weight loss.

- Be aware that your spouse may be undermining your weight loss effort, and don't get sucked into it.

GET THE SCOOP ON...
Food obsessions vs. eating disorders ▪
Binge-eating disorder ▪ Bulimia ▪
Anorexia ▪ Getting help

Eating Disorders Aren't Just for Skinny People

Chapter 12

It almost always starts with a diet. "It's a gradual thing, an obsession that slowly grows. I was always careful about what I ate, then at a certain point I just stopped eating. I enjoyed the hunger because it made me feel powerful; I'd conquered it," explains Melinda (her full story is at the chapter's end). It doesn't matter if you're 250 pounds or 100 pounds; if you're on a diet you can develop an eating disorder. At the higher weights it involves bingeing; at the lower weights, semi-starvation and bingeing and purging. So it's not just skinny teenagers who have eating disorders; don't think you're off the hook because you're overweight. In fact, somewhere between 5 and 30 percent of obese people have an eating disorder called binge-eating disorder.

With emaciated models and actresses as our aesthetic role models, it's a wonder no more than an estimated eight million Americans have eating disorders. "Actually, the cult of thinness is more a

❝
Today's ideal is taller and thinner than most of the female population. It is also contrary to the nature of the female body, which normally carries a fat content of 25 percent and is resolutely pear-shaped. As a result, women go to great lengths to reshape their bodies. We agree to be fixed. If this were a Greek play, it would be a tragedy.
—Vivian Hanson Meehan, President, ANAD (National Association of Anorexia Nervosa and Associated Disorders)
❞

maintaining factor than a causing factor. These illnesses get started because of developmental issues and are fed (ironically) by the cult of thinness," explains Adrian Brown, MD, a prominent Washington, D.C.–based psychiatrist specializing in eating disorders and Medical Director of the Eating Disorders Program at Georgetown University. Later on in the chapter, I'll show you how Brown and her colleagues around the country can help you leave the cult and the eating disorder through therapy, nutrition counseling, and in some cases, medications.

When do your food habits become a "disorder"?

Maybe you occasionally eat a pint of Häagen-Dazs when you feel stressed out. Or you're uncomfortable eating in front of some people. Do you have an eating disorder? Not necessarily. The key is, do your behaviors impact your mental, social, or physical well-being? Two of the leading researchers in the eating disorders field—Christopher G. Fairburn and B. Timothy Walsh—define eating disorders as "a persistent disturbance of eating or eating related behavior that results in the altered consumption or absorption of food and that significantly impairs physical health or psychosocial functioning." That definition's pretty broad; the disordered eating in the first part of the definition could mean starving, vomiting, bingeing, or fearing and avoiding certain foods. The second part is essentially about how it affects you: Has the eating pattern left you malnourished, depressed, or caused heart damage?

The psychological community has given only two eating disorders precise definitions: anorexia nervosa and bulimia nervosa. And they're working on another one: binge-eating disorder. But many of the eight million or more Americans with eating disorders don't make the cut for these precise definitions but still have serious and life-threatening illnesses.

To get an idea of whether your relationship with food constitutes an eating disorder, take the Eating Attitudes Test that follows. This test was developed and scientifically validated by David Garner, Ph.D., a prominent eating-disorder researcher. While this test does not determine whether you have a specific eating disorder, it can give you a sense of whether you're headed for trouble. **If you score greater than 20, then you should seek a professional consultation with someone who understands eating disorders.** In a study of 534 women and 186 men who filled out the questionnaire, of those who scored above 20, a third had clinically significant eating concerns or weight preoccupations. Of the higher scorers, 20 percent considered to have a "partial syndrome" went on to develop full-blown eating disorders when contacted 12 to 18 months later.

Please check a response for each of the following statements:

EATING ATTITUDES TEST

Always	Usually	Often	Sometimes	Rarely	Never	Score
1. Am terrified about being overweight.						
☐	☐	☐	☐	☐	☐	____
2. Avoid eating when I am hungry.						
☐	☐	☐	☐	☐	☐	____
3. Find myself preoccupied with food.						
☐	☐	☐	☐	☐	☐	____
4. Have gone on eating binges where I feel that I may not be able to stop.						
☐	☐	☐	☐	☐	☐	____
5. Cut my food into small pieces.						
☐	☐	☐	☐	☐	☐	____

	Always	Usually	Often	Sometimes	Rarely	Never	Score
6. Aware of the calorie content of foods I eat.	☐	☐	☐	☐	☐	☐	_____
7. Particularly avoid food with a high carbohydrate content (i.e., bread, rice, potatoes, etc.).	☐	☐	☐	☐	☐	☐	_____
8. Feel that others would prefer if I ate more.	☐	☐	☐	☐	☐	☐	_____
9. Vomit after I have eaten.	☐	☐	☐	☐	☐	☐	_____
10. Feel extremely guilty after eating.	☐	☐	☐	☐	☐	☐	_____
11. Am preoccupied with a desire to be thinner.	☐	☐	☐	☐	☐	☐	_____
12. Think about burning up calories when I exercise.	☐	☐	☐	☐	☐	☐	_____
13. Other people think I'm too thin.	☐	☐	☐	☐	☐	☐	_____
14. Am preoccupied with the thought of having fat on my body.	☐	☐	☐	☐	☐	☐	_____
15. Take longer than others to eat my meal.	☐	☐	☐	☐	☐	☐	_____
16. Avoid foods with sugar in them.	☐	☐	☐	☐	☐	☐	_____
17. Eat diet foods.	☐	☐	☐	☐	☐	☐	_____
18. Feel that food controls my life.	☐	☐	☐	☐	☐	☐	_____
19. Display self-control around food.	☐	☐	☐	☐	☐	☐	_____
20. Feel that others pressure me to eat.	☐	☐	☐	☐	☐	☐	_____
21. Give too much time and thought to food.	☐	☐	☐	☐	☐	☐	_____
22. Feel uncomfortable after eating sweets.	☐	☐	☐	☐	☐	☐	_____
23. Engage in dieting behavior.	☐	☐	☐	☐	☐	☐	_____
24. Like my stomach to be empty.	☐	☐	☐	☐	☐	☐	_____

25. Have the impulse to vomit after meals.
☐   ☐   ☐   ☐   ☐   ☐   _____

26. Enjoy trying new foods.
☐   ☐   ☐   ☐   ☐   ☐   _____

Total score   _____

How to Score the EAT Test

For the first 25 questions, give yourself the following score for each answer (put under "Score" in the right-hand column of the test):

Response	Score
Always	3
Usually	2
Often	1
Sometimes	0
Rarely	0
Never	0

Score the last question (number 26) as follows (put the number under "Score" in the right-hand column of the test):

Response	Score
Always	0
Usually	0
Often	0
Sometimes	1
Rarely	2
Never	3

Total up all the individual scores for each question. As mentioned in the introduction to this test, if you score over 20, you may have an eating disorder and should schedule a counselling session with an eating-disorders specialist.

That binge high

We've all gotten stuffed out of our minds at Thanksgiving or left a brunch buffet in pain. You could call it a binge, but it's not the worrisome type. And that's not the way I'm using the word "binge" in this chapter. Eating disorder bingeing is different from benign bingeing. The two tip-offs to disordered bingeing are that you eat a large quantity of food and you feel out of control while doing it. That out-of-control feeling is the main thing distinguishing a binge from a simple episode of overeating or mere indulgence.

People with bulimia, binge-eating disorders, and other types of disordered eating that involve bingeing, regularly eat 1,000 to 2,000 calories at once or within a two-hour time period. That's what's typical, but binges can reach 30 times your daily calorie needs, hitting 20,000 or more calories. Here's what goes on during a binge, paraphrased from *Overcoming Binge Eating* (The Guildford Press, 1995), an excellent self-help book by Christopher Fairburn, MD.

- **Pleasure/disgust.** The pleasure you initially get from the taste and the "up" sensation of a binge usually turns to disgust and revulsion.

- **Compulsive stuffing.** Food is scarfed down, often stuffed in the mouth and chewed almost mechanically, or barely chewed. Often bingers drink lots of water to wash it down, which makes them feel even more bloated afterward.

- **Agitation.** Bingers feel desperate, driven by the powerful force of their craving, and may pace or wander around during the binge. Getting food is of paramount importance causing people to steal food from others or from stores or to take it from the trash, causing feelings of shame and disgust.

- **Altered state.** People report going into a trance-like state, where eating seems automatic as if it's not really you doing it. Or, to not think about what they are doing, people may distract themselves with TV or loud music.

- **Secretiveness.** Often they eat normally—or even less than normal—in front of others but binge in private.

- **Loss of control.** Some get this sense before a binge, some as they start to eat, and for others it happens once they realize they've eaten too much. After years of bingeing, the lack of control may fade, as people become resigned that bingeing is part of their life. So they plan their binges into their schedule in the most convenient way possible. This may seem like control, but it's not: They still can't stop bingeing, and can't stop eating once they begin.

Binge-eating disorder

If you binge, you may very well have an eating disorder, even if you don't meet the complete checklist for the two binge disorders defined by the American Psychiatric Association: binge-eating disorder and bulimia (defined later in this chapter). People with binge-eating disorder binge frequently, but they don't drastically cut back on calories, or vomit, or abuse laxatives to compensate.

Official definition

Binge-eating disorder hasn't yet received official full-fledged psychiatric disorder status with the

American Psychiatric Association as has anorexia and bulimia, but it's getting close with the status of "research criteria." Here's the full-blown disorder (adapted from the American Psychiatric Association's Diagnostic and Statistical Manual of Mental Disorders):

■ Recurrent episodes of binge eating. An episode of binge eating is characterized by the following:

1. Eating, in a discrete period of time (e.g., within any two-hour period), an amount of food that is definitely larger than most people would eat under the same period of time and in similar circumstances.

2. A sense of lack of control over eating during the episode (e.g., a feeling that one cannot stop eating or control what or how much one is eating).

■ The binge-eating episodes are associated with three (or more) of the following:

1. Eating much more rapidly than normal

2. Eating until feeling uncomfortably full

3. Eating large amounts of food when not feeling physically hungry

4. Eating alone because of being embarrassed by how much one is eating

5. Feeling disgusted with oneself, depressed, or very guilty after overeating

■ Marked distress regarding binge eating is present.

■ The binge eating occurs, on average, at least two days of the week for six months.

■ The binge eating is not associated with the regular use of inappropriate compensatory behaviors (e.g., purging, fasting, excessive exercise) and does not occur exclusively during the course of anorexia or bulimia.

As you can imagine, binge-eating disorder can make you very fat and make weight loss impossible. However, according to Fairburn, only about half are overweight (the rest must have amazing metabolisms). Researchers don't know how many obese people have binge-eating disorder; studies show that it affects about 30 percent of obese people seeking treatment in university weight loss programs. "And it may affect 3 to 5 percent of obese people in the general population. Although many more than that binge, without having the full-blown disorder," according to Marsha Marcus, Ph.D., Associate Professor of Psychiatry and Psychology, and Director of the Behavior modification program at Western Psychiatric Institute and clinic at the University of Pittsburgh. Marcus is a leading authority on this still-understudied disorder. Unlike anorexia and bulimia, in which the overwhelming number of cases are female, a fourth to a third of those with binge-eating disorder are men.

"The more extreme the obesity, the more likely people binge or have binge-eating disorder," says Marcus. One study found that while 10 percent of mildly overweight people (BMIs of 25 to 28, see Chapter 1) were bingers, 40 percent of those with BMIs of 31 to 42 had the problem. In studies comparing binge eaters to equally obese people who don't binge, the bingers reported becoming obese at an earlier age, dieting early on, and having more episodes of gaining and losing a lot of weight.

> **"**
> The worship of the willowy supermodel has become a cult, and the parent of even the scrawniest six-year-old will know that she is quite likely to come home from school announcing that she is starting a diet. . . . In recommending weight loss to our patients, there is a possibility that we may sometimes do more harm than good.
> —William Jeffcoate, MD, City Hospital, Nottingham, UK in "Obesity is a disease, food for thought," *The Lancet* (a British medical journal), March 21, 1998.
> **"**

What it does to you

During a binge, especially a big one, you can get a whopping stomach ache. Sometimes the stomach presses up on the diaphragm leaving you feeling breathless. In rare cases, the stomach gets overstretched and tears: If you feel severe abdominal pain while bingeing you've got to stop and go to the emergency room—a ruptured stomach can be fatal.

Over the long haul, binge-eating disorder can make you fat; not just because of the binges but because people typically overeat in between. And, in turn, being overweight increases your risk for getting all the medical conditions listed in Chapter 1, such as heart disease, cancer, and diabetes.

Bulimia nervosa (bulimia)

Bulimia and binge-eating disorder share the same out-of-control binges, but from there, bulimia parts company in three important ways:

1. Bulimic binges are followed by purging (vomiting or laxatives) and/or excessive exercise.

2. Instead of being overweight, many with bulimia remain at a normal body weight.

3. Dieting strictly between episodes of bingeing and purging is common.

Eventually, half of those with anorexia (defined later in the chapter) develop bulimia. Bulimia typically begins in adolescence, but shame can prevent women from seeking help until they reach their 30s or 40s. By this time this deeply ingrained eating habit is difficult to treat.

Official definition

Here's the official definition adapted from the American Psychiatric Association's Diagnostic and

Statistical Manual of Mental Disorders (remember, you could still have a serious eating disorder even if you don't make the entire checklist):

- Recurrent episodes of binge eating. An episode of binge eating is characterized by both of the following:

  1. Eating, in a discrete period of time (that is, within any two-hour period), an amount of food that is definitely larger than most people would eat under the same period of time and in similar circumstances.

  2. A sense of lack of control over eating during the episode (that is, a feeling that one cannot stop eating or control what or how much one is eating).

- Recurrent inappropriate compensatory behavior in order to prevent weight gain, such as self-induced vomiting, misuse of laxatives, diuretics, enemas, or other medications; fasting; or excessive exercise.

- The binge eating and inappropriate compensatory behaviors both occur, on average, at least twice a week for three months.

- Self-evaluation is unduly influenced by body shape and weight.

- The disturbance does not occur exclusively during episodes of anorexia nervosa.

This definition of bulimia is broken down into two types: (1) "Purging": regularly vomiting or misusing laxatives, diuretics, or enemas. (2) "Nonpurging": fasting or excessively exercising.

A key element in bulimia is that feeling of being out of control, of being swept up by the binge and

Unofficially . . .
Columbia University researchers found that women with bulimia eat 81.5 calories per minute compared to the 38.4 calories per minute speed of women without eating disorders.

unable to walk away before finishing the box of cookies or the quart of ice cream. (One of my patients told me that she once ate a pound of raw bacon, unable to wait long enough to cook it.) But while they last, binges can induce a temporary high, or at least make a person feel better than the depressed, distressed, or anxious state that typically precedes—and triggers—the binge. That's why the condition is so self-perpetuating; the source of relief from stress is the disease itself, which becomes psychologically addicting. Purging isn't just a guard against what's called "a morbid fear of becoming fat"; it also relieves the incredible discomfort you feel from downing thousands of calories. Binges can reach up to 30 times the normal calorie level for a day—20,000-plus calories—stretching stomachs to the max.

What it does to you

As you can imagine, bingeing, vomiting, and laxative abuse can have some pretty unpleasant side effects. While some are very serious, bulimia, unlike anorexia, is rarely fatal.

- **Effects of stomach acid in vomit.** Over the years it wears down tooth enamel, sometimes to the point of exposing nerves of the teeth, so that teeth must be pulled. Also the acid can inflame the esophagus and burn the part of the hand used to induce vomiting.

- **Electrolyte abnormalities.** The body maintains a certain level of electrolytes—sodium and potassium—for proper nerve and muscle function, including heart beat. Vomiting and laxatives cause dehydration and electrolyte loss; over 50 percent of bulimic patients have electrolyte abnormalities. This can cause abnormal heart rhythms and low blood pressure, and it may damage heart valves.

- **Swollen glands.** For reasons that are not completely clear, the salivary glands swell up, giving a chipmunk appearance. It's probably due to over stimulation of the glands from the vomiting.

- **Gastrointestinal complications.** When you use lots of laxatives, the intestines "forget" how to work, and constipation results. A more serious, potentially fatal GI complication is a ruptured stomach. A possible cause: A person is unable to vomit after a particularly large binge because of pressure changes in the gut.

- **Depression.** About half of those with bulimia are also depressed. As for which came first, the depression or the bulimia, research indicates that the bulimia drives the depression more than the other way around.

- **Petichae.** Broken capillaries around the eyes from the pressure induced during vomiting.

- **Glycemic disturbances.** Caused by changing levels of blood sugar and the hormone insulin.

Anorexia nervosa (anorexia)

It's the most serious of eating disorders because you are, literally, starving yourself. The intense preoccupation with body weight and shape and relentless pursuit of thinness wreaks physical and mental havoc. The two most risky times of life to develop it are puberty and around college time when leaving home for the first time.

About 1 percent of young women have anorexia. The disease has been around long before Twiggy.

Watch Out!
Don't be fooled
into thinking
that taking birth
control pills
can ward off
anorexia-induced
osteoporosis.
Studies show
that while the
pills may improve
bone density in
some cases, in
general, they
don't prevent
osteoporosis.

One of the first reliable medical reports of anorexia dates back to a 1698 medical textbook describing an 18-year-old girl who stopped getting her period due to "a multitude of cares and passions of her mind." And the 16-year-old boy who "fell gradually into a total want of appetite, occasioned by his studying too hard and the passions of the mind." Sporadic reports of the disorder appeared in the medical literature over the ensuing centuries, but it wasn't until this century that the disease was thoroughly defined.

As I mentioned with the binge-related disorders, you may still have a life-threatening eating disorder even if you don't tick off every point in the official definitions. For instance, if you meet all the criteria spelled out in the following section for anorexia, except you still get your period, most eating disorder specialists would still say you fit the bill.

Official definition

Here's the full-blown syndrome (as adapted from the American Psychiatric Association's Diagnostic and Statistical Manual of Mental Disorders):

A. Refusal to maintain body weight at or above a minimally normal weight for age and height (e.g., weight loss leading to maintenance of body weight less than 85 percent of that expected, or failure to make expected weight gain during period of growth, leading to body weight less than 85 percent of that expected).

B. Intense fear of gaining weight or becoming fat, even though underweight.

C. Disturbance in the way in which one's body weight or shape is experienced, undue influence of body weight or shape on self-evaluation, or denial of the seriousness of the current low body weight.

D. In postmenarchal females, amenorrhea, i.e., the absence of at least three consecutive menstrual cycles. (A woman is considered to have amenorrhea if her periods occur only following hormone, e.g., estrogen, administration.)

The definition is further divided into two types: "Restricting," in which the person simply limits food, but doesn't binge and purge (or misuse laxatives, diuretics, or enemas to get rid of the food) or "Binge-Eating/Purging," which is as it sounds. About 50 percent of people with anorexia binge.

What it does to you

▪ **Heart damage.** Your heart and other organs and muscles need a particular balance of electrolytes—sodium and potassium—to function properly. The disordered eating patterns create electrolyte imbalances and other nutrient imbalances that slow heart beat and shrink the heart muscle. The heart condition can lead to sudden death.

▪ **Brain damage.** Starved of nutrients, brain cells eventually die. For instance, brain cells need fat. Fat is an integral part of the protective coating of each brain cell, and healthy nerve coatings are essential for the flow of communication between nerves. Typically, those with anorexia are on extremely low-fat diets; years of this can cause permanent damage to brain cells.

▪ **Halts menstruation (amenorrhea).** Body fat is critical for sex hormone production, and when body fat gets too low, women don't produce enough estrogen and other hormones to have menstrual cycles. Men with anorexia lose sexual interest. If anorexia hits before puberty, it delays it, and girls don't develop breasts or menstruate. After puberty, the low hormone levels can prevent pregnancy and damage the fetus if the anorexia persists during pregnancy.

- **Osteoporosis.** This bone-thinning disease is one of the more devastating and irreversible side effects of anorexia. Osteoporosis is usually a disease of aging, where bones become thin and brittle and break easily, and victims may become wheelchair-bound. It strikes mainly women, although men get it. It hits women after menopause, when estrogen levels dwindle; estrogen helps build and maintain bone. Anorexia creates a premature low estrogen state. Also, high levels of the stress hormone cortisol present in anorexia contribute to bone erosion.

- **Gastrointestinal complications.** Fasting and laxative use both cause constipation. Although rare, bingeing can rupture the stomach, which can be fatal.

- **Suicide.** This disease is just as tough on you psychologically as physically. Of all the psychiatric illnesses, anorexia nervosa has the highest death rate and the highest suicide rate. Suicide is one of the most common causes of death from eating disorders.

Getting help

Unfortunately, there's still lots of shame attached to psychological disorders, which prevents people from going in and getting help. But remember, the sooner you get treatment, the better your chances for complete recovery. Early treatment is especially critical in the case of anorexia.

The basics

Treatments vary according to the disorder and its severity. But there are some common procedures and players involved. First is a complete physical exam by a medical doctor, usually an internist. This rules out any other illness and lets you know how serious a toll the eating disorder has taken on your body. Usually, the doctor recommends outpatient treatment, but if you're in grave medical condition hospitalization will be recommended. The doctor should ask about (and if not, you should volunteer):

1. Your menstrual history, because amenorrhea (the absence of menstrual periods) is a symptom of anorexia.

2. Techniques used to control weight, such as dieting, bingeing, vomiting, laxative abuse, diuretic use, diet pills, emetics (drugs that induce vomiting), diet pills or other appetite suppressants, chewing and spitting out food before swallowing, fasting, and excessive exercise.

Then there is psychological or psychiatric evaluation and counseling and treatment. What's critical here is that the psychiatrist or psychologist is trained and experienced in treating eating disorders. The particular psychological approach isn't as important as how good the therapist is. The most popular treatment approach, and one with some decent research behind it, is "cognitive-behavioral therapy." The theory behind this therapy is that the eating disorder is fueled by a set of beliefs and characteristics such as self-worth hinging upon your shape and weight, low self-esteem, and perfectionism. These ways of thinking lead to fear of fatness and strict control over what goes into your stomach. When that tight control snaps, bingeing follows; the binges are the extreme reaction to starving or going "off" the diet. In typical all-or-nothing thinking of eating disorders, having one slice of cake means "I'm bad, I'm weak," which spirals into an "I've blown it so I might as well go all the way" binge.

Since there are so many ways of conducting therapy, I can't tell you how yours will or should go, or even what approach is most constructive. If it's cognitive-behavioral therapy, you'll typically go through these stages:

1. Regaining control over eating and establishing regular meal patterns.

2. Addressing the fear of fatness, perfectionism, and other ways of thinking that got you into the disorder in the first place.

3. Exploring background issues that contribute to the eating disorder.

4. Working on maintaining the new ways of thinking and eating, with an emphasis on preventing relapse.

On your first visit, you may fill out one of the standardized written tests that will give you and the therapist a sense of the severity of the disorder. One of these is the Eating Attitudes Test, presented earlier in the chapter.

Then you should go for weekly sessions of one-on-one counseling, perhaps bolstered with group therapy.

Nutrition counseling is also important. Seeing a nutritionist will do more than straighten out your diet, it will help straighten out your head. You see,

---

I Feel Fat

"My patients always tell me they're afraid of getting fat, or that they 'feel' fat," says Adrian Brown, MD, a Washington, D.C.–based psychiatrist specializing in eating disorders. When she asks them what "fat" means, they get quite befuddled. "You know, *fat*, I know it when I see it," they finally respond.

Brown will probe further, "Does one more pound make you fat?"

"No,"

"Five pounds?"

"Yes."

"At five more pounds are you really fat?" questions Brown.

"Well, I'll *feel* fat," they typically respond.

Brown wants her patients to understand the difference between feeling fat and being fat. "Fat isn't a feeling," she reminds them. But anger at your controlling father, or anxiety about going away to college, now those are feelings. "Feelings like anger and fear catch hold of their underlying anxiety about their weight and fuel it," she says. "When you address the feelings, they are able to look at the weight issue more realistically."

---

eating disorders, especially anorexia and bulimia, essentially cause malnutrition. And that malnutrition can, literally, prevent you from thinking straight, making you too irritable and distracted to get much out of your psychotherapy.

A registered dietitian (RD) who specializes in eating disorders is always the safest bet in terms of a

Watch Out!
A 1998 national survey by the Calorie Control Council found that 41 percent of dieters say that one reason their diets fail is because they often binge on their favorite foods.

solid nutrition background, but more important than the RD after the name is the experience in eating disorders. Given the choice between an RD with no eating disorders experience and another type of health professional seasoned in treating eating disorders (such as a registered nurse (RN) or a nutritionist who doesn't have an RD), I'd opt for the veteran.

A nutritionist should help normalize your diet and, in the case of adolescents, make sure the diet is adequate for growth. Hand-in-hand with promoting a normal diet he or she (they're usually shes) should help bring you back to a normal way of eating and thinking about food and help you get back in touch with hunger and fullness cues. As with psychotherapy, there are many different approaches that are effective, so I can't tell you how your nutritionist should go about achieving these goals. That said, there are two tools that a good nutritionist should use: a diet history and a food (or diet) record (or diary). In the diet history you tell the nutritionist your eating patterns and body weight fluctuations dating back to childhood. Over the course of the treatment, you should keep a food record of everything you eat, when you eat it, and how you were feeling at the time.

Medication is also an option. Clinicians got the idea of using drugs to treat eating disorders when they noticed that people with eating disorders share many symptoms of other psychological disorders—such as depression or anxiety—that respond well to medication. Drugs aren't always prescribed, but they can be very useful in some cases. "Drugs are no substitute for psychotherapy, but in some cases they can be very helpful at the beginning of treatment," says psychiatrist Adrian Brown. "They can help get symptoms under control quickly while you work on the underlying issues," she explains. In general, the research shows that medications work much better on bulimia than anorexia.

Make sure you're getting your prescription from a psychiatrist versed in prescribing and monitoring antidepressants or else a psychopharmacologist (someone trained at dispensing antidepressants or other "psychoactive" medications). Psychologists aren't permitted to prescribe drugs but can work collaboratively with a psychopharmacologist.

Finding treatment

Check local hospitals or university medical centers for an eating disorders clinic. These organizations can help you find a treatment program and will send you information on eating disorders:

The National Eating Disorders Organization (NEDO)
6655 South Yale Avenue
Tulsa, OK 74136
(918) 481-4044
website: www.laureate.com

An education, prevention, and treatment resource center. Can provide information on what to look for in a good program. Helps guide you through possible treatment options in your local area as well as nationally.

National Association of Anorexia Nervosa and Associated Disorders (ANAD)
Box 7
Highland Park, IL 60035
(847) 831-3438
(847) 433-4832 (fax)
e-mail: anad20@aol.com

66

I have a demon inside of me, dancing on my soul. It feeds on my insecurity and shame . . . hungry for a fight . . . I try to wish him away, I try to eat him away, I try purging him out . . . From the play *Body Loathing . . . Body Love,* by Jessica Weiner (see ACT-Out Ensemble under "Finding treatment" for more info).

99

A nonprofit educational and self-help organization "dedicated to alleviating eating disorders." The group provides counseling, doctor and treatment facility referrals, and sponsors self-help groups with chapters in 46 states and 15 foreign countries.

American Anorexia Bulimia Association, Inc. (AABA)
165 West 46th Street, Suite 1108
New York, NY 10036
(212) 575-6200
(212) 278-0698 (fax)
e-mail: AmAnBu@aol.com
website: members.aol.com/amanbu

A nonprofit organization dedicated to preventing eating disorders through advocacy, research, and as a resource for those with eating disorders and their families. They give referrals for doctors and treatment facilities.

Eating Disorder Awareness and Prevention
603 Stewart Street, Suite 803
Seattle, WA 98101
(206) 382-3587
website: members.aol.com/edapinc

A nonprofit information clearinghouse that provides educational resources on eating disorders and their prevention for schools, health professionals, community organizations, and individuals. The organization sponsors several specific educational eating disorders programs and activities, including Eating Disorders Awareness Week (EDAW) and a Puppet Project for Schools.

The ACT-Out Ensemble

Not a support group in the traditional sense, the ACT-Out Ensemble offers support through theater performance. Sponsored by Indiana University and Purdue University, the group travels the country performing *Body Loathing . . . Body Love,* by Jessica Weiner, a collection of powerful monologues and dialogues that tell stories of eating disorders. The performances are followed by an audience participation discussion led by Weiner (a recovered exercise bulimic) accompanied by a local eating disorders professional. You can book the group in your church, theater, community center, corporation, or other space by calling Jessica Weiner or L.E. McCullough at (317) 278-2530. Or write to: Jessica Weiner, 401 East Michigan Street, Indianapolis, IN 46204.

Binge-eating disorder treatment specifics

In addition to the general info on treatment outlined in the preceding section, here are some particulars for those of you with binge-eating disorder. Whatever the treatment, you know it's working if you're bingeing less often and finally stop bingeing altogether. You know the treatment *worked* if you remain binge-free.

- **Psychotherapy.** Besides the cognitive-behavioral approach, other forms of therapy may be useful, including self-help groups such as Overeaters Anonymous.

- **Nutrition.** Along with a psychotherapist, a nutritionist may come in handy to help you get the diet part on track and lose some weight.

- **Medication.** In some cases, medication, most often antidepressants, are helpful. "Antidepressants can help if the person is also

Bright Idea
Overcoming Binge Eating, by Dr. Christopher Fairburn (Guilford Press, 1995) is a must for anyone who binges. The book helps you understand your problem and offers a step-by-step treatment program. Fairburn is a leading researcher in the eating disorders field.

depressed, but sometimes they have an anti-binge effect even with non-depressed patients," observes University of Pittsburgh's Marsha Marcus. But drugs are no panacea; sometimes they stop working after a while. However, as the research into this disorder evolves, more effective drug treatment may emerge.

Bulimia treatment specifics

Count on all your treatment to be outpatient unless the condition has gotten really out of hand and you're at medical risk; at that point you may have to be hospitalized. In addition to the general treatment information in the preceding section, here are some things to keep in mind:

Psychotherapy. So far, the research favors cognitive-behavioral therapy. According to Fairburn, cognitive-behavioral therapy reduces episodes of bingeing and purging by 70 percent, and a third to half of patients stop bingeing altogether. You should be in treatment at least four to five months, going once or twice a week. Studies that track patients six months to six years post-treatment show that the changes made from this therapy really stick.

Although much more research has been done on the effectiveness of psychodynamic and family therapy in anorexia than bulimia, the preliminary studies show these approaches (described later under "Anorexia treatment specifics") and group therapy may also be useful in bulimia.

Another type of therapy that has proven successful is interpersonal therapy. Interestingly, this works entirely opposite to cognitive-behavioral therapy (CBT); instead of focusing on the eating disorder, this therapy ignores it completely. You and the therapist discuss nothing of food, weight, diet, but speak exclusively about your relationships or lack of relationships. This is an option to consider if CBT isn't working.

Antidepressant medication. Research into a variety of types of antidepressants shows that the drugs reduce the frequency of binges, improve mood, and reduce the preoccupation with body shape and weight. Interestingly, the antidepressants aren't necessarily alleviating depression. "An equal number of depressed and non-depressed people with bulimia are helped by the drugs, so it's not depression that's being targeted," says Adrian Brown. It may be appetite suppression and increased levels of serotonin that are helping suppress symptoms, she speculates.

But antidepressants are no panacea. There's no evidence that the benefits from the drugs are sustained after you stop taking them. So, psychotherapy is still the mainstay of therapy, with or without drugs. And for non-depressed people with bulimia, the general recommendation is to try psychotherapy first; if it isn't working, then it may be appropriate to combine the therapy with medication.

Anorexia treatment specifics

Since anorexia is a more stubborn condition, and more life-threatening, the treatment is more intense and takes longer—it may take years of weekly psychological counseling sessions—than therapy for bulimia or binge-eating disorder. Getting your weight back up is critical to treatment. The "anorexia paradox" is that patients want to feel better without doing the one thing that will do it: getting back up to a safe weight. There are no dependable statistics on recovery rates, but, according to Oxford University's Christopher Fairburn, "All that can be reasonably said is that the majority of patients with

Timesaver
After you end your eating disorder treatment program, be vigilant against relapse. As soon as you start slipping back (that is, losing weight if you're recovering from anorexia, or bingeing if you're recovering from bulimia or binge-eating disorder) do something about it. Do the lapse recovery techniques you learned in therapy or go back and talk to your therapist. Don't hope it goes away . . . act quickly.

Moneysaver
If you're enrolled in college, see whether the student health services offers eating disorder treatment. The counselors may be well qualified and treatment cost may be paid for by the school.

anorexia nervosa recover although it may take some years." However, be warned: The longer you have it, the harder it is to treat and recover from.

Psychotherapy. While cognitive-behavioral therapy (CBT) seems to be the approach of choice in treating anorexia, other forms of psychotherapy may work just as well as long as you're in the hands of an experienced and competent therapist specializing in eating disorders. While CBT has proven to work for bulimia, the research is muddier for anorexia, with no one form of therapy clearly superior to the others. However, until better research paints a clearer picture, it's generally assumed that CBT is best. In addition to changing the beliefs that cause and drive the anorexia, therapy also involves getting the patient to understand that starvation is the cause of the unpleasant side effects such as irritability, lack of concentration, preoccupation with food, and depression.

Two other forms of therapy are considered useful in treating anorexia: psychodynamic therapy and family therapy. Psychodynamic therapy focuses less on normalizing eating behavior and more on psychologically understanding and strengthening the patient in other ways (which, hopefully, will ultimately fix the eating disorder). In family therapy the patient either comes in with her parents or other close family members, or the same therapist sees the patient and family members separately.

Nutrition. It's critical that you start eating more food right away because in the malnourished anorexic state, you're in no condition to process what's happening in therapy. The goal is to normalize your eating patterns and to move up to a healthy weight. The dietitian will help reintroduce high-calorie "forbidden" foods you've crossed off your list.

Hospitalization for anorexia

While anorexia is always dangerous, some cases are so immediately life-threatening that doctors want their patients checked into a hospital. The hospital should have a team that includes doctors, psychologists, nurses, and nutritionists trained and experienced at handling the disease. According to Manfred M. Fichter writing in *Eating Disorders and Obesity* (Brownell and Fairburn, The Guilford Press, 1995), hospitalization is warranted when:

- Medical complications arise such as anemia, stomach rupturing or bleeding (from bingeing), fainting, and blood electrolyte (sodium and potassium) imbalances, which can cause heart problems.

- The patient is suicidal.

- The outpatient treatment isn't working, or there is a temporary crisis.

- There isn't a decent outpatient option in the area.

- The patient persists in fasting and bingeing; sometimes the hospital environment disrupts the patient's patterns.

- The patient needs to be separated from his or her family either to provide a break when he or she feels overburdened and stressed, or when the family or partner is threatening the patient's well-being.

- A patient in denial needs to be confronted.

Medication

The hope that medications could help speed up weight gain in anorexia by improving mood and/or appetite didn't pan out in the research. One reason

Bright Idea
To find eating disorder specialists (psychotherapists, nutritionists, MDs, and treatment centers) call ANAD at (847) 831-3438 or NEDO at (918) 481-4044 (more on these organizations under "Finding treatment," in the preceding section).

that those with anorexia don't respond to psychoactive drugs as might be predicted is that the malnutrition has altered the way their brain cells respond to drugs. With anorexia, drugs seem to be most useful *after* weight restoration, in the relapse prevention period. Studies are now underway evaluating a class of antidepressants called serotonin reuptake inhibitors, which increase the amount of the brain chemical serotonin, linked to improved mood and appetite.

What causes eating disorders?

Like obesity, eating disorders seem to spring from a mixture of genetics, biochemistry, and environment. The environmental aspect is pretty clear: Twiggy, Kate Moss, and every fashion ad you've ever seen. But most women who are not thin don't have eating disorders (at least not full-blown ones). That's where the genes and biochemistry kick in. Some experts believe that eating disorders are just a late-20th-century way of expressing a mental illness that manifested itself in other ways in other eras— what fainting was for Victorians, for example. In this schema, psychological and physiological disturbances are being played out in a fairly culturally acceptable way: being thin.

The impossible ideal

As the fashion model aesthetic ideal (5'7" or taller and around 100 pounds) spreads throughout the world, so do eating disorders. Argentina is experiencing an anorexia epidemic, with hospitals full of young girls. (The country is also plastic surgery happy, an obvious tie-in.) The scientific literature documents cases of young women from countries where plumpness-is-prettier, such as Arab countries, who develop eating disorders when they immigrate to thin-is-in industrialized countries like England.

Being slender has come to symbolizes success, competence, willpower, and sexual attractiveness. So it's almost your duty as a good citizen to try and achieve the ideal figure. The media/advertising complex relentlessly drives this message home, convincing us that if we only used the right cosmetics, the right diet, the right plastic surgery, we could mold ourselves into this ideal. And if we can't (and very few people are genetically capable; that's why there are only a handful of supermodels—genetic mutations—in the world) then the inescapable message is that we're failures. But we can fight that message; see the advice on accepting less-than-skinny in Chapter 9.

And, by the way, the sexual attractiveness part is way overblown, according to a now-classic study performed at the University of Pennsylvania. Male and female undergrads were shown the drawings in Figure 12.1 and asked to pick body types in their own sex that they considered a) ideal, b) attractive to the opposite sex, and c) close to their own shape. In addition, they were asked to pick a body type of the opposite sex that they found most attractive. As you can see in Figure 12.1, women guessed wrong (skinnier) about the female figure most attractive to men. And their ideal female form was quite a bit thinner than the average female participating in the study. Interestingly, women's and men's choices for the ideal male figure and the figure of the average man participating in the research were very close. No wonder men don't get anorexia or bulimia! All right they do, but at a minuscule rate compared to women.

Figure 12.1
Mean ratings by
women (top) and
men (bottom) of
current figure,
ideal figure, and
figure most
attractive to the
opposite sex;
mean ratings by
men of the
female figure
they find most
attractive (top,
labeled "other
attractive") and
equivalent mean
ratings by
women on the
bottom.
*Adapted from
"Use of the
Danish Adoption
Register for the
Study of Obesity
and Thinness"
by A. Stunkard,
T. Sorensen, and
F. Schulsinger,
in* The Genetics
of Neurological
and Psychiatric
Disorders, *edited
by S. Kety, 1980,
p. 119. Used with
permission.*

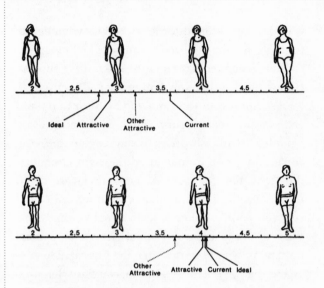

Psychological links

Eating disorders run in families; it's unclear how much blame goes to genes or biochemistry and how much to the harsh societal standard for thinness being reinforced at home. Mommy's constant dieting or her obsession about her little girl's weight and appearance or critical remarks from daddy and brother about her weight have—no surprise—been linked to an increased risk for developing eating disorders.

Or it could be, that like so many psychological diseases, eating disorders are rooted in genetically passed down altered brain chemistry because people with eating disorders do have altered chemistry. Some of the chemical imbalances are caused by the disease itself; for instance, malnutrition starves your brain of the necessary materials to build the brain chemicals. Weight loss, semi-starvation, and bizarre diet patterns can cause poor concentration, depression, obsessive thinking, irritability, and impulsiveness even in "normal" people.

But in people with eating disorders, the seeds of the disease exist beforehand. People with eating disorders commonly have many of the following traits:

1. feelings of ineffectiveness
2. low self-esteem
3. lack of autonomy
4. obsessiveness
5. introversion
6. poor relationship skills
7. social anxiety
8. dependence
9. perfectionism
10. poor impulse control
11. conflict avoidance
12. vulnerability to substance abuse

These people are more likely to be in psychological pain. They also have a higher lifetime rate of psychiatric disorders including anxiety and mood and personality disorders. Depression affects about half of those with eating disorders; the research indicates with anorexia, the eating disorder brings on the depression, while with bulimia, it's more likely that the person was depressed beforehand. And obese binge eaters have more psychological dysfunction and symptoms, such as depression, than obese non-binge eaters. One study found that binge eaters are about 13 times as likely to have a history of major depression. Bingeing gets worse during times of depression, and depressed binge eaters have more severe bingeing than binge eaters who are not depressed. Many bulimics also struggle with alcohol and drug addiction and compulsive

> At 100 pounds, ballerina Gelsey Kirkland was still not thin enough for famed choreographer George Ballanchine, who thumped on her chestbones and said, "Must see the bones. Eat nothing."

Unofficially . . .
Eating disorders
afflict eight mil-
lion Americans.
That's 5 percent
of adolescent
and adult women
(15 percent of
women have
some form of
disordered eating
even if it's not a
full-blown eating
disorder) and
1 percent of
men. One thou-
sand women die
each year from
anorexia.

stealing. Bingeing, starving, or vomiting, though painful, may be a way to block out feelings that are even more painful. Bingeing may be a way of coping with anxiety, depression, or other problems; that "binge high" temporarily blocks out the pain.

While sexual abuse is not necessarily a cause of eating disorders, the research indicates that more people with eating disorders have sexual abuse in their backgrounds than those without eating disorders, especially in cases of bulimia. That abuse can cause low self-esteem and intense shame. "Women recovering from sexual abuse use food to build a barrier against their shame and memory. This can take the form of compulsive eating and bingeing," says playwright Jessica Weiner.

Sufferers of anorexia are often described as "perfect" children, compliant and helpful. For many the emotional problems arise from separation anxiety and difficulty with identity and with sexual maturation. During puberty, starving is a way of halting or staving off sexual maturation: Without body fat, breasts stop growing, and the menstrual cycle shuts down.

Who gets eating disorders?

Eating disorders are mainly a disease of affluent societies that ascribe to the thin beauty aesthetic. It used to be thought that only upper-middle-class white girls got eating disorders because they were the ones who showed up in hospitals where researchers collect their data. But studies that look beyond the patient population find that all of the socioeconomic rungs are affected. The research now suggests that binge eating is just as common in blacks as whites.

About 90 percent of those with anorexia and bulimia are adolescent girls and young women. The particularly hard hit professions are fashion models and dancers (big surprise!) as well as certain athletes such as skaters and gymnasts. Hard to tell which came first, whether the proclivity to being anorexic attracts people to some of these professions, or if the professions drive the disease. And while anorexia and bulimia are overwhelmingly women's disorders, about a quarter to a third of those with binge-eating disorder are men.

Did your diet make you do it?

Most eating disorders start with a diet. While dieting won't cause an eating disorder in most people, it can be the trigger in susceptible individuals, either because of their biochemistry, psychological history, or any of the traits mentioned earlier. For instance, obsessive-compulsive tendencies common in those with anorexia mean they will become very "good" dieters, taking dieting to its ultimate extreme. Being able to control her hunger may be an empowering thrill for a young woman with low self-esteem, a sense of being ineffective, and fears of maturity.

Dieting is considered a major culprit in binge-eating. The common chain of events goes like this: overeating from an early age, dieting in response, then bingeing in response to the deprivation induced by dieting. In that case, the overeating since childhood could be psychological or could be genetically induced. The genetic/biological explanation goes like this: People who are genetically inclined to be overweight fight it by dieting, which in turn makes them hungry, preoccupied with food, and feel like failures if they don't achieve a usually

66

Dieters tend to think along narrow lines—what they ate and didn't eat—and minimize other things. An A on a term paper may make them happier for a minute, then the next thought is 'but I overate.' You've got to think about your strengths and accomplishments—write a strength on a sticker, put it in a very visible place around your house and look at it.
—Edward Abramson, Ph.D., professor at California State University at Chico and author of *Emotional Eating* (Jossey-Bass, 1998).

99

Success Story: "Melinda"

My friend Melinda (fake name, real person, real story) bowls you over with her personality, energy, wit, and beauty. A dancer and choreographer, it's a pleasure just to watch her walk across a room. But 16 years ago she couldn't even make if up the stairs; at 5'9" and 85 pounds, she finally collapsed from her anorexia and was hospitalized.

Her story is classic: Put in ballet schools from age nine, "I was always in front of a mirror, dancing, looking at my body, striving for perfection," she recounts. "At puberty, I watched other girls getting breasts and hips; it was my worst nightmare." Always careful about what she ate, she gradually ate less and less and at age 14, "I just stopped eating. My stomach shrank to the point where I'd feel absolutely stuffed on a cup of tea and a tomato." If she did eat a meal, she'd throw it up.

"It's a real feeling of empowerment; you have complete control over your body. I enjoyed the hunger because it made me feel powerful; I'd conquered it," she says. While it was a thrill to hear that she was too thin, she also didn't believe it. "I was brainwashed into thinking I'm fat, so I just didn't believe them. I thought they were just saying it because they were jealous and wanted me to be fat."

Over the next year or so she got progressively weaker, her muscles withered to the point where she had to stop dancing, and her "mind shut down." She doesn't even remember her collapse, hospitalization, and the weeks following. "I remember when I started gaining back the weight. It's easy to get anorexic; what's hard is relearning how to eat. The worst thing was putting on weight. I tried not to look at myself in the mirror, if I did I'd cry."

"I didn't feel better for years and years. The recovery is hard." Although she never slipped back into anorexia, Melinda admits, "I still don't have a normal relationship with food; food is frightening. I still feel fat." (She's very slender—a size 2, maybe 4). "What I've done is learn to live with my irrationality and to cultivate the rational part of me that understands I'm not fat while the irrational part always thinks I am." Her most helpful aid: the scale. "The scale is the truth. If I eat a big dinner, or think I'm fat, I run upstairs and weigh myself and see I'm still okay." (She stays at 120 plus or minus three pounds.)

Melinda's recommendation for those who are in the throws of an eating disorder: Get involved in something that will take your mind off it, something outside yourself. For her it was dance (although double-edged, because dance contributed to the disorder). "And don't expect the recovery to be easy, it takes years. But you'll learn so much about yourself, about obsessive behavior, about control."

impossible goal weight, so they give up and binge. Supporting that theory is that many with binge-eating disorder were overweight as children.

I'm not going to tell you getting out of an eating disorder is easy. As you can see from Melinda's story, which follows, your relationship to food may always be an uneasy one. The earlier you get help the better your chances for a complete recovery. If you're still in the clear, remember that restrictive diets are eating disorder catalysts, the non-depriving way of eating recommended in this book is a safer bet.

Just the facts

- Just because your eating disorder doesn't meet all the official criteria doesn't mean you don't have a serious illness.

- Overweight people can have eating disorders; a typical one is binge-eating disorder, which can be treated with therapy and drugs.

- Research shows bulimia can be successfully treated with a few different types of psychotherapy and medications.

- Anorexia is the most serious and life-threatening disorder, requiring long-term therapy.

- Treatment approaches may vary; what's key to treatment is that the clinician is seasoned at treating eating disorders.

- The roots of eating disorders go further than fashion model emulation, reaching into underlying biochemical, social, and genetic causes.

Get Moving

GET THE SCOOP ON...
Exercise and weight loss ▪ Exercise and
better health ▪ Exercise nutrition ▪
Making a good fitness fit

PART V

Chapter 13

You've Got to Keep Moving

The thing about exercise, guys, is that it's always better than you think. In fact, once you get into it—even just daily walks—you'll start feeling deprived if you *can't* exercise. While even exercise addicts have those drag-themselves-to-the-gym days, for the most part exercise is fun once you've made a good exercise match. And boy, will you feel good—good like you haven't felt since you were a teen. That every-cell-alive feeling, that doubling of energy, that pride when you look at the new curve of your arm, that relief when you're older and you still have your balance, your bone mass, and the strength to carry in the groceries.

If you haven't been in a pair of shorts in a decade or so, the idea of exercising may seem as remote as permanent weight loss. And maybe that's why: It really does take exercise to keep the weight off. Maybe not to lose the initial pounds, but zillions of studies keep showing that you gotta move to maintain that loss. In the past two decades of the great

American Weight Gain, where we jumped from 25 percent to 33 percent obesity, our calorie intake didn't go up that much. So it's got to be that we've slacked off on the other side of the equation.

In my interviews for the preceding chapters, I tried to get the experts focused on diet, but before long they were talking exercise. "We're not working it off. People used to eat 3,000 calories a day and lose weight. We sit in front of the TV, put wheels on luggage, and don't require PE in most public schools," complains David Kritchevsky, Ph.D., Professor at the Wistar Institute in Philadelphia and professor emeritus in biochemistry at the University of Pennsylvania. "I ascribe to the GOYA principle: Get Off Your Ass," he says bluntly.

Next chapter gets into the how-to of exercise. This one will make you an offer you (hopefully) can't refuse: exercise and shed more body fat to increase your life span and reduce your chance of getting the diseases that bring down most Americans.

At the end of the day, or at the end of the weight loss, one motivator that propels people through a lifetime of weight maintenance is doing it for themselves: to nurture their bodies and to feel good. Not to get into a bikini in two months or because their boss tells them to shape up. That's why I'm diverting from the subject of weight loss for much of this chapter; I want to give you reasons to exercise that go beyond your clothing size.

Outside beauty

Fat or thin, you'll look better if you exercise. And soon you start looking better—even before you lose the weight. And I'm not just talking rosy glow; I mean your butt, your torso, your arms, your thighs, the whole thing. I watch the overweight men and women in the exercise studio I go to—the ones who've been at it a few months. They've still got some fat to lose, but their bodies are getting firmer, they carry themselves with grace, they look better in their clothes. Then there's the enhanced weight loss. And, a real shot at the holy grail—weight maintenance.

Exercise and weight loss

Dieters who don't exercise, eat your hearts out. Here are the bonuses you're missing.

- You can double or triple your fat loss. It's true that you'll lose body fat by cutting calories only, but you'll also lose a lot of muscle. Several studies found that about 60 percent of what's shed from people on very-low-calorie diets who were not exercising was muscle and water. But add exercise to the weight loss and you can actually *gain* muscle; so what you're losing is really fat.

- You become a more efficient fat-burner. As your body gets used to the fact that you are regularly exercising, it adapts by burning fat more easily. Think of your body fat as coal. Instead of a few people half-heartedly shoveling coal into a furnace, as you become more fit, you gather legions of coal-shovelers sending more fat, more quickly to fuel your bout on the treadmill, your jog, or your laps at the pool.

- You'll probably be less hungry. Various studies have noted an appetite suppressing effect of exercise. Some reports suggest that exercise specifically reduces your appetite for high-fat foods.

Watch Out!
While exercise normally means getting fitter and healthier, in excess, it can be symptomatic of an eating disorder. Over-exercising to burn calories, in essence, accomplishes the same thing as semi-starvation or purging after a binge. In fact "exercise bulimics" don't vomit, they exercise off their binges.

Moneysaver
Don't waste your money on sports drinks; plain water is just as good for replenishing fluids lost in sweat. Don't be sold by claims that the drink's sodium and sugar helps you absorb fluid faster and replaces electrolytes; eating a meal within three hours of exercising does the same. During very strenuous exercise, athletes may need sugar for a pick-me-up; they can get it cheaper in diluted fruit juice.

■ You'll burn more calories while you're sleeping, sitting, lying down, or doing very light activity. That's because your new, improved muscle mass demands more fuel to nourish and maintain, so you're always burning more calories keeping it happy. You can jack up the amount of calories you burn at rest by 15 percent. That's a lot.

■ And, of course, the obvious: You're burning fat while you exercise. As you'll see in the next chapter, you can burn a heck of a lot of calories doing certain types of exercise.

Will Java Jolt Your Fat Cells?

My friend just called to tell me the latest "fat-burning" prescription from her personal trainer: Arrive at workout in the morning with nothing in her stomach but a caffeine pill. And then no food until two hours after working out. Needless to say she's jittery and irritable at work until she finally gets lunch. And, needless to say, I didn't approve of the skipping breakfast part. But is there something behind this prescription?

Studies have shown that a pre-exercise slug of caffeine (the amount in $2^1/_2$ cups of coffee) raises blood levels of free fatty acids (building blocks of fat) higher than if you exercised without caffeine. This implies that the body is breaking down body fat at a higher rate. Also, studies show that people last longer and work harder at the same exercise after taking caffeine. In one study, getting the equivalent of two cups of coffee helped runners go 15 more minutes before exhaustion; in another, cyclists getting the caffeine equivalent of one cup of coffee were able to last 29 percent longer. It appears that caffeine makes exercise seem easier, so you don't fatigue as quickly.

Whether all this translates into significant fat-burning is debatable. "Yes, caffeine picks up your metabolism a little bit, but in terms of fat-burning, it's fairly inconsequential," says Charles Kuntzleman, Ed.D., an exercise physiologist and Director of the Blue Cross/Blue Shield of Michigan Fitness for Youth program. "A better approach is to do a few extra repetitions and build up muscle mass; that'll also raise metabolic rate," he advises.

Unless caffeine seems to make a real difference for you, I'd avoid it. If you're doing it for energy, remember, somewhere in the middle of your workout, your body's own stimulants kick in, like adrenaline and epinephrine. And while caffeine is a real energizer for some, it leaves others feeling jittery. And after the caffeine high, you're likely to crash, zapping you of the energizing effects of exercise.

So, how much sweat is it going to take to shed that body fat? Sorry, there's no pat prescription: It's very individual, hinging on your metabolic rate (how fast you burn calories) and your calorie intake. Consider this example given in Chapter 3: Let's say your body needs 1,800 calories a day to keep you at your current weight. Eat 1,600, and your body will have to reach into those fat stores for the extra 200 (if you weren't exercising it would be dipping into both the fat and muscle stores for energy). Or, increase your exercise by burning 300 calories a day, and your body's got to dip even further into those fat stores. Now 500 calories of fat are being dragged out of storage. Keep this up and you'll lose about a pound of fat a week (a pound of body fat is 3,500 calories). To find out what 300 calories worth of exercise looks like, check out the "Burn, baby, burn" chart. But remember, each of you has a different metabolic rate, so you may burn more or fewer calories than posted on the chart. Still, the chart provides a good rough guide.

Exercise and weight maintenance

Nothing beats exercise for maintaining your weight loss, confirmed a recent review of 493 studies of weight loss and weight maintenance published over the past 25 years. The review, written by researchers at George Washington University Medical Center, found that in most studies people lost about the same amount of weight on diet alone compared to diet plus exercise, but check back on them a year later and the ones who were exercising kept off more of the weight. (And most certainly, there was lots more body fat in weight lost through the diet/exercise combo.)

Exercise was at the top of the "how I did it" list of the hundreds of successful maintainers in the ongoing National Weight Control Registry study, discussed in Chapters 1 and 11. (The registrants have kept off an average of 66 pound for 5½ years.) Women report getting an average of 2,670 calories' worth of exercise per week; men 3,490. In that study 282 people relied on what is considered "medium intensity" exercise; their top picks were cycling, aerobics, walking or running on a treadmill (sounds high-intensity to me!), and hiking or backpacking.

The reason exercise is so critical to maintaining your weight loss is because it compensates for the more sluggish metabolism you inherit post-pound shedding. As I mentioned in Chapter 11, the more weight you lose, the more your metabolic rate usually falls after weight loss. According to prominent weight loss expert Thomas Wadden, Ph.D., Director of the Weight and Eating Disorders Program at the University of Pennsylvania School of Medicine, "caloric needs probably drop about 10 calories for every pound lost. That means if you lost 40 pounds, you could be burning 400 fewer calories than before you lost the weight." Instead of having to deprive yourself of 400 calories daily (an entire meal!), if you exercise you can burn them off and reap all the health rewards to boot. Although exercise requirements are individual, research suggests that you need about three hours of aerobic exercise per week or 1,500 calories to keep off the weight you lost.

Exercise combats age-related muscle loss

If you've hit your 40s, you know what this is all about: a natural age-related decline in muscle mass, called sarcopenia (from the Greek *sarco* for "flesh" and *penia* for "loss"). Muscle deteriorates by about 5 to 10 percent per decade; from their 20s to their 70s, on average, people lose about 30 percent of their strength and 40 percent of their muscle size. But exercise, particularly strength training, can to a great extent prevent sarcopenia and reverse it once it's begun. So says Miriam Nelson, Ph.D., a Scientist at the Nutrition Research Center on Aging

Unofficially . . .
In a dramatic "it's never too late" story, 10 men and women aged 86 to 96 increased their strength by an average of 175 percent and scored 48 percent higher on tests of walking speed and balance. They did it by lifting weights three times a week for eight weeks as part of a Tufts Center on Aging study.

Bright Idea
If you quit smoking, take up exercise. An ongoing Harvard University study tracking 121,700 women found that over a two-year period, women who quit but didn't change their exercise habits gained five pounds more than those who continued smoking. But quitters who exercised gained only about $2^1/_2$ pounds.

ACSM's 30 Minutes for Health

In a report published in the *Journal of the American Medical Association,* the American College of Sports Medicine (ACSM), a well respected and reputable scientific organization promoting physical activity research and education, made the following points about exercise. Keep in mind our earlier advice, however, that you may need even more exercise to lose weight and maintain your loss.

▪ "Every U.S. adult should accumulate 30 minutes or more of moderate-intensity physical activity over the course of most, preferably all, days of the week." And that's just for overall fitness and health; they're not talking specifically about weight maintenance. The ACSM suggests expending about 200 calories during that 30 minutes, with activities such as walking briskly (see Table 14.1 for calories expended during various exercises).

▪ The more you exercise, the greater the benefits. And, according to the ACSM report, "evidence suggests that amount of activity is more important than the specific manner in which the activity is performed (i.e., mode, intensity, or duration of the activity bouts)."

▪ It doesn't have to be structured exercise: "The recommended 30 minutes of activity can be accumulated in short bouts of activity: walking up stairs instead of taking the elevator, walking instead of driving short distances, doing calisthenics, or peddling a stationary cycle while watching television. Gardening, housework, raking leaves, dancing, and playing actively with children can also contribute to the 30-minute-per-day total if performed at an intensity corresponding to brisk walking. Those who perform lower-intensity activities should do them more often, for longer periods of time, or both."

- The report goes on to say, "People who prefer more formal exercise may choose to walk or participate in more vigorous activities, such as jogging, swimming, or cycling for 30 minutes daily."

(Source: *Journal of the American Medical Association,* January, 1995.)

at Tufts University, and author of *Strong Women Stay Young* and *Strong Women Stay Slim* (Bantam, 1997 and 1998, respectively). Nelson's books (highly recommended) are based on years of research developing exercise programs for post-menopausal women.

Inner beauty

The list of life-extending, disease-preventing aspects of exercise just keeps getting longer. In addition to helping you lose weight and keep it off, there are many more benefits that your body will thank you for.

First, exercise reduces risk of heart disease and stroke. The type of heart disease that exercise helps stave off is the coronary heart disease—clogged and hardened arteries that supply the heart muscle with blood, oxygen, and nutrition. A heart attack occurs when blood can't get to the heart muscle; a stroke is when blood can't flow to the brain (either because of narrowed arteries or because of a clot clogging the way). Coronary heart disease is the primary killer of Americans, causing one in every five deaths. Stroke accounts for one in every $14^1/_2$ deaths and is the leading cause of long-term disability in this country.

People who are physically inactive are up to two-and-a-half times more likely to develop heart disease, according to the American Heart Association. That's about the same degree of risk conferred by high cholesterol, high blood pressure, and cigarette smoking. While exercise can directly strengthen the heart muscle, it's heart disease–preventive effects are largely indirect (most of the same things apply to stroke):

- Lowered blood pressure (high blood pressure is a major contributor to heart disease). Regular exercise lowers both types of blood pressure (systolic and diastolic) by 10 points. On the flip side, being sedentary increases your risk for developing high blood pressure by 30 to 50 percent.

- Increased blood flow to the heart muscle. The body adapts to regular exercise by dilating blood vessels that lead to muscles (including the heart), sending in more blood, oxygen, and nutrients.

- Improved blood fat profile. High levels of the "bad" cholesterol-containing particles (LDL) and another blood fat called triglycerides raise your risk of heart disease. Exercise lowers both these blood fats. At the same time it raises HDL, the "good" cholesterol-containing particles, which send cholesterol out of the body.

- Increased insulin sensitivity (see the "diabetes" discussion later in this chapter). Not only does increased insulin sensitivity lower your risk for developing diabetes, but it lowers your risk for heart disease.

A second benefit of exercise is that it cuts down on your overall risk for cancer. In particular, it seems most protective against cancers of the breast, prostate, and colon—all major killer cancers. Here's what the research shows:

- **Breast cancer.** A few studies have found that physically active women cut their risk of developing breast cancer down to 20 to 42 percent over sedentary women. Although the reasons exercise helps prevent breast cancer are still under investigation, it appears that it cuts back on at least two risk factors: obesity and estrogen. Actually these risk factors are linked because obesity increases levels of circulating estrogen, and estrogen is a breast cancer trigger. Several studies support the overweight/breast cancer link. Those who stayed the slimmest were at lower risk for breast cancer in a Harvard study tracking 95,256 nurses. The more weight gained the riskier; accumulating 44 to 55 pounds after age 18 increased risk by 40 percent. On the estrogen front, exercise may occasionally block ovulation and decrease estrogen output. There is preliminary evidence that other cancers that are triggered by estrogen,

Unofficially . . .
According to the National Heart, Lung and Blood Institute, the average HDL ("good" cholesterol-containing particles, which send cholesterol out of the body) for men is about 45 mg/dL, for women 55 mg/dL. (The mg/dL notation stands for milligrams per deciliter, an efficient way for researchers to measure particles in a given quantity of blood. A deciliter is 1/10 of a liter.) The higher the better; below 35 mg/dL and your risk of heart disease goes up. In general, studies putting people on exercise regimens report a 10 to 20 percent increase in HDL in response to an exercise program.

such as cancer of the ovary, endometrium, cervix, and vagina, are also reduced in physically active women.

▪ **Colon cancer.** Studies show that people who get the most physical activity throughout their lives have the lowest risk of developing colon cancer. These studies indicate that people getting the most exercise have about 60 percent reduced risk of colon cancer compared to sedentary people. Although the reasons aren't clear, one theory is that exercise stimulates intestinal muscles to excrete waste more quickly, decreasing the time cancer-causing substances come in contact with the colon. Also, physical activity strengthens the immune system, which helps fight off cancer.

▪ **Prostate cancer.** Several studies comparing physically active men to sedentary men show that the active men have about half the risk of developing prostate cancer. However, several other studies show no link, so the jury's still out. These studies are difficult to interpret because prostate cancer takes decades to develop, and it's hard to tell at what stage in life the exercise is protective. If the link pans out, researchers speculate that exercise may protect by reducing blood levels of the male hormone testosterone. In a similar way that estrogen promotes breast cancer, testosterone promotes prostate cancer, and several studies show that physically active men have decreased testosterone levels.

In addition to providing the two benefits just discussed, exercise has also been shown to be effective in derailing diabetes. With 10.5 million diagnosed (and perhaps another 5.3 million who don't know they have the disease), we're experiencing a diabetes epidemic, according to Frank Vinicor, MD, MPH, director of the Center for Disease Control's Diabetes Division. About 95 percent of cases are Type II diabetes, the type you develop later on in life, as an adult, and the type that can usually be cured by diet and exercise. Diabetes is the seventh leading cause of death in the U.S.; it also causes blindness, can lead to the amputation of limbs, and is linked to heart disease. Diabetics have out-of-control blood sugar because of malfunctions of the hormone responsible for controlling blood sugar, insulin. Whereas Type I diabetics may not produce insulin at all, Type II diabetics either produce too little of the hormone, or the body doesn't respond to it properly (a condition called "insulin resistance"). While we depend on blood sugar for energy, too much damages organs.

An excess of body fat, particularly belly fat, decreases your body's ability to use insulin, making you insulin resistant. Being overfat also strains the pancreas, an organ that makes insulin, slowing down production of the hormone. "Physical inactivity along with overeating, particularly in persons who may have a genetic predisposition, are the main causes of Type II diabetes," says Vinicor. "So it stands to reason that becoming physically active is perhaps the most important way to prevent or reverse the disease" he advises. Exercise helps the condition directly by removing some glucose from the blood to use for energy during and after exercise, lowering blood glucose levels. Also, it helps reduce the increased risk of heart disease in people with diabetes.

> **"**
> Because physical activity is so directly related to preventing disease and premature death and to maintaining a high quality of life, we must accord it the same level of attention that we give other public health practices that affect the entire nation.
> —Acting Surgeon General Audrey F. Manley
> **"**

But heed this warning: *Always consult with your doctor* before embarking on an exercise regimen. Diabetes may have put you at increased risk for heart disease. In that case you have to work your way into fitness gradually to avoid straining the heart. Also, exercise can send blood sugar too low, especially if you're taking diabetes medication. Again, don't step up your level of physical activity without checking with your physician.

Exercise also counters osteoarthritis. Being overweight places undue stress on knee, spine, and hip joints, wearing away cartilage, the bone-like substance that makes up joints. This worn-down cartilage is osteoarthritis, which ranges in severity from mild stiffness and joint pain to severe pain and disability. As mentioned in Chapter 1, if you're obese, dropping 10 to 15 pounds cuts the risk of getting osteoarthritis by half. Exercise not only helps prevent osteoarthritis, by keeping your weight down, but it's also a treatment. In a University of Maryland School of Medicine study, 48 overweight women with knee osteoarthritis walked a treadmill three times a week, up to 45 minutes per session. They also met with a nutritionist weekly to help them follow a reduced-calorie, 30-percent-fat-calorie diet. Six months later the women had lost an average of $15^1/_2$ pounds each, and most had a lot less knee pain. Using something called the Womach pain score, 40 percent of the women reported only half as much pain. A third of the women experienced a 50 percent improvement in functions such as walking up stairs. And compared to when they began the study, on average, the women walked 15 percent farther on a six-minute walking test. And, by the way, it's thought that exercise doesn't cause osteoarthritis unless you have a previous injury.

Watch Out!
As many as 250,000 deaths a year in the United States— about 12 percent of total deaths— are attributed to a lack of regular physical activity. (Source: the 1998 Heart and Stroke Statistical Update, American Heart Association.)

And while we're on the subject of bones, exercise is also known to protect against osteoporosis. You might think of bone as a permanent, unchanging structure, particularly once you've reached your full adult height. But, like other tissues, our bones are constantly taking in nutrients, creating new bone and destroying old bone in a process called "remodeling." As we age, we lose calcium from bone faster than we can put it in. In women, this bone loss accelerates at a frightening pace during the six to eight years of menopause, then slows down. (Estrogen replacement therapy can slow down this loss.) Women entering menopause with bones in good calcium shape can withstand the loss, but those with low bone-calcium reserves are at high risk for developing osteoporosis, a disease resulting from calcium-poor, brittle bones. More than 28 million Americans, mostly women, are at high risk of developing osteoporosis. Osteoporosis weakens bones, making them very susceptible to breaking.

In addition to getting enough calcium throughout life, exercise is also a major player in preventing osteoporosis. The type of exercise that does your bones the most good is called "weight-bearing"— movement that forces you to work against gravity such as walking, jogging, racquet sports, hiking, aerobic dance, and stair climbing. A U.S. Department of Agriculture study of 238 women past menopause found that those who habitually walked about a mile a day had denser bones and a slower rate of bone loss than women of the same age who were sedentary. Other research shows that lifting weights also helps preserve bone. These exercises stimulate bone growth; the benefits last as long as you keep up the activity.

Timesaver
Don't have time
this week to
fit in both an
aerobic workout
and strength-
training? Do
both at once
with an interval
training class
that alternates
between a few
minutes of aero-
bics and a few
minutes of
weights, bands,
or other forms
of strength
training.

If you have osteoporosis, you should exercise, but you must get the okay from your doctor first. The doctor, or a specialist in physical medicine, should help you design an appropriate exercise regimen that will safely preserve bone, but also will strengthen your back and hips and maintain flexibility.

After all of exercise's benefits I've just ticked off, it *better* stave off the biggie: death. Not permanently (yet!), but the research certainly shows that more active people live longer than less active people. That was the conclusion of a recent review of the major longevity/exercise studies worldwide, done by researchers at the department of medicine at Brigham and Women's Hospital in Boston.

How much longer? Depends on the study. One of the authors of the review, Ralph S. Paffenbarger, Jr., MD, was also a researcher for the College Study, which tracked alumni from Harvard and the University of Pennsylvania (mainly men) who entered college between 1916 and 1950. The 19,000 or so alumni, now ranging in age from 62 to 100, have been answering periodic questionnaires about their health habits. Those who burned over 1,500 calories worth of exercise per week lived two years longer than those who were sedentary, or went from active to sedentary. Even those who took up exercise much later in life—at 75 to 84—lived almost a year longer than their non-exercising counterparts. As Paffenbarger points out in his book *LifeFit* (Human Kinetics, 1996), nine more months of life may not sound like much, but it's almost a 10 percent increase in longevity when you hit 90. But please, don't wait until you're old to do it; in the College Study, those who were physically active earlier added more years to their lives.

A study tracking 1,405 Swedish women for 20 years found that those who were somewhat active lowered their risk for dying by 28 percent in comparison to the inactive women in the study, and those who had active jobs or exercised regularly were 56 percent less likely to die during the time period of the study.

And you don't have to gain those extra years with lots of sweat, according to a University of Virginia study linking walking to longevity in retired men aged 61 to 81 years. Over a 12-year period, there were twice as many deaths among men who walked less than a mile daily compared to those who walked more than two miles daily.

Improved mood

Now here's an immediate exercise payoff: a better mood. If exercise is going to prolong life, you might as well be happy about it, right? It's a positive cycle: Exercise makes you feel good; when you feel good you're more likely to stay on track and keep exercising. You'll also get a better night's sleep if you exercise.

"The antidepressant effect of exercise is proving stronger than we thought," says Tuft's Miriam Nelson. "Strength training (weights) and aerobic exercise both fight depression," confirms Nelson. "We're not sure what's at work, but in our research into strength training, we've seen that when depressed people become fitter and stronger so does their self-esteem and self-confidence," says Nelson. She notes that it doesn't seem to matter whether you go at it alone or in a group setting; the mood improvements happen either way.

Bright Idea
Exercise is the most successful strategy to change a bad mood, and it was rated fourth in raising energy and reducing tension in a *Journal of Personality and Social Psychology* study. The conclusions came from a survey of 410 people (including 102 college students) and 26 psychotherapists.

University of Montana fitness expert Brian Sharkey, Ph.D., in his book *Fitness and Health* (Human Kinetics, 1997) offers the theories on why exercise is such an upper:

- **Positive coping strategy.** When you can cope better, you feel more in control and happier. Instead of using food or drugs to combat stress, you're using exercise, the healthiest stress reliever out there. And once you feel like you've mastered the skill or sport, you tend to do better at it, and, most importantly, stick with it. Writes Sharkey: "It has even been suggested that this enhanced *self-efficacy*, defined as a sense of one's ability to organize and execute actions required to achieve designated outcomes, may generalize to other areas of performance."

- **Exercise improves self-esteem.** You're taking control over your health, losing weight, looking good; it's bound to boost your confidence. Sharkey says that middle-aged men participating in fitness programs report enhanced sex lives.

- **Biochemical boosts.** One of the much-touted claims of exercise is that it hikes up levels of endorphins, "feel-good" brain chemicals, responsible for a runner's high. Yes, exercise does hike up blood levels of endorphins, says Sharkey, but the research hasn't proven one way or another that they correspond to brain levels. Meanwhile, these circulating endorphins seem to be acting as natural pain killers. Running actually seems easier after 20 minutes; that's when the endorphins kick in. And, Sharkey notes, exercise induces other biochemical effects such as improving the body's responsiveness to insulin and providing a better balance of hormones and brain chemicals that fight depression. The temporary effects of exercise— a raised body temperature and feeling relaxed—has a tranquilizing effect. One study found that a single bout of walking reduced tension as well as a tranquilizer.

Eating for exercise

Unless you're getting into exercise in a big way— working out strenuously for more than an hour a day—you don't need to do anything differently than follow the Food Guide Pyramid advice in Chapter 4, keeping your consumption of fat low, whole grain complex carbohydrates high, and protein moderate. The only big difference is that you get to eat more food than if you were just cutting calories without exercise. That means moving up the range of servings for some of the pyramid groups. For instance, before you started exercising, six servings of low-fat grain-based foods were probably plenty. But add three or more hours of aerobic exercise weekly and you can eat eight or 10 servings—it all depends on your metabolism and how hungry you feel. Remember, fat stays low; but there are some carbohydrate and protein nuances that may enhance your performance.

Nutritional nuances for the exerciser

One such nuance has to do with carbohydrates. You've probably heard of athletes "carb-loading" before their event, filling up on pasta and bread in order to fill their body's carbohydrate stores, called glycogen, to the max. During very intense bouts of

Unofficially . . .
Lifelong exercise may lower your risk of developing Alzheimer's disease, according to a Case Western Reserve University study of people in their mid- to late 70s. Compared to a group of 126 Alzheimer's patients, a group of 247 healthy people reported getting significantly more exercise from age 20 through 59. The exercise boost still came through even after scientifically controlling for differences in age, gender, and education.

exercise, such as sprinting or racing, the body relies on glycogen for fuel. It's when the glycogen runs out that athletes "hit the wall" and performance drops off. As you get in better shape, your muscles can store 20 to 50 percent more glycogen. Carb-loading simply means eating 60 to 70 percent of calories from carbohydrates in the days preceding an event. Endurance athletes (like marathoners) also benefit from sipping fruit juice or another sweetened beverage while exercising to keep sugar (glucose) available for energy.

What if you're not running any races? Then you don't have to worry about increasing carbs beyond the 55 to 60 percent that you'll get when you follow the pyramid-style diet outlined in Chapter 4. Unless you're a serious athlete relying heavily on glycogen, during low-intensity exercise (i.e., walking), body fat's your main fuel, not carbohydrates. Medium-intensity (jogging) activity uses up a combo of body fat and glycogen. Complex carbs not only contribute to your glycogen stores, but that pasta and bread fuels your walks and workouts by slowly releasing glucose into your blood stream, giving you a steady supply of energy (explained in Chapter 4).

Another "nuance" has to do with protein. Nope, those tins of protein powder won't make you look like the guys with gigantic muscles pictured on the labels. It's the exercise myth that won't die, this idea that athletes and body builders need lots of protein. Yes, we do tear down muscle as we exercise and then need protein to build it back up. But that's easily taken care of by a normal diet. Predictably, companies are cashing in on the misinformation; a pound of powder cost $12 to $18 in my local health food store—for that price you could get salmon flown from Washington state (probably a better protein

> **"**
> Carbohydrates are important for not only endurance athletes but also those who train hard day after day and want to maintain high energy. If you eat a low-csarbohydrate diet, your muscles will feel chronically fatigued. You'll train, but not at your best. (Source: *Nancy Clark's Sports Nutrition Guidebook,* 2nd ed., Nancy Clark, MS, RD Human Kinetics, 1997). (By the way, this is a great book for anyone serious about working out and nutrition.)
> **"**

source). Many of the protein powders also contain carbohydrates, apparently to help restore glycogen. I can think of a lot of tastier ways of getting my carbs. To be fair, there is some research showing that powders containing specific amino acids (structural components of protein) may be useful for body builders, but there's other research showing no effect. And the current consensus is that this stuff isn't needed at all by recreational exercisers, runners, dancers, or other athletes that aren't focused on building big muscles.

Too much protein and too little carbohydrate and you'll feel sluggish. Plus, it's unhealthy; diets high in animal protein may raise your risk of cancer, and diets high in red meat may raise blood cholesterol and/or cause iron overload in susceptible people. On the other end of it, skimping on whole grain breads, cereals, and grains means missing out on B vitamins, minerals, and fiber.

It's not only too much protein that's a problem; some of us are getting too little. On the one extreme are the steak, burger, and protein shake-guzzling football players or bodybuilders, with the bagel-pushing, protein-shy, fat-phobic ballet dancers and runners on the other. Dancers, runners, and other athletes avoid animal protein for fear that it contains fat and causes weight gain; another fallacy because many animal-based foods, like turkey breast, are virtually fat-free. So you've got to strike a balance, and that balance is outlined for you in Chapter 4 in the section on the Food Guide Pyramid.

Since you are tearing down and building up muscle when you start getting serious about exercise, your protein needs come up a little. But not much, unless you turn into an athlete. According to

Watch Out!
While there is some evidence that protein powders may be useful for body-builders, for the rest of us, protein powders are a rip-off, particularly those that push single amino acids (components of protein) such as arginine, ornithine and leucine. You get these amino acids when you eat a piece of chicken, beef, or fish, for a lot cheaper.

Nancy Clark's Sports Nutrition Guidebook, here's what you need:

TABLE 13.1   HOW PROTEIN NEEDS INCREASE WITH EXERCISE

	Grams of protein per pound of body weight
Current RDA* for sedentary adult	0.4
Recreational exerciser, adult	0.5–0.75
Competitive athlete, adult	0.6–0.9
Growing teenage athlete	0.8–0.9
Adult building muscle mass	0.7–0.9
Athletes restricting calories	0.8–0.9
Maximum useable amount for adults	0.9

(Source: *Nancy Clark's Sports Nutrition Guidebook,* 2nd ed., Nancy Clark, MS, RD. Copyright © 1997 by Nancy Clark. Excerpted with permission of Human Kinetics, Champaign IL, (800) 747-4457).

* RDA means "Recommended Dietary Allowance," a recommendation put out by the National Academy of Sciences and generally accepted by the scientific community.

To calculate your protein needs, simply multiply your body weight by the grams of protein that fit your exercise category. For instance, if you go to the gym and work out on the treadmill, stair machine, or another aerobic machine or take a strenuous aerobic-type class four or five days a week, you are a pretty serious recreational exerciser. Going toward the top of that 0.5 to 0.75 range, let's pick 0.7. Supposing that you weigh 140 pounds, multiply 140 × 0.7 = 98 g of protein. Now look at the following table and see how easy it is to get that and more protein on a very normal diet—no protein shakes necessary. And by the way, this day comes to 1,835 calories, 23 percent of calories from protein, 17 percent of calories from fat, 60 percent from carbohydrates:

	g protein
Breakfast	
1 cup skim milk	8
1 cup raisin bran	5
1 glass orange juice	1
banana	1
Snack	
1 ounce low-fat cheddar	9
2 rye crackers	2
Lunch	
2 cups lentil soup	18
Caesar salad	2
2 slices whole grain bread	6
1/2 cup frozen yogurt	3
Snack	
12 oz. skim milk latté	13
1 graham cracker spread with a total of 1 teaspoon peanut butter	2
Dinner	
5 oz. fillet of fish	25
1$\frac{1}{2}$ cups of steamed vegetables with lemon and fresh herbs	4
$\frac{1}{2}$ cup rice	3
cup of strawberries topped with 2 tablespoons whipped cream	1
	———
	103 g

Bright Idea
Take advantage of the speaker phone and get up and move around during calls. Standing burns more calories than sitting down. From the Shape Up America! website (www. shapeup.org).

As you probably noticed, except for the fish, this day was otherwise lacto-vegetarian (dairy included). You can get all the protein you need on a vegetarian diet; You'll make it a lot easier on yourself by including dairy and eggs. Remove these from the diet, and you'll be eating a lot of beans, tofu, soyburgers and soymilk.

Vitamin requirements that increase with exercise

Do you need more vitamins as you become more physically active? Probably, slightly, but it appears that you don't have to go out and buy supplements to get them.

Supplement manufacturers really push B vitamins for "energy." The promises on the labels of B-complex vitamins look mighty enticing, but they're bogus. True, three B vitamins are especially critical to producing energy: thiamin (B1), riboflavin (B2), and vitamin B6. And studies do show that exercisers may need a little more of these than sedentary folks because more energy is needed to fuel exercise. However, these Bs are easy enough to get through a balanced diet. Here are the best food sources:

- **Thiamin.** Enriched cereals and bread and beans
- **Riboflavin.** Eggs, lean meats, milk, broccoli, and enriched breads and cereals
- **B6.** Chicken, tuna, beans, cereals, and brown rice

As you can see, these are the types of foods that hold up the pyramid; so a pyramid-style diet à la Chapter 4 should provide all the B vitamins you need. Perhaps if you were subsisting off cola and rice and exercising like mad, you'd need to supplement with extra B vitamins, but after reading this far, I know you're not going to do that.

Supplement manufacturers are also hoping we buy into the idea that exercisers need to supplement with antioxidants. These nutrients fight disease-causing substances called free radicals that are formed in the body in the presence of oxygen. Antioxidants are vitamins C and E, beta-carotene, and the mineral selenium (and there's a whole host of non-vitamin or mineral antioxidants). In typical fashion, the supplement manufacturers seize on preliminary research and leap to conclusions not yet borne out by the science. And think about it: Exercisers wouldn't be living longer and healthier lives if the exercise/free radical connection was so dangerous.

It's true that exercise increases free radical formation. Since you're inhaling so much oxygen during aerobic exercise, and free radicals are formed in the presence of oxygen, your body manufactures more free radicals. Free radicals are also accumulating from the breakdown products of other substances that spike during exercise, such as epinephrine and lactic acid.

But there's still no scientific consensus on whether exercisers need to supplement with antioxidants. Right now, according to the current state of research, you light- to medium-intensity exercisers don't need to. There may be a case for "ultra-endurance" athletes, whose' bodies really take a pounding, to supplement with antioxidants, but that's still far from a consensus opinion. Also, it's been speculated that "weekend warriors," those who exercise hard only once a week, might benefit. Since they're not exercising regularly, their bodies haven't adapted with a souped-up antioxidant defense system. Still, without scientific consensus, I'd wait before taking antioxidants in levels beyond what I recommended in Chapter 5.

Where to begin

If you're a fairly recent exercise dropout, at least you know what you do and don't like. That's going

66

Bitter Orange jump-starts the Qi (vital source) to make the energy circulate quickly during workouts. Puerarin in Kudzu dilates blood vessels and directs efficient blood oxygen supply to the muscles. Chinese Knotweed helps muscles recover more efficiently due to its 'blood-activation' properties (anti-inflammatory). (Source: An Internet advertisement for an herbal supplement.) (This could be proven one day, but it hasn't been scientifically substantiated yet.)

99

Unofficially . . .
Regular exercisers recover more quickly than non-exercisers from the temporary hearing loss that happens after you're exposed to a loud noise, according to a study published in the "Medicine & Science" column in *Sports and Exercise*. It could be that fitter people are able to provide energy more quickly to the hair cells of the ear, which are involved in the recovery of hearing.

to help you develop a better system this time around. And if it's been years or even decades since you've done anything more than walk through the mall, you're going to have to reacquaint yourself with exercise. It's a good time to go back, there's so much more to choose from and so many more qualified instructors to help you, as you'll see in the next chapter.

Walking should be your starting place, advises Charles Kuntzleman, Ed.D., an exercise physiologist and Director of the Blue Cross/Blue Shield of Michigan Fitness for Youth program. So, unless you have severe knee problems, or any other condition that prevents you from walking, here's Kuntzleman's prescription for easing back into it:

- **Get into calorie balance by walking.** Maybe you won't lose much weight at first, but with enough walking, you'll stem the weight gain. And, it'll start preparing your body for the stronger stuff. Kuntzleman asks his clients to walk, not do any other exercise, for three to six weeks. Do it six or seven days a week, starting at 10 to 15 minutes. If you're in better shape, go longer, but don't overdo it. Ideally, you should work up to 45 to 50 minute walks. "If they can stick with it, I know they are committed. And, in the mean time, they've strengthened their leg muscles and their heart for more vigorous exercise."

- **Ease into fat-burning exercises.** Keep walking, but start replacing some of the walking time with "fat-burning" exercises such as biking, swimming, aerobic dance, jumping rope, cross-country skiing, and treadmill and stair-stepping machines (not that walking isn't fat-burning, but these activities will get you there faster). At first, shave 10 minutes off your walking and replace it with one of these activities. Do this about four days a week. Gradually increase the time you spend on the fat-burners until you reach about a half hour, four times a week. Meanwhile, walk at least 15 minutes six to seven times a week.

According to Kuntzleman (and supported by research and echoed by his colleagues) 30 minutes of fat-burning exercise four times a week, supplemented by walking, should be the minimum goal of people who want to shed body fat. If you want to do more, that's great; you'll get an even bigger fat loss and will reap even more health rewards.

Meet your exercise match
Take the PAR-Q test below, look back at the exercise section of the readiness quiz in Chapter 2, and keep the following in mind when deciding how best to get back into it:

- **Health concerns,** such as heart condition or diabetes. The general rule of thumb is if you're over 40 and have been sedentary, get a physical from your doctor, especially if you're overweight. These conditions will usually not prevent you from exercising, but may mean you have to start more slowly.

- **Your body.** Bad knees? Then a high-impact exercise class isn't for you, but swimming or cycling may be fine. Think of what will suit you best physically so you don't get into something hurtful. But don't automatically assume you can't do something. For instance, even if you're very weak, you can try a "body sculpting" class that uses free weights. You simply pick up the

> 66
> Strength training is so important for women because pound for pound, we have less muscle mass than men. We live longer and need that strength.
> —Miriam Nelson, Ph.D., a Scientist at the Nutrition Research Center on Aging at Tufts University, and author of *Strong Women Stay Young and Strong Women Stay Slim* (Bantam, 1997 and 1998, respectively).
> 99

one or two pound weights or use no weights for
the first few classes. Don't worry, you'll quickly
work up to heavier weights.

- **The indoor/outdoor factor.** If you're cooped up
all day and night, and long to be outdoors,
think about hiking, walking, cycling, and an outdoor pool. If nature's too messy for you or dangerous (many neighborhoods are, especially in
the evening), then you'll do fine in a gym or
exercise studio, or even walking the mall.

- **Accessibility.** Even though that gym on the
other side of town may be $100 cheaper per
year, it'll turn out to be a huge waste of money
if you don't go because you don't feel like making the haul across town. Spend a little more for
a gym near your office or home.

- **The drill sergeant problem.** Since 1985, I've had
a lifetime membership to a gym with several outlets in Washington, D.C., where I live. I haven't
paid a dime for it in all the ensuing years. And I
haven't stepped foot in it since 1991. I just
couldn't stand the aerobic instructors, their
barking, their awful music, their unimaginative,
awkward, or dangerous routines. Instead I pay
to take classes at the exercise studio in my neigh-
borhood because of the great instructors. So,
don't be put off by one bad exercise class experience. Instead, shop around; there are great
instructors out there.

- **Boredom.** Mix it up—take water aerobics once
a week, a body sculpting class once or twice
weekly, get on the exercise bike three times a
week. In other words, keep it varied so you don't
burn out on any one thing.

Incidental exercise

It's speculated in serious scientific circles that fidgeting—you know, a nervous wiggling of the foot, fingers drumming on the table, getting up and pacing, is one of the things that keeps people lean. Fidgeters are skinnier than non-fidgeters. The larger point is that short hits of movement throughout the day really do add up. So that advice that you've seen a million times—parking the car at the far end of the lot, taking the stairs instead of the elevator, walking 10 to 15 minutes to a lunch spot instead of going to the cafeteria downstairs—*really works*. At the end of the day (literally) that stuff adds up, perhaps in the hundreds of calories.

Safety screening

Before going and getting 'em, tiger, take this widely used Physical Activity Readiness Questionnaire (PAR-Q) below, developed by the Canadian Society for Exercise Physiology. PAR-Q gives you a sense of whether you need to get a physical before increasing your physical activity.

PAR-Q and You

Regular physical activity is fun and healthy, and increasingly more people are starting to become more active every day. Being more active is safe for most people. However, some people should check with their doctor before they start any form of exercise.

If you're planning to become more physically active than you are now, start by answering the following questions. If you're between the ages of 15 and 69, PAR-Q will tell you if

continued

---

you should check with your doctor before you start. If you are 69 years of age, and you are not used to being active, check with your doctor.

Common sense is your best guide when you answer these questions. Please read the questions carefully and answer each one honestly. Check Yes or No.

	Yes	No
1. Has your doctor ever said that you have a heart condition *and* that you should only do physical activity recommended by a doctor?	☐	☐
2. Do you feel pain in your chest when you do physical activity?	☐	☐
3. In the past month, have you had chest pain when you were not doing physical activity?	☐	☐
4. Do you lose your balance because of dizziness or do you ever lose consciousness?	☐	☐
5. Do you have a bone or joint problem that could be made worse by a change in your physical activity?	☐	☐
6. Is your doctor currently prescribing drugs (for example, water pills) for your blood pressure or heart condition?	☐	☐
7. Do you know of *any other reason* why you should not do physical activity?	☐	☐

If you answered yes to one or more questions: Talk with your doctor *before* you start exercise and before you have a fitness appraisal. Tell your doctor about the results of this questionnaire and which questions you answered yes to.

■ You may be able to do any physical activity you want—as long as you start slowly and build up gradually. Or, you may need to restrict your activities to those which are safe for you. Talk with your doctor about the kinds of activities you wish to participate in and follow his or her advice.

▪ Find out which community programs are safe and helpful for you.

If you honestly answered no to *all* questions:
You can be reasonably sure that you can:

▪ Start becoming much more physically active—begin slowly and build up gradually. This is the safest and easiest way to go.

▪ Take part in a fitness appraisal. This is an excellent way to determine your basic fitness so that you can plan the best way for you to live actively.

Delay becoming more active:

▪ If you are not feeling well because of a temporary illness such as a cold or a fever. Wait until you feel better.

▪ If you are or may be pregnant. Talk to your doctor before you start becoming more active.

Please note: If your health changes so that you then answer *yes* to any of the above questions, tell your fitness or health professional. Ask whether you should change your physical activity plan.

Informed use of the PAR-Q: The Canadian Society for Exercise Physiology, Health Canada, and their agents assume no liability for persons who undertake physical activity, and if in doubt after completing this questionnaire, consult your doctor prior to physical activity.

Just the facts

- Sure you'll lose weight by just cutting calories, but you'll lose lots more body fat—and have a better chance of keeping it off—if you also exercise.

- Living two years longer and staving off the major killers of Americans comes courtesy of increased physical activity.

- A bunch of studies all show it: Exercise is a fantastic mood-elevator.

- Unless you're a really hard-core exerciser/athlete, let the food guide pyramid be your guide.

- Start gradually, take into consideration your tastes and health, and you'll wind up with an exercise program you can stick with.

GET THE SCOOP ON...
Getting started ▪ Fat-burning exercise ▪
Strength-building exercise ▪ Staying limber ▪
Making it safe ▪ Getting the most
muscle for your money

Getting Physical

To really make a big, fat dent in your weight, there's no way around it, you've got to exercise. Diet alone just isn't going to cut it for most of you, especially if you've been heavy most of your life. To outwit those genetics you're gonna have to get out there and walk, hop on a treadmill or bike, swim . . . it really doesn't matter as long as it burns calories.

But calorie-burning isn't what keeps you coming back to the gym. Once you get into exercise, it becomes all about the way it makes you feel: the higher energy level, the better mood, the sense of control over your life. If you read Chapter 13, you know exercise also jacks up your odds for a longer and healthier life.

This chapter gives you a feel for the various types of exercise out there and helps you make the right exercise match. It's also about how to get reliable help and how to buy reliable equipment.

Please check with your doctor before starting any new exercise regimen. The PAR-Q test in Chapter 13 will help you get a sense of whether you need to get a doctor's go-ahead.

Getting started

Watch Out!
Within two weeks of slacking off on exercise you lose many of its benefits; they disappear alto-gether within two to eight months if you don't get back into it, according to 1996 Surgeon General's Report on Physical Activity and Health.

Even if you've been exercising, it's probably not been enough of the right type if you're reading this book. Here are some suggestions on how much you need and how to go about getting it.

What works out very nicely is that the heavier you are, the more calories you burn while exercising. If you don't fall into one of these weight ranges, just estimate. These calories are based on an hour spent on the activity. Going down this list, think about how much time you actually spend and adjust the numbers appropriately. Also, if you work out more intensely than the levels here, then assume you're burning even more calories.

TABLE 14.1   BURN, BABY, BURN

Calories Burned Per Hour If You Weigh:	138–148 lbs	149–159 lbs	182–192 lbs	193 or more
dancing (aerobic)	420	445	515	540
gardening (weeding, hoeing, digging, etc.)	365	390	450	470
golf: a. twosome 9 holes in 1½ hours (carrying clubs)	360	380	440	460
b. twosome 9 holes in 1½ hours (pulling clubs)	315	335	385	405
hiking w/a 20 lb. pack, 3½ mph	360	300	440	465
sex (energetic)	285	300	350	365
stationary bike, resistance sufficient to get pulse rate to 130, 10 mph	400	420	490	515

Calories Burned Per Hour If You Weigh:	138–148 lbs	149–159 lbs	182–192 lbs	193 or more
treadmill: a. 3 mph	285	300	350	365
b. 4 mph	330	345	405	520
walking: a. 2 mph	175	185	215	225
b. 3 mph	285	300	350	365
c. 4 mph	330	345	405	420
d. 5 mph	525	555	645	675
running: a. $5^1/_2$ mph	620	655	760	795
b. 7 mph	660	700	810	850
swimming, 35 yards per minute	510	540	630	655

Adapted from *Diet Free!*, by Charles T. Kuntzleman, EdD. (Arbor Press, 1981). For a complete chart (more activities, more body weight ranges), order the book by calling Fitness Finders at (800) 789-9255. Adapted with permission.

How much is enough?

Prescriptions vary, but to lose weight it looks as though you need to burn somewhere between 300 and 500 calories daily, or 2,000 in a week. That translates to about an hour of aerobic exercise a day (aerobics will be defined later in this chapter). You could spend that hour in an aerobics class or taking a brisk walk, or you can accumulate it in shorter bouts throughout the day (don't make them shorter than 15 minutes). As you can see from the Physical Activity Pyramid in Figure 14.1, you should have a baseline amount of daily routine exercise, and on top of that, calorie-burning aerobic exercise.

And, of course, you've got to phase exercise in gradually and get the okay from your doc, especially if it's been a while since you've exercised. Here's a phase-in strategy from Richard B. Parr, Ed.D, FACSM, a professor of exercise science in the Department of Health Promotion and Rehabilitation

Bright Idea
Vary your workout. Yes, things will seem a lot more comfortable and easy once you train your body to run, swim, do push-ups, and so on. But that also means you stop burning as many calories; challenging yourself with new exercises trains new muscles and, in the process, uses up more calories.

at Central Michigan University and chairperson of the American College of Sports Medicine's Professional Education Committee:

Phase I: If you've been sedentary for a while, exercise 20 minutes, seven days a week for a two-week period. If you're out of shape, don't exercise vigorously; a medium-paced walk is a good start.

Phase II: Same drill, but for 40 minutes.

Phase III: You've worked up to 60 minutes, seven days a week.

To maintain your weight loss it appears that you need to burn about 200 to 400 calories daily—a minimum of 30 minutes of aerobic exercise daily.

While daily exercise is ideal, you can, of course, skip a day here and there. "If you take a day off, enjoy it. If people can exercise 80 percent of the time, they'll be successful at weight loss. But if they exercise every day, they'll lose the weight more quickly," advises Parr.

Mapping out your strategy

Even 20 minutes may seem like a lot if you've been out of the exercise habit. In that case, you'd probably benefit from setting short and long-term exercise goals. Goals motivate, clarify your strategy, and you can look back and assess your progress. Here are some ideas:

Short Term:

- Visit gyms and exercise studios until I find one I'm comfortable with.
- Talk to my doctor about starting an exercise program.

- Start walking _____ minutes daily. (You fill in the blank depending on your level of fitness. See Kuntzleman's prescription in Chapter 13.)

- Try one or more _____ classes. (Again, you fill in the blanks: aerobic dance, water aerobics, and so on.)

Long Term:

- To walk a mile in _____ minutes. (Choose a number that is three-fourths to half the time it currently takes you.)

- To do _____ push-ups. (Double or triple your current number.)

- To swim laps for _____ minutes. (Double or triple (or more) your current minutes.)

- To run an upcoming 5K race in six months.

- To bike _____ miles.

- To take two strength-training classes and three aerobics classes weekly.

Staying motivated

For some hints on staying motivated, I went to the person who keeps me going back to her workout classes: Rachel Posell, an AFAA-certified professional aerobics instructor and co-owner of Work It!, a much-acclaimed exercise studio in Washington, D.C. Here are her tips:

- Think of exercise as an energizer. "People tell me that they're too tired to exercise, but I tell them that they are too tired *not* to exercise. If everyone knew what it felt like to regularly exercise, they'd be doing it every day, all day," says Posell.

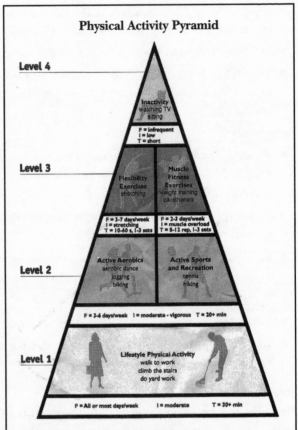

Figure 14.1 Physical Activity Pyramid.
(Source: Corbin, C. B., and R. Lindsey, Fitness for Life *(4th edition, Scott, Foresman/Addison-Wesley, 1997), and from Corbin, C. B., and R. P. Pangrazi, "Physical Activity Pyramid Rebuffs Peak Experience." ACSM's Health and Fitness Journal 2(1), 12–17, 1998. Used with permission.)*

Here's a nifty overview of how much exercise you should be getting, developed by Charles B. Corbin, Ph.D., and Robert P. Pangrazi, Ph.D., two professors at Arizona State University's Department of Exercise Science and Physical Education. The FIT prescription written underneath each area of the pyramid stands for frequency, intensity, and time you should spend on the activities. If you're trying to lose weight, your ultimate goal is the higher end of the ranges given in the pyramid (but work up to this gradually).

Level 1: The pyramid's base contains activities you do as part of your daily routine. For people with active jobs, such as mail carriers, these activities really add up. If you've got a sedentary job, compensate by doing things like walking from a farther bus stop, taking the stairs instead of the elevator, raking leaves; in other words, come up with "natural" ways of getting some exercise. If you stop at level one, you'll be meeting the minimum healthy exercise criteria, but it's unlikely you'll burn enough calories to make much of a dent in your weight.

Level 2: Active aerobics and/or active sports. For more activities, see the "Aerobic exercise" section in this chapter. Moving up to this level of the pyramid will help you really burn that body fat.

Level 3: These exercises will help add muscle and improve flexibility. No, they won't burn many calories, but they enhance your weight loss—and overall health—in indirect ways that will be explained later in this chapter.

Level 4: Obviously, you shouldn't spend to much time at this top level. Of course, you do need to rest and relax, but spending endless hours in front of the tube is what's doing in many an American.

- Write your exercise "appointment" down in your calendar, just as you would a doctor's appointment ("Hopefully then you won't need to go to the doctor," Posell quips).

- Cross-train, meaning exercise in different ways, take a variety of different classes so you don't get bored, and, just as importantly, so you use different muscles.

- Get a workout partner, someone who'll go with you. "It makes it more fun; you encourage each other if someone's not in the mood. And it's safer, especially if you go running."

- While you're working out, don't space out, really focus on what you're doing. You should be engaged, interested, not looking at the clock. Plus, you get better results. "People tend to think that just showing up is good enough. By concentrating, you do the exercise better. For instance, when you're doing abdominal crunches think about the abdominal muscles lifting you up. If you space out, you may wind up just lifting your shoulders and not getting the abdominal workout you came in for."

- In class, look at yourself in the mirror. "This is especially important for new exercisers who can't tell if they're in good form." You'll feel more engaged and get more out of the workout.

Aerobic exercise

These are the exercises that will really dig into that body fat, burning it off to fuel your workouts. It's called "aerobic" because the way your body creates energy while doing these exercises requires oxygen as an essential last step in a complex biochemical process. Previous steps in that process use body fat and blood sugar or stored carbohydrate called glycogen.

When the exercise gets too strenuous, you can no longer take in enough oxygen to meet your energy demands, and that complex energy-producing process gets backed up and produces a substance called lactic acid. That's the stuff that makes your muscles feel tired, legs feel too heavy to walk or jog. When lactic acid starts to form, you're passed aerobics into an anaerobic exercise mode, which isn't nearly as efficient a way to create energy. You'll feel that inefficiency in the form of labored breathing and heavy muscles.

During an aerobic workout, you burn a higher percent of body fat at the lower end of the target heart rate (about 60 percent of maximum heart rate—see the "Target Heart Rate" box later in the chapter). At that point you're burning about 50 percent fat and 50 percent carbohydrate, according to Edmund Burke, Director of the Exercise Science program, University of Colorado at Colorado Springs, and editor of *Precision Heart Rate Training* (Human Kinetics, 1998). But as your exercise intensity and length of workout—and target heart rate—increases, you're burning a smaller percentage of fat. For instance, says Burke, move up to the 80 percent of maximum heart rate zone, and you use about $2/3$ carbohydrate and $1/3$ body fat for fuel. But you're better off working at that higher target heart rate because you're burning more *total* calories. And, says Burke, you've cut deep into your glycogen stores, so that pasta you eat after your workout won't turn to fat, but will be used to replenish glycogen stores. And, of course, working at a higher target heart rate improves your cardiovascular fitness. "So,

Watch Out!
Energy bars may
simply add
unwanted calo-
ries. While these
bars are useful
on hikes and
long bike rides
where you don't
want food to
weigh down your
backpack and
possibly spoil in
the heat, they
are otherwise
unnecessary. If
you do use them,
sub them in for a
snack or part of
a meal. Don't
have them
on top of your
regular diet.

TARGET HEART RATE

The exercise experts have figured out a safe, effective exercise heart rate that you should eventually work up to. It's called, appropriately, your "target heart rate," and it's the number of beats per minute at which you are working hard, but not dangerously hard, and burning a lot of calories. It's based on something called maximum heart rate; the number of beats per minute you reach after very strenuous, exhaustive activity such as running hard for as long as you can. Maximum heart rate drops with age, so the formula for calculating it hinges on your age. Here's how you calculate it:

Your maximum heart rate = 220 – your age

Target heart rate = 60 – 80% of your maximum

Example: You're 35 years old. 220 – 35 = 185

Maximum heart rate for your age: 185
60% of 185 (.6 × 185) = 111
80% of 185 (.8 × 185) = 148
Target exercise heart rate = 111 – 148

You can either spring for an electronic heart rate monitor, found in sporting goods stores, or you can learn to take your own pulse. A good book on how to use heart rate monitors to get the most out of your workout is *Precision Heart Rate Training*, by Edmund R. Burke, ed. (Human Kinetics, 1998).

Here's how to take your pulse:

1. On your left hand, wear a watch that indicates seconds. During the most intense part of your workout, pause.

2. Bend your right arm, holding out your right hand, palm up.

3. Touch index and middle fingers of your left hand to the base of your right thumb.

4. Slide your two left fingers down slightly from the base of the right thumb, past the bones of your right wrist, and find a slight hollow dipping down off the tendons.

5. You'll feel the heartbeat there. Press firmly and count the number of beats for 15 seconds. Multiply by 4 and you've got your heart rate. Now compare to the target heart rate chart.

NOTE: Do not check your pulse by pressing on the carotid artery in your neck. This can cut off blood flow to the brain and may cause fainting!

Age	Maximum Heart Rate (beats/minute)	Aim for this Exercise Range		
		60%	70%	80%*
20	200	120	140	160
25	195	117	137	156
30	190	114	133	152
35	185	111	130	148
40	180	108	126	144
45	175	105	123	140
50	170	102	119	136
55	165	99	116	132
60	160	96	112	128
65	155	93	109	124
70	150	90	105	120
75	145	87	102	116
80	140	84	98	112

* As you get in better shape, head for the higher end of the range to burn more calories and improve cardiovascular fitness.

Bright Idea
There are many good exercise books that give you detailed, structured walking regimens (and solid advice and prescriptions for other forms of exercise); here are just a *few*: *Fitness and Health,* by Brian J. Sharkey (4th ed., Human Kinetics, 1997); *Fit Over Forty* by James Rippe, MD (William Morrow & Co, 1996); *ACSM Fitness Book* (2nd Edition, Human Kinetics, 1992).

as you get in better shape, work up to a more intense level of aerobic workout," Burke recommends.

The amount of aerobic exercise you need depends on your metabolic rate, your diet, and other genetic and hormonal factors. But in general, you need about an hour a day to lose weight, a half hour or more a day to maintain the weight loss. You can accumulate this in a daily bout of aerobic exercise, or in shorter bouts throughout the day. I've listed the more common and convenient types of aerobic exercises. For the number of calories burned doing these exercises, see Figure 14.1 earlier in this chapter.

Walking works

Treadmill a turnoff? Stair climber scary? Relax, you can always walk. It takes a little longer this way, but walking is an effective fat-burner. In fact, if you've been out of the exercise game a while, walking is all you *should* do, according to fitness expert Charles Kuntzleman, Ed.D., Director of the Blue Cross/Blue Shield of Michigan Fitness for Youth program. Check out his walking prescription in Chapter 13 under "Where to begin."

Fitness walking is a faster pace than strolling, but obviously not as fast as running or jogging. If you've been basically sedentary for a while, you might want to start out at a slower pace—more of a stroll. Build up to a fitness walk, which uses the arms. Walk with a straight back, head up, shoulders relaxed.

Even a little walking can make a real dent long-term. Let's say you don't do anything diet-wise or exercise-wise except take two 15-minute walks every day. Assuming that burns an extra 100 calories daily (this will vary according to your size and metabolism), by the week's end you've burned an extra 700 calories. Over a month, that's 3,000 calories. Now a pound of fat is 3,500 calories, so you've burned off nearly a pound a month with very little effort. Over a year, those two 15-minute walks will make you 10 pounds lighter.

Doing it right. Unless you've got joint problems in your legs, walking is safe. And don't think those problems necessarily exclude you from walking. Check with your doctor; walking may be therapeutic. The right way to walk is to hit the ground, heel first, then roll through and push off with the ball of your feet to the toes. Walk straight and tall; don't bend forward or you may wind up with neck, lower back, and hip problems. Arms should swing close to your sides.

Gear. Invest in a good shoe designed for fitness walking. To get your heart rate up, you'll be walking more quickly than a typical stroll, placing a little more stress on the ankle, knee, and hip joints, so you need a shoe that supports and cushions. You might think a running shoe would be even more supportive but it's not, according to James M. Rippe, MD, in *Fit Over Forty* (William Morrow & Co, 1996). "The soft materials in a jogging shoe required to cushion the higher forces of jogging are not needed for fitness walking and, in fact, make it difficult to provide the stiff sole needed to support the foot properly during the forward rolling motion of the walking stride," Dr. Rippe advises.

Wear loose, comfortable clothing that won't constrict arm or leg movements. In cooler weather, layer and peel off clothing as you get warmer, then put the clothes back on as you cool down.

Unofficially . . .
According to a
survey by the fit-
ness organization
IDEA, between
1996 and 1997
the following
areas of fitness
grew in popu-
larity: yoga (up
24%); ballroom
dancing and bal-
let (up 22%);
walking (up
19%); circuit
training
(up 17%); Tai
Chi (up 16%)
and other martial
arts (up 15%).

Happy hiking

On a flat terrain, hiking's about as strenuous as fitness walking. But add a mountain trail and a 20-plus-
pound backpack and you can double your calorie
expenditure.

Doing it right. As with the other exercises, start slowly
to warm up, and do some mild stretches (deeper
stretching after you've warmed up). Water is particularly critical, especially when you're hiking in hot
weather. Drink water—not soft drinks, fruit juices,
or other caloric beverages; they aren't very hydrat-
ing. Most people require a gallon per day, more in
very hot or cold weather. And when it really gets hot,
avoid hiking during the early afternoon if possible.

Gear. Pick boots that fit and break them in doing
small hikes or walks. Boots vary according to terrain,
so buy an appropriate pair. You can get away with
your gym shoes for hikes on fairly smooth terrain
lasting no more than about two hours

In addition you'll need a compass, flashlight,
backpack, food, water . . . For a detailed inventory of
hiking gear and what to put in the backpack, get a
good book or go to www.teleport.com/~walking/
gear.shtml. Look under "Advice on Gear and Lists of
Essentials."

Running/jogging

If you haven't been running in a while, you're going
to feel it the first few times. To minimize the ache,
alternate short bouts of running with longish bouts
of walking. Gradually increase the running and
decrease the walking until you can run for about
20 minutes straight. Some of you shouldn't run: If
you're very overweight or have problems with leg
joints, skip it and do one of the other types of aerobic exercise.

Doing it right. Don't go too fast when you just start out. You know you're going at a safe pace when you can still carry on a conversation; if you're too out of breath to speak fairly normally, slow down.

Run with your head up (not only for good form but to make sure you don't crash into anything), chest open, and try not to arch your back too much; this causes lower back pain. Arms remain close to the body, hands cupped, not clenched. As with walking, your heel touches first, and you roll through to the toes.

Gear. Running shoes should be softer and more flexible than walking shoes. The test: The shoe should bend in half at the ball of the foot. The least you can spend and still get a good shoe is probably $40 to $50; more expensive doesn't necessarily mean better quality. Avoid the discount shoe outlets unless you go in knowing which shoes you want and see them at a lower price. As for clothing, what you'd wear for walking is fine for running, too.

Swimming

While you can get a good workout swimming in the ocean or a lake, it's easier to get a consistent workout in a pool. Pools make it simpler to measure progress (I did 10 more laps than last week!). Since it's a virtually zero-impact sport, it's gentle on the joints and great for people with arthritis or knee injuries. And it's the one exercise that's actually easier if you have more body fat; you don't have to expend so much energy staying afloat. Don't get discouraged if you tire quickly at first; swimming gets easier as you perfect your technique. If you're rusty, take one or two refresher sessions with a swim coach or certified water exercise instructor (see "Evaluating instructors," later in the chapter).

Timesaver
Don't have time this week to do both aerobic and strength training workouts? Try a class that combines the two, with short bouts of aerobics interspersed with a few minutes of strength training. And keep walking.

Doing it right. As with other aerobic exercises, start with a warm-up and cool-down (slow, easy laps). Varying your strokes (crawl, breaststroke, backstroke, and butterfly) will give you a more complete workout. Fewer, longer, and more powerful strokes are better than lots of short strokes. Kick from the hips, not the knees, creating froth, not splashes.

Gear. A secure-fitting swimsuit (one piece for women). Fins are fun, propel you much more quickly, and make beginners feel more powerful. But they don't give you as strenuous a workout, so don't keep them on long. Goggles are absolutely necessary, not only to keep out chlorine, but to help you see so you don't crash into other swimmers.

Classes

I'm one of those that can't get motivated to step foot in a gym or exercise studio unless I take a class. A good class, that is, with an inspiring, creative instructor, not a drill sergeant. The classes listed below are what you'll typically find. Remember, *quality varies;* don't be turned off for good if you get a bad instructor. In fact, if you're like me and classes are important, the quality of the instructors should be a major factor in picking a gym (see "Exercising good sense with your dollars," later in the chapter).

Water exercises. Just what is sounds like: exercising in a pool. I'm putting this at the top of the list not because it's the biggest calorie-burner, but because it's a great way to ease into exercise if you're very overweight. It's easy on the joints, and you'll feel graceful. If you're very body conscious, there is the other-people-seeing-me-in-a-swimsuit problem, but once you're in the pool your body is somewhat obscured by water. It's also a lifesaver for anyone recovering from a knee injury or another injury or condition requiring a low-impact workout.

While usually not quite as strenuous (or calorie-burning) as land-based exercises, exercising in water can give you a decent workout and is a very good way to tone the quadriceps, the front thigh muscles. Here's a description of what's out there from United States Water Fitness Association (USWFA), an organization that promotes water exercise and certifies instructors:

- **Water walking/jogging.** Using many types of steps and arm moves in waist- to chest-deep water.

- **Water aerobics.** Full-body rhythmic moves for 20 minutes or more in shallow or deep water. Purpose is to provide cardiovascular benefits.

- **Water toning/strengthening training.** Movement of upper and lower body using water resistance and/or equipment to strengthen, firm, and sculpt the muscles.

- **Flexibility training.** Large moves using full range of motion and full body stretches.

- **Water therapy and rehabilitation.** Procedures in the water implemented for specific clinical purposes.

- **Water yoga and relaxation.** Gentle, easy-flowing movement with the water as a relaxation medium.

- **Deep water exercise.** Movements of any speed done where feet do not touch bottom. Flotation belts and devices are used.

- **Deep water jogging/running.** Simulating land jogging and running at a depth where the feet

Bright Idea
Want to try water exercising on your own? The non-profit United States Water Fitness Association sells three videos on water walking, exercising in your home swimming pool, and deep water exercise. To order: USWFA, PO Box 3279, Boyton Beach, FL 33424.

do not touch the bottom of the water. Flotation belts and devices are used with various drills, methods, and running styles.

- **Wall exercises.** Using the pool wall for support to isolate various parts of the body.

- **Water fitness equipment.** Professional products especially designed for water toning, strengthening, and endurance work. They create interest and add resistance and support.

- **Stretching.** Specific slow movements done and held for a time after warm-up and at the end of the workout to stretch the hard-worked body muscles and help prevent soreness.

Gear. A bathing suit that won't fall off you and aquatic shoes that protect your feet from rough pool bottoms.

Aerobic dance. These classes can vary from basically calisthenics-to-music to highly choreographed classes with fancy footwork and creative routines. Don't worry if it's confusing at first, you'll get the hang of it. After a while you'll learn the set of core "moves" used by aerobics teachers everywhere, making it easier to pick things up when you get a new teacher. High-impact aerobics, so popular in the 1980s, have been largely replaced by better-for-your-joints low-impact or high/low (alternates) aerobics.

Doing it right. The class should begin with a warm-up and end with a cool-down. If high impact moves—jumping, hopping, jump-kicks, and so on—are part of the routine, the instructor should also give the class low-impact alternatives.

Gear. Go to an athletic shoe store and ask for aerobics shoes, which should support both lateral (side-to-side) and front-to-back movement. As far as what else to wear: anything easy to move in. Shorts and a T-shirt are fine, as are long or short leggings. Women definitely need a supportive exercise bra as there's lots of jiggling going on.

Step. Step aerobics, bench aerobics, bench stepping or aerobic stepping are all terms for a type of exercise involving choreographed stepping up and down on a platform to music. The higher the platforms, the more calories you burn. You can adjust the height on most platforms.

Doing it right. First-timers should always set their platforms as low as possible: four, maybe six inches. Step is considered "high-fitness, low-impact," and that's true unless the instructor has you leaping around a lot. Remember, you can always choose to step up and down instead of leaping; a good instructor should give you the lower-impact alternatives (if not, ask for them). Those of you with knee problems should consult your doctor before taking step. (For instance, I don't have the greatest knees, but I've done okay with step as long as I keep the platform low.) Place your entire foot on the bench to absorb shock and reduce risk of Achilles tendonitis, which can happen when heels hang over the platform edge. As with all aerobics classes, begin with a warm-up and end with a cool-down.

If you haven't ever taken a choreographed aerobics class, I wouldn't start with step. First give your coordination a tune-up with regular aerobics classes. Once you're comfortable making those moves, then go for step. It's not that the routines in step classes are so much more complicated, it's that you're simultaneously learning the whole stepping motion along with a routine. Don't worry, if I can get it (after a while, mind you), so can you.

Watch Out
Make sure your exercise classes are performed on a good floor. Cement floors covered by a carpet are not good; they can damage knees and other joints. Wood floors, especially suspension floors, are kindest.

Bright Idea
If you sprain
your ankle,
remember RICES:

Rest
Ice
Compression
Elevation
Stabilization

Gear. Same as for aerobic dance. You can buy shoes specific for step, but aerobics shoes are just fine. Don't wear running shoes: The flat overhang on the side of the shoes and the deep waffled soles can get caught on the step.

Calories burned per 45 minutes to an hour in class will vary greatly depending on the height of the bench and your body weight (the more you weigh, the more you burn). But extrapolating from one study, you can burn, depending on your body weight, about 340–519 calories in a 45-minute session using a six-inch platform. On an eight-inch platform, 355–560; and on a 10-inch platform, 375–614 calories.

Spinning. This can be a mega-calorie burner depending on how you push yourself. Everyone's on his or her own stationary bike, with the instructor's bike in the front, facing the class. To revved-up music, your (hopefully) revved-up instructor leads you through a simulated outdoor workout ("Picture yourself going up a hill, the trees are rushing by . . ."). The instructor suggests when to pick up the pace and increase the tension on your bike. But, ultimately, you've got the controls on your bike, so you can go at your own pace. (In honor of you readers I took my first spinning class last night. Tough, but doable if you're not totally out of shape and you can swallow your pride and not try to keep up with experienced spinners.)

Doing it right. The class should start with a warm-up and end with a cool-down. You shouldn't be pedaling backward or standing straight up on the pedals—these moves are dangerous. However, hovering over the seat in a squat is fine.

Gear. You want to distribute the pressure along your entire foot, so the best shoes to wear are biking shoes, which have a stiff sole. Running shoes are the worst because the flexible soles tempt you to bend your foot, placing all the stress on the balls of the foot. A stiff cross-trainer shoe also works, and an aerobics shoe, while not ideal, is okay. Wear what's comfortable; biking shorts and a T-shirt are best.

In one study, six "spinners" burned between 7.2 and 13.6 calories per minute for an average of 475 calories expended for a 45-minute class. (The study was sponsored by Mad Dogg Athletics, the group that certifies spinning instructors; the researchers are respected exercise physiologists.)

Martial arts. Karate and Tae Kwon Do are particularly aerobic. Tai Chi and Aikido are more strength- and balance-building.

Other calorie-burning classes include:

- **Line dancing or country-robics.** Doing country-western dancing to country-western music can be a good workout depending on how much the instructor pushes you.

- **Funk and hip-hop.** On the other end of the musical spectrum, this part dance, part aerobics class is set to the latest dance club music. Some are highly choreographed, requiring lots of coordination, while others are simpler. Calorie-burning also depends on the intensity of the workout.

- **Boxing or kick-boxing.** You get a boxer's training without having to really box, just mock-spar with your instructor (at least in a safe class). Boxing classes use sandbags. Kick-boxing, which focuses mainly on kicking, may not use sandbags. It's an intense workout, developing coordination and muscle power.

- **Slide.** You don nylon booties over your gym shoes, get up on your own slick board, and slide side-to-side (booties and board provided by the club). Looks easy, but it's hard work, great for developing inner and outer thigh muscles.

Aerobic exercise machines

Watch Out!
Walkers, also called striders or gliders, are machines with two platforms for your feet, which are connected to swinging legs which offer resistance as you walk. According to *Consumer Reports,* walkers may get your heart rate up, but won't tone your muscles much.

You can get a great workout and burn lots of calories on exercise machines, as you can see in Figure 14.1, earlier in this chapter. It's particularly satisfying to watch yourself progress from five minutes on the easiest setting to 15 minutes at a harder setting. To keep from getting bored, and to work out different muscles (you burn more calories when you "surprise" your muscles), switch machines. For instance, do the treadmill one day, the stair climber the next. And, if you like exercise classes, alternate them with machine days. Here's a list of common gym or home standbys:

- **Exercise bike.** Depending on how you set the pedaling resistance, your workout can be light to heavy in intensity. If you've got back problems, try recumbent seats that support your lower back sort of like a chair. Some come with lever handlebars that you pump for toning arms and increasing the intensity of the workout. Keep in mind that outdoor cycling is also a great workout, particularly if you've got to pedal up hills. Get a model you're comfortable with; being bent over like a racer can be a strain on the back. And yes, those hard, slim seats are supposed to shape to your rear, but go for the bigger ones if they're more comfortable. And, of course, always wear a helmet.

- **Treadmill.** Again, depending on the setting, the workout ranges from light to heavy. Those that vary the terrain, simulating hills and interspersing sprints, make things more interesting and challenging.

- **Stair climber or stair steppers.** Depending on how you adjust the stepping height or resistance, your workout will range from light to intense. Stair climbers may have a calorie-burning edge over treadmills and bikes. According to *Consumer Reports,* you'll get a better, more natural workout on "non-linked" steps, those that don't automatically push one step up as the other goes down.

- **Rowing machine.** While treadmill and stair climbers develop lower body muscles, rowing machines tone both lower and upper body. Again, depending on resistance and speed, your workout will range from light to intense. These can strain the knees and back if you're not positioned properly.

- **Cross-country ski machines.** These also tone the whole body, and, as you can now predict, your workout will range from light to intense depending on resistance and speed.

- **Elliptical exercisers.** A cross between a stair climber and a cross-country ski machine. You stand on two platform pedals; you pump one up and down, the other back and forth. May be too strenuous a workout if you're not in reasonable shape. These machines develop leg and butt muscles. As of press time, *Consumer Reports* gave the thumbs down to home versions of this machine, saying they break easily. Maybe round two will be better quality.

Strength training

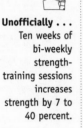

Unofficially . . .
Ten weeks of bi-weekly strength-training sessions increases strength by 7 to 40 percent.

I've tried a lot of different types of exercise over the years, but I didn't even consider weightlifting; I thought it was just for Schwarznegger wannabes. But over the last year, I've become addicted to my strength-training class and have seen results. It's empowering to carry really heavy groceries home without putting them down every block and thrilling to see limbs looking more toned. And the class—more women than men—is surprisingly non-competitive. Some are using five-pound weights to do arm curls, others 25 pounds, and no one cares or even seems to look.

While strength training (weightlifting or using bands and the body for resistance) isn't a mega-calorie burner like aerobic exercise, with bi-weekly sessions, it'll help out your weight loss effort in more subtle ways:

- Strength training builds muscle, which in turn slightly increases metabolic rate, so you burn a few more calories even at rest.
- Since you're building muscle, the weight your losing is truly body fat.
- You'll start looking more toned even before you lose much body fat.
- Your improved balance and strength carries over to your aerobic exercises.

And there are all the health-related goodies recounted in the previous chapter: a guard against osteoporosis, blood sugar stabilizer, and a reversal of the natural age-related decline in lean body mass.

Two myths that need to be busted before you continue:

- No, your muscles will not turn to fat if you stop lifting weights. They'll just wither down to their former unconditioned state.

- Sorry guys, unless you have a body that readily puts on muscle, you won't end up looking like Schwarznegger. Men will get bulkier, how much so depends on genetics. And women, you'd have to quit your jobs and work out all day and have the right genetics in order to get big and bulky. What'll happen instead is that you'll look slimmer as the muscles get toned.

There are entire books dedicated to the ins and outs of strength training. Here's an overview:

Your body "weight"

You don't always need equipment: Lifting your own body can build quite a bit of muscle. Think not? Try to do 10 push-ups if you haven't worked out your arms in a while. Or pull-ups, or a series of squats. Don't rely entirely on your body as a weight; it's limiting and gets boring quickly. But pull out those moves when you're traveling, had to go to something *really important* and missed your weight-training session, and as an adjunct to your regular weight-training. And there's one move that you really don't need paraphernalia for: abdominal crunches.

Free weights, tubes, and bands. Free weights are simply weights that you pick up, not part of a machine. Dumbbells are the shorter ones, while barbells or body bars are the long ones that you grip with both hands. With some, you slide on plates of

One of the most remarkable trends in recent years is the growth in strength train-ing. Participation by females [in 1996] more than doubled since 1987, from 7.4 million to 16.8 million. The number of males who used free weights climbed 52% over the same period, from 17.1 million to 26 million. (Source: "Tracking the Fitness Movement," a 1997 report from the Sporting Goods Manufacturers Association.)

various weights; others are one solid, unchangeable weight. You can do a seemingly endless variety of exercises using free weights, alone or in a class.

A stretchy rubber tube, with or without handles at each end, and a band—literally a huge thick rubber band, will tone nearly every muscle group. Instead of relying on the weight itself, you pull or push against the tension of the band or tube.

Reps is jargon for repetition, the number of times you execute a complete motion, for instance one rep of an *arm curl* is beginning with the dumbell hanging at your side, bringing it up to chest level, and back down again. To build bigger muscles and get as strong as you can, you need to do fewer reps using heavier weights. To tone muscles and develop the kind of strength that will help you carry in the groceries and pick up a toddler, you do more reps with lighter weights. As your trainer or instructor will remind you, the last rep or two you do—whether it's the fifth or the 25th, should be a real effort. Otherwise, your weights are too light.

Doing it right. If you decide to lift weights alone, get some professional help the first few sessions. Hire a personal trainer or get a certified instructor at the gym to show you the ropes (see "Evaluating instructors" later in the chapter for who's qualified). Otherwise, you could end up not getting much out of your workout, or worse yet, truly hurt yourself. Likewise with the tubes and bands. And if you're using very heavy weights, get someone to *spot* you (act as a safety net to catch the weight before it crushes you). Alone or in a class, always warm up, and at some point, either after each exercise or at the end, stretch the muscles you've worked so they don't get tight.

Gear. Comfortable clothing, similar to aerobics wear. You don't need those big abdominal support

Safe Stretching

Stretch too quickly when you're not warmed up, or make a wrong move, and you could wind up with a pulled muscle. Do it right, and you'll make important gains in range of motion and help prevent sore muscles from your aerobic and strength-training workouts.

Unsafe/Incorrect	Instead
Deep stretching before a workout	Warm up first by doing a lighter version of your workout, then do light stretching. At the end of the workout do the deep stretching, once the muscles are very warmed up.
Bobbing and jerking stretches	"Static" stretching, slowly moving into the stretch, then holding it and relaxing into it.
Full head rolls	Tilt head from side to side.
Touching your toes, legs straight, then coming up quickly	Before coming up, bend knees, support yourself by placing hands on thighs, round up slowly.
Deep knee bends	Half knee bends, sticking your butt out, knees shouldn't stick out further than your toes.

belts unless you're body-building and lifting very heavy weights.

Weight machines. They do the same thing as free weights, and you don't need as much training. Once you learn to adjust the weights and position yourself properly by adjusting the seats or height, you've pretty much got it. Still, I'd have a certified trainer guide you through the *circuit* (where members go from one machine to another in order) the first time around. Various machines work out specific muscles such as the back of legs (hamstrings), shoulders, back, buttocks, and biceps. By

Moneysaver
Before buying an exercise video, go to the video store and rent it. Rent a few more, and buy the one that suits you best.

Unofficially . . .
In case you hadn't heard: You can't spot reduce. Sure, doing abdominal crunches will tone your stomach, but it won't get rid of belly fat. That comes with eating less and burning more calories.

completing the entire circuit you've worked out most major muscle groups.

Stretching and flexibility

The connective tissue that coats muscles is what limits your flexibility (your limbs' range of motion). But over time, certain exercises stretch the connective tissue allowing you to reach past your toes, or do any number of things you never thought possible. Stretching exercises combat the age-related decrease in flexibility. Following a stretching book or video, you can do it at home or take a class or try yoga. Yoga poses, which you hold for seconds to minutes, not only make you more flexible, they are a wonderful way to improve balance. And the stress-relieving meditative exercises I learned from yoga carry over into my everyday life.

Exercise safety

Done correctly and safely, exercise will put more zip into your life than you thought possible. However, injuries can occur; these tips will help you avoid potential hazards:

Stay hydrated

It ain't called calorie-burning for nothing; as you burn those calories your internal body temperature rises. Your body cools itself off by dissipating heat through the skin in the form of sweat. As the sweat evaporates you cool down. Great system, but there's one problem: As you sweat you get dehydrated, and after a while, dehydration can cause muscle cramps, dizziness, and confusion. Advanced heat exhaustion can be fatal. To counter all these effects, go into your workout well hydrated. Drink water all day before the workout (a test of good hydration is passing clear-colored urine). And drink 8 to 10 ounces of water

10 to 20 minutes before the workout. If you feel parched during the workout, take a break to get some water.

Warm-up

Before you push yourself hard, start slowly. Taking five minutes to gradually increase your heart rate, breathing, and body and muscle temperature prepares enzymes and muscle fibers for what's coming so your body functions better. Doing some light stretching during the warm-up period (reserve the "deeper stretching" for cool-down when muscles are more limber) may reduce your chances of pulling something.

Cool-down

In the last five minutes of your workout, slow things down. For instance, go from running to walking, from vigorous to easy cycling. The cool-down's effects on heart rate and blood pressure will help you avoid post-exercise light-headedness and clear the lactic acid buildup more quickly.

Pull back a little when you're pregnant. While exercise can make pregnancy a more pleasant experience and give you more stamina for labor, overdoing it can be dangerous for you and the fetus. Whether you're simply continuing your pre-pregnancy regimen or just starting out, *first get the okay from your obstetrician.* Some experts suggest cutting your workouts back to about two-thirds of your normal intensity. Be particularly careful to avoid dehydration and overheating. And stay away from these activities altogether: scuba diving, waterskiing, rock climbing, hang gliding, snowmobiling, and martial arts that involve throwing and contact. Also, outdoor bicycling, downhill or cross-country skiing, and ice-skating have a high accident potential; you might want to put these on hold until after delivery.

Exercising good sense with your dollars

Just like the diet industry, the exercise biz is fraught with potential rip-offs. Before joining a gym or studio, hiring a personal trainer, or plunking down dough for home exercise equipment, read on.

Evaluating instructors

Anyone can get up there and teach an exercise class or offer their personal training services, which means, you could get in the hands of someone who hasn't a clue to safe, effective exercise. By insisting upon certified instructors and personal trainers, you reduce that risk. Here are a list of reputable certifying organizations (there may be others, but these are the ones that my sources were most comfortable with):

> Aerobics and Fitness Association of America (AFAA)
>
> American Alliance for Health, Physical Education, Recreation and Dance
>
> American Athletic Training Association
>
> American Council on Exercise (ACE)
>
> American College of Sports Medicine (ACSM)
>
> American Physical Therapy Association
>
> International Association of Fitness Professionals (IDEA)
>
> Cooper Institute for Aerobics
>
> National Academy of Sports Medicine (NASM)
>
> For water exercise:
>
> Aquatic Exercise Association (AEW)
>
> United States Water Fitness Association (USWFA)
>
> YMCA

Watch Out!
"A good personal trainer will prevent you from doing too much, too soon. While a little soreness is expected after sessions, you'll know you should switch trainers if you're virtually crippled for days after."
—Rachel Posell, Co-owner of Work It!, an exercise studio in Washington, D.C.

Hiring a personal trainer

If you've never even stepped into a gym, the idea of hiring your own personal trainer may seem a bit extravagant and glamorous. But there are very good reasons to do so, as you'll see in the following list. And at $25 to $100 a pop ($50 is average for Washington, D.C., where I live), you may not be able to afford many sessions. That's okay, sometimes just one session is all you need.

- **Equipment savvy.** In just one or two sessions (you can meet the trainer at your gym or use one of the club's trainers) you can map out a good exercise regimen and learn to use the equipment safely.

- **Motivation.** It's hard to not show up when you're paying someone and know he or she is waiting for you.

- **You need to work around an injury.** The trainer can develop a regimen that doesn't stress out your knee, hip, back, or whatever else you're favoring.

- **Prepping for an event.** You don't want to ruin your ski trip, bike ride, or run because you didn't get your muscles in shape. A trainer can point out the best training exercises and provide a little extra motivation.

- **Improving a medical condition.** My friend was diagnosed with osteoporosis (a bone-thinning disease) last year. A year of strength-training with a personal trainer plus aerobics classes (along with the bone-building drug Fosamax), and her doctor was amazed at how much bone she'd built.

Bright Idea
Change your
exercise shoes
every 500 miles
or six months.

▪ **You've plateaued.** You're exercising regularly, but your weight has plateaued and you still want to lose more. A personal trainer can push you a little beyond your usual level and reinvigorate your weight loss.

Don't get gypped by a gym

So many people join gyms and don't use them. To avoid falling into that group, make sure you've made a good match from the get-go. Here are some tips:

▪ If you like exercise classes and aren't too crazy about exercise and weight machines, don't join a real gym. Find a good exercise studio and pay by the class (a series of classes is usually cheaper). Then consider a gym.

▪ The gym or studio should be clean and not smelly.

▪ It shouldn't be too crowded. Visit during the hours you're most likely to go and check for these signs of overcrowding: lines to use the equipment and sardine-packed classes.

▪ Try to talk them into letting you take a class for free before joining.

▪ Facilities. Do they have a decent variety of equipment? Does the equipment look fairly new (not too many "Out of Order" signs?)? Is the exercise class schedule diverse? Do they offer classes you want to take and at the right time?

▪ Instructors. Ideally, they should all be certified (see "Evaluating instructors" earlier in the chapter).

▪ Pull some members aside and get their scoop on the place.

- Comparison shop. Go to several different gyms or studios.

- Location, location. If you have to drive across town to get there, you'll think of dozens of excuses not to go. Even if you have to pay a little more, join one near your home or office.

- Atmosphere. Gyms tend to attract types: tattooed muscle builders, more women, more men, gay men, heteros on the make, seniors. . . . Get the feel of the place and make sure you're comfortable there.

- What do you actually get for your money? Unlimited use? Access to personal trainers? Showers? Towels? Get the details.

Before you sign up

Before your signature graces the dotted line, consider these tips from the *Consumer's Resource Handbook,* put out by the U.S. Office of Consumer Affairs:

"When you are considering whether to join a health club, be cautious of:

- Joining clubs that have not opened—they might never open.

- Low-cost "bait" ads—many switch you to expensive long-term contracts.

- Promises that you can cancel anytime and stop paying—check the written contract for the terms of membership and any other promises.

- The fine print—many low-cost ads and contracts severely restrict hours of use and services.

- Signing long-term contracts—consumer protection agencies report that many consumers quit using the club within a few months.

Unofficially . . .
Gardening is good exercise. A study published in *Medicine and Science in Sports and Exercise* found that you expend just as many calories trimming shrubs or trees, mowing the lawn, weeding, planting, carrying and chopping wood, and shoveling as you do doing other intense aerobic exercise.

- Automatic monthly billing to your charge card or debit from a checking account—these are easier to start than to stop.

- Unbelievably low one-time fees with no monthly dues.

- Read the contract carefully before you sign. Is interest charged for a payment plan? Are all promises in writing?

- Check with your local or state consumer agency or Better Business Bureau for any laws in your state, cancellation rights, or complaints against the company."

Success Story: John P.

"I was heavy for the first time in junior high, and from then on my weight fluctuated up and down," says John, a 47-year-old manager. "But two years ago I discovered exercise, and the weight's been down ever since."

Before exercise, he lost weight through dieting, often with the help of commercial weight loss programs including Jenny Craig and Nutri/System. He'd lose weight but gain it back. Then, with no change in diet, he got into spinning (exercise classes on a stationary bike described in this chapter). "With spinning the weight seemed to melt off, I lost 30 pounds in four months and it hasn't come back in two years."

"When I started exercising, everything else kind of fell into place. I eat better, and I can relax a little about eating and enjoy it more because I know I burn it off." The

CHAPTER 14 ▪ GETTING PHYSICAL   443

> exercise has also helped him cope with the
> stress of managing four offices spread across
> the country, which means lots of travel. Both
> at his main office in Washington, D.C., and on
> the road, he makes time for exercise. He calls
> ahead to see where there's a spinning class in
> the city he's traveling to. "If the president of
> the company comes to town, he knows to
> schedule meetings around my lunch hour
> exercise time," John laughs. He adds: "The
> key is to change the way you typically think
> about weight loss, to get rid of the notion of
> dieting. I've learned to live with low-fat foods,
> and now I don't miss the high-fat ones. But if
> I really want something fattening, I occasion-
> ally get it."

Do your homework on home exercise equipment

Your starting point: *Consumer Reports* or other
favorite consumer magazine. Their teams test
machines for durability and give you a good sense of
the type of workout you'll get. Check out the library
for back issues from the past year, or check the
Consumer Reports website: www.consumerreports.org.
Also, a wonderful resource on buying and using the
equipment is *Complete Home Fitness Handbook*,
Edmund R. Burke, editor (Human Kinetics, 1996).

Then go to a top-notch fitness specialty store
where the salespeople really know their stuff. (It's
doubtful that you'll find someone that knowledge-
able at a K-Mart or sporting goods store.) Go to at
least two different stores selling different brands
of equipment. Before limiting yourself to a price

range, let them tell you the difference between the more and less expensive treadmills, stair climbers, or other machines so you know just what you're getting. These stores have more of a vested interest in making you happy than a store that sells everything; a bad reputation could hurt them, and they want repeat customers.

The electronic gadgets that come with exercise equipment, such as digital calorie readers, are lots of fun, but if they add a lot to your bill and nothing to your workout, resist them.

Just the facts

- Build up strength and endurance gradually and stay motivated.
- You've got a big choice in fat-burning exercises.
- Strength building complements fat-burning exercises.
- Stay flexible, but do it safely.
- Avoid injuries and overexertion when you exercise.
- Insist on qualified instructors, and don't get ripped off by the exercise biz.

Recommended Reading List

T hese are not exhaustive lists, but a compilation of quality books I've come across.

Losing/maintaining weight

Many of these are described in Chapter 7.

Choose to Lose, by Ron and Nancy Goor
(Houghton Mifflin, 1995).

The Complete Idiot's Guide to Losing Weight,
by Susan McQuillan with Edward Saltzman
(Alpha Books, 1998).

The Diet-free Solution, by Laurel Mellin
(HarperCollins, 1998).

Eating on the Run, by Evelyn Tribole, MS, RD
(2nd ed., Leisure Press, 1991).

The LEARN® Program for Weight Control,
by Kelly Brownell (7th ed., American
Health Publishing, 1997).

Living Without Dieting, by John P. Foreyt, Ph.D., and
G. Ken Goodrick, Ph.D. (Warner Books, 1994).

*Now That You've Lost it: How to Maintain Your Best
Weight*, Joyce D. Nash (Bull Pub. Co., 1992).

Thin For Life, and *Eating Thin for Life*, both by Anne
M. Fletcher, M.S., R.D. (Houghton Mifflin, 1994
and 1997, respectively).

Losing weight: more exercised focused

*Get Real: A Personal Guide to Real-Life Weight
Management*, by Daniel Kosich (Idea Press, 1995)
(more exercise-driven).

Living With Exercise, Steven Blair (American Health,
1991).

Strong Women Stay Slim, by Meriam E. Nelson
(Bantam, 1998).

Exercise books (not necessarily weight loss)

ACSM Fitness Book, by The American College of
Sports Medicine (2nd ed., Human Kinetics, 1992).

The Bodywise Woman, by Judy Mahle Lutter and
Lynn Jaffee (Human Kinetics, 1996).

Fit Over Forty, by James M. Rippe
(William Morrow and Co., 1996).

Fitness and Health, by Brian Sharkey
(4th ed., Human Kinetics, 1997).

Lifefit, by Ralph S. Paffenbarger, Jr., and Eric Olsen
(Human Kinetics, 1996).

The Rockport Walking Program, by James M. Rippe
and Ann Ward (Prentice Hall Press, 1986).

Strong Women Stay Young, and *Strong Women Stay
Slim,* by Miriam E. Nelson (both Bantam, 1997 and
1998, respectively).

Other useful nutrition books
(not necessarily weight loss)

*The American Dietetic Association's Complete Food
and Nutrition Guide,* by Roberta Larson Duyff
(Chronimed, 1996).

The Complete Idiot's Guide to Eating Smart, by
Joy Bauer (Alpha Books, 1996).

Eat More, Weigh Less, by Dean Ornish
(HarperCollins, 1993).

Eating on the Run, by Evelyn Tribole
(2nd ed., Leisure Press, 1992).

Monthly Nutrition Companion, The American
Dietetic Association (Chronimed, 1997).

Nancy Clark's Sports Nutrition Guidebook, by Nancy
Clark, MS, RD (2nd ed., Human Kinetics, 1997).

6 Weeks to Get Out the Fat, American Heart
Association (Times Books, 1996).

Lean/healthful cooking

Eater's Choice and *Choose to Lose,* by Ron and
Nancy Goor (both Houghton Mifflin, 1995).

Eating Thin for Life, by Anne Fletcher
(Houghton Mifflin, 1997).

Everyday Cooking with Dr. Dean Ornish, Dr. Dean
Ornish (HarperCollins, 1996).

Moosewood Restaurant's Low-Fat Favorites
(Clarkson Potter, 1996).

Head books

Afraid to Eat. Children and Teens in Weight Crisis,
by Frances M. Berg (Healthy Weight Publishing
Network, 1997).

The Beauty Myth, by Naomi Wolf (Double Day,
1992).

Body Traps, by Judith Rodin (Quill, 1993).

*The Dance of Anger: A Woman's Guide to Changing the
Patterns of Intimate Relationships,* by Harriet Goldhor
Lerner, Ph.D. (Harper and Row Publishers, 1985).

The Diet-free Solution, by Laurel Mellin
(HarperCollins, 1998).

*Intuitive Eating: a Recovery Book for the Chronic Dieter:
Rediscover the Pleasures of Eating and Rebuild Your
Body Image,* by Evelyn Tribole and Elyse Resch
(St. Martin's Press, 1995).

Living Without Dieting, by John P. Foreyt, Ph.D., and
G. Ken Goodrick, Ph.D. (Warner Books, 1994).

Tailoring Your Tastes, by Linda Omichinski
and Heather Wiebe Hildebrand (Tamos Books,
Inc., 1995).

Self-esteem Comes In All Sizes, by Carol Johnson
(Main Street Books, 1996).

When Women Stop Hating Their Bodies, by
Jane R. Hirschmann and Carol H. Munter
(Fawcett Columbine, 1995).

Eating disorders

*Emotional Eating: What You Need To Know Before
Starting Another Diet,* by Edward Abramson
(Jossey-Bass, 1998).

Fasting Girls: The History of Anorexia Nervosa,
by Joan Jacobs Brumnerg (Plume, 1989).

Overcoming Binge Eating, by Christopher Fairburn
(The Guilford Press, 1995).

Overcoming Overeating, by Jane R. Hirschmann and
Carol H. Munter (Fawcett Books, 1998).

Newsletters (general nutrition, not specifically weight loss)

Environmental Nutrition
P.O. Box 420235
Palm Coast, FL 32142-0451
(800) 829-5384

Nutrition Action Health Letter
Center for Science in the Public Interest
1875 Connecticut Ave., NW, Suite 300
Washington, DC 20009
(800) 237-4874

Tufts University Health and Nutrition Letter
P.O. Box 57857
Boulder, CO 80328-7857
(800) 274-7581

**University of California at
Berkeley Wellness Letter**
Health Letter Associates
P.O. Box 420235
Palm Coast, FL 32142
(800) 829-9080

Resources

Organizations

General nutrition information (including weight control info)

American Dietetic Association
The largest association of nutrition professionals
and certifying body for registered dietitians.
(800) 366-1655 (for their Consumer Nutrition Hot
Line) (900) CALL-AN-RD, or (900) 225-5267, (for
customized answers to your nutrition questions;
the cost is $1.95 the first minute and $.95 each
additional minute)
website (for food and nutrition information and a
referral to a registered dietitian in your area):
www.eatright.org

Center for Science in the Public Interest
A Washington D.C.–based consumer nutrition
advocacy group and publishers of *Nutrition Action,*
a monthly newsletter.
(202) 332-6718
website: www.cspinet.org

Mayo Health Oasis
website: www.mayohealth.org (click on diet and
nutrition for advice from the venerable Mayo
Clinic)

Tufts University Nutrition Navigator
A website that rates other nutrition websites.
website: http://navigator.tufts.edu

Weight Control Information Network (WIN)
Part of the National Institutes of Health.
1 WIN Way
Bethesda, MD 20892-3665
(301) 984-7378 or (800)-WIN-8098
fax: (301) 984-7196
website: www.niddk.nih.gov/health/nutrit/win.htm

www.quackwatch.com
A website run by health professionals that alerts
the public to health frauds and scams.

For specific diseases

American Cancer Society
1599 Clifton Road, NE
Atlanta, GA 30329
(404) 320-3333 or (800) ACS-2345, or (800)
227-2345
website: www.cancer.org/pandes.html

American Diabetes Association
1660 Duke Street
Alexandria, VA 22314
(703) 549-1500
website: http://diabetes.org/professional.htm

American Heart Association
7272 Greenville Avenue
Dallas, TX 75231
(214) 373-6300
website: http://207.211.141.25

American Institute for Cancer Research
1759 R Street, NW
Washington DC 20009
(800) 843-8114
website: www.aicr.org

American Lung Association
1740 Broadway
New York, NY 10019
(212) 315-8700
website: www.lungusa.org/index2.html

Cancer Research Foundation of America
1600 Duke Street
Alexandria, VA 22314
(703) 836-4412 or (800) 227-CRFA
website: www.preventcancer.org

National Institutes of Health
Bethesda, Maryland 20892
(301) 496-4000
website (for specific institutes, such as National
Cancer Institute or National Heart, Lung and
Blood Institute): www.nih.gov/icd

National Osteoporosis Foundation
1150 17th Street, NW, Suite 500
Washington DC 20036
(800) 223-9994
website: www.nof.org/Welcome.html

Weight control information

**National Institutes of Health's Weight
Information Network (WIN)**
A government office supplying print and video info.
1 WIN Way
Bethesda, MD 20892-3665
(800) WIN-8098
website: www.niddk.nih.gov/NutritionDocs.html

Shape Up America!
A national campaign to reduce obesity led
by former Surgeon General C. Everett Koop.
website: www.shapeup.org

Self-help groups
See Chapter 6 for more details.

Overeaters Anonymous (OA)
(505) 891-2664
website: www.overeatersanonymous.org

Take Off Pounds Sensibly (TOPS)
(800) 932-8677
website: www.tops.org

Commercial diet programs
See Chapter 6 for more details.

Jenny Craig
(800) 435-3669
website: www.jennycraig.com

Nutri/System
(800) 321-THIN
website: www.nutrisystem.com

Weight Watchers
(800) 651-6000
website: www.weightwatchers.com

Support organizations for eating disorders
See Chapter 12 for more details.

The ACT-Out Ensemble
c/o Jessica Weiner
401 East Michigan Street
Indianapolis, IN 46204
(317) 278-2530 (Jessica Weiner or L. E.
McCullough)

**American Anorexia Bulimia
Association, Inc. (AABA)**
165 West 46th Street, Suite 1108
New York, NY 10036
(212) 575-6200
fax: (212) 278-0698
email: AmAnBu@aol.com
website: members.aol.com/amanbu

Eating Disorder Awareness & Prevention
603 Stewart Street, Suite 803
Seattle, WA 98101
(206) 382-3587
website: http://members.aol.com/edapinc

**National Association of Anorexia Nervosa
and Associated Disorders (ANAD)**
Box 7
Highland Park, IL 60035
(847) 831-3438
fax: (847) 433-4832
email: anad20@aol.com

**The National Eating Disorders
Organization (NEDO)**
6655 South Yale Avenue
Tulsa, OK 74136
(918) 481-4044
website: www.laureate.com

Outside the U.S.

Canada
Bulimia, Anorexia Association
3640 Wells Street
Windsor, Ontario N9C 1T9
(519) 253-7545

National Eating Disorder Information Centre
200 Elizabeth Street
College Way
Toronto, Ontario M5G 2C4
(416) 340-4156

United Kingdom
Eating Disorders Association
Sackville Place
44 Magdalen Street
Norwich
Norfolk NR3 1J3
01603-621414

Non-dieting/size acceptance organizations

Healthy Weight Network
402 South 14th Street
Hettinger, ND 58639
(701) 567-2646
fax: (701) 567-2602
website: www.healthyweightnetwork.com

Network for Size Esteem
P.O. Box 9404
New Haven, CT 06534-0404
website: 75773.717@compuserve.com

Radiance: The Magazine for Large Women
(in Barnes and Noble and other magazine stands)
telephone and fax: (510) 482-0680
website: www.radiancemagazine.com/index.html

Size Acceptance Website
www.bayarea.net/~stef/Fatfaqs/size.html

Vegetarian organizations

Vegetarian Awareness Network
(800) 548-3438

Vegetarian Resource Group
PO Box 1463
Baltimore, MD 21203
(410) 366-VEGE
website: www.vrg.org

Exercise

The following national organizations, or their state
or local affiliates, promote physical activity and
many will send you information.

Aerobic and Fitness Association of America
15250 Ventura Boulevard, Suite 200
Sherman Oaks, CA 91403
(818) 905-0040
website: www.aerobics.com/10000.asp

**American Alliance for Health, Physical
Education, Recreation & Dance**
1900 Association Drive
Reston, VA 20191
(703) 476-3400

American College of Sports Medicine
P.O. Box 1440
Indianapolis, IN 46206-1440
(317) 637-9200

American Council on Exercise
5820 Oberlin Drive, Suite 102
San Diego, CA 92121
(619) 535-8227
website: www.acefitness.org

American Running and Fitness Association
4405 East-West Highway, Suite 405
Bethesda, MD 20814
(301) 913-9517

Arthritis Foundation
1330 West Peachtree Street
Atlanta, GA 30309
(404) 872-7100

Association for Worksite Health Promotion
60 Revere Drive, Suite 500
Northbrook, IL 60062-1577
(708) 480-9574

Bicycle Federation of America
1506 21st Street, NW, Suite 200
Washington, DC 20036
(202) 463-6622

Campaign to Make America Walkable
1506 21st Street, NW, Suite 200
Washington, DC 20036
(202) 463-6622

**IDEA-International Association
of Fitness Professionals**
6190 Cornerstone Court East, Suite 204
San Diego, CA 92121
(619) 535-8979

**International Health, Racquet &
Sportsclub Association**
263 Summer Street
Boston, MA 02210
(617) 951-0055

League of American Bicyclists
749 North 26th Street
Philadelphia, PA 19130
(215) 232-7543

**National Association for Sport
and Physical Education**
1900 Association Drive
Reston, VA 20191
(703) 476-3410
website (to support the availability of quality
sports physical education programs in schools):
www.aahperd.org/naspe/naspe.html

**National Association of Governors' Councils
on Physical Fitness and Sports**
201 S. Capitol Avenue, Suite 560
Indianapolis, IN 46225
(317) 237-5630

National Bicycle and Pedestrian Clearinghouse
1506 21st Street, NW, Suite 210
Washington, DC 20036
(800) 760-6272

National Coalition for Promoting Physical Activity
P.O. Box 1440
Indianapolis, IN 46206-1440
(317) 637-9200

National Gardening Association
180 Flynn Avenue
Burlington, VT 05401
(802) 863-1308

National Recreation and Park Association
P.O. Box 6287
Arlington, VA 22206
(800) 626-6772

National Strength & Conditioning Association
P.O. Box 38909
Colorado Springs, CO 80937-8909
(719) 632-6722
fax: (719) 632-6367
website: www.colosoft.com/nsca/menu.htm

National Youth Sports Safety Foundation
3335 Longwood Avenue, Suite 202
Boston, MA 02115
(617) 277-1171

Shape Up America!
6707 Democracy Boulevard, Suite 306
Bethesda, MD 20817
(301) 493-5368
website: www.shapeup.org/sua/index.html

Sierra Club
85 Second Street, 2nd Floor
San Francisco, CA 94105
(415) 977-5500
website: www.sierraclub.org

Sporting Goods Manufacturers Association
200 Castlewood Drive
North Palm Beach, FL 33408-5696
(561) 842-4100

U.S. Disabled Athletes Fund, Inc.
2015 South Park Place, Suite 180
Atlanta, GA 30339
(770) 850-8199

United States Water Fitness Association, Inc.
P.O. Box 3279
Boynton Beach, FL 33424
(561) 732-9908
fax: (561) 732-0950
website: www.emi.net/~uswfa/

Walkable Communities
320 South Main Street
High Springs, FL 32643
(904) 454-3304

Wellness Councils of America
7101 Newport Avenue, Suite 311
Omaha, NE 68152
(402) 572-3590

Young Men's Christian Association (YMCA)
101 N. Wacker Drive
Chicago, IL 60606
(312) 977-0031

Young Women's Christian Association (YWCA)
726 Broadway
New York, NY 10003
(212) 614-2700

Walking/hiking websites
http://walking.miningco.com
http://www.webwalking.com/hiking.html
http://www.ava.org

Menus for You

Need a little structure to kick off your weight loss? Use this plan to create your own low-fat days (it's adapted from an article I wrote for a 1998 issue of *Family Circle*). For each, fat comes to about 20 percent of calories. You've got thousands of possible combinations with these 10 breakfasts, 10 lunches, 10 dinners, 10 high-calcium snacks, and 10 snack snacks. If your daily menu is based on three of these meals and one each of the two types of snacks, you'll average about 1,400 calories—for most of you, dropping calories any lower will slow your metabolism. Or use the meals as models, substituting similar foods that you like better. The main thing is to keep the fat level low.

Here's how to make the most of this plan:

- If you're exercising regularly, 1,400 is almost certainly too low (you'll know if you're hungry and/or losing more than two to four pounds the first week and more than $1^1/_2$ pounds per week starting at the third week). Either add another snack or slightly increase portions in the meals until you no longer feel hungry and are losing weight at an appropriate rate.

- Take a standard multivitamin/mineral tablet along with this plan. Although these meals are high in nutrients, it's hard to get all your vitamins and minerals on anything under 2,000 calories.

- Make sure you get at least one of the high-calcium snacks daily (if you are lactose intolerant, substitute nonfat Lactaid milk or calcium-fortified nonfat or low-fat soy milk). Your other snack can come from either the high-calcium list or the other snacks list.

- If you've got a sweet tooth, check out the "Tiny Treats" box in Chapter 10 for sweet nearly-nothin's you can slip in daily.

Ten breakfasts, averaging 335 calories

In these recipes and the ones that follow I usually don't mention salt and pepper. Season to taste.

1. $1/2$ large whole grain bagel with 1 Tbsp. cream cheese.

   $1/2$ pink grapefruit.

   1 cup skim milk (plain or as part of a coffee).

2. 2 whole-grain waffles topped with $1/2$ cup nonfat vanilla yogurt and $3/4$ cup strawberries.

3. 1 cup bran cereal flakes with 1 sliced banana and 1 cup skim milk.

4. Crispy french toast: 2 slices oven-baked whole wheat bread. Mix 1 egg with 2 Tbsp. skim milk and $1/4$ tsp. each vanilla and cinnamon. Soak 2 slices bread in egg mixture. Either bake on a vegetable oil–sprayed cookie sheet at 350° for

10 to 12 minutes OR grill on a heavy bottomed, nonstick skillet sprayed with vegetable oil over medium heat. Cook for 2 minutes, flip, and cook another minute. Top with $3/4$ cup berries of your choice.

1 cup skim milk (plain or as part of a coffee).

5. Toasted whole grain English muffin with 1 tsp. of butter.

   $3/4$ cup orange juice.

   1 cup skim milk (plain or as part of a coffee drink).

6. 1 cup cooked oatmeal topped with a sliced apple sprinkled with cinnamon.

   1 cup skim milk (part with the oatmeal, rest in cup).

7. Mushroom scrambled eggs: In a nonstick skillet sautée $1/3$ cup sliced mushrooms in 1 tsp. canola oil. Add one egg and one egg white, scramble).

   2 slices whole wheat toast with 1 tsp. butter

   $1/2$ cup calcium-enriched orange juice.

8. 2 buckwheat pancakes (about four-in. diameter) topped with 1 Tbsp. syrup and $3/4$ cup blueberries (or fruit of your choice).

   1 cup skim milk (plain or as part of a coffee).

9. Tomato-feta omelet: Combine 1 egg and 1 egg white and 1 tsp. water. Cook omelet in 1 Tbsp. canola oil; fill with $1/2$ a tomato, diced, and 1 Tbsp. crumbled feta.

   1 slice whole grain toast with a tsp. of butter or soft margarine.

   1 cup of skim milk (plain or as part of a coffee).

10. Small bran muffin (approx. $2^3/_4$-in. diameter, $1^1/_2$-in. high)

    $3/_4$ cup strawberries.

    1 cup skim milk (plain or as part of a coffee).

Ten lunches averaging 345 calories

1. Smoked salmon sandwich: Smoked salmon (2 oz.), watercress ($1/_4$ cup), and sun-dried tomato (3 slices) on whole wheat.

   $1^1/_2$ cups fruit salad.

2. Spinach salad with turkey, apple, and blue cheese: Toss 3 cups spinach with $1^1/_2$ tsp. each olive oil and lemon juice, top with 1 cup chopped apple, 1 oz. smoked turkey, and 2 Tbsp. crumbled blue cheese.

   1 slice crusty whole grain bread.

3. Bean burrito with salsa and 1 Tbsp. shredded cheddar (approx. $1/_2$ cup refried beans, flour tortilla).

   small vegetable salad with 2 Tbsp. dressing.

4. Bean and tuna salad: Combine $1/_2$ cup canned, rinsed white beans with $1/_4$ cup drained tuna in water, a sliced tomato, $1/_2$ sliced red pepper, $1^1/_2$ tsp. olive oil, 1 tsp. lemon juice, 1 to 2 tsp. chopped fresh basil or $1/_2$ tsp. dried. Serve with a rye cracker.

5. Curried garbanzo couscous: In $1^1/_2$ tsp. olive oil, sautée 2 Tbsp. onion, add $1/_2$ a chopped green pepper, $1/_3$ cup canned, rinsed garbanzo beans, and $1/_2$ tsp. curry powder. Heat a few minutes, adding water if needed. Serve with $3/_4$ cup cooked couscous (cook using no more than $1/_2$ tsp. butter or oil).

Yogurt/cucumber raita: Combine $1/3$ cup plain, nonfat yogurt with $1/4$ cup finely diced cucumber and $1/4$ tsp. dried mint.

6. Peanut butter ($1^1/2$ Tbsp.) and jelly (2 tsp.) sandwich.

   1 carrot.

   1 red pepper, sliced.

7. Salad bar special: $1/3$ cup garbanzo or other beans, $1^1/2$ cup plain greens, 1 Tbsp. chopped egg or shredded cheese, 1 cup broccoli or other chopped vegetable, 1 Tbsp. regular dressing or 2 Tbsp. reduced-cal dressing

   2 slices whole grain bread.

8. Lentil or minestrone soup ($1^1/2$ cups).

   small green salad topped with 2 tsp. regular dressing or 4 tsp. diet dressing.

   7 crispbread crackers (fat free).

   1 cup grapes.

9. Chicken wrap, weighing approximately 9 oz. (3 oz. chicken, salsa, grilled and/or fresh vegetables).

10. Grilled low-fat cheese ($1^1/2$ oz.) and sliced tomato sandwich on whole wheat.

    1 cup fruit salad.

Ten dinners averaging 440 calories

1. Convenience dinner: 280 to 300 cal light frozen dinner containing chicken, fish, or beef with rice or pasta.

   vegetables crudites (2 cups vegetable sticks) dipped in 2 Tbsp. Ranch dressing.

2. Seafood risotto with steamed zucchini risotto (makes two servings): Heat $1^1/2$ tsp. olive oil in

a heavy-bottomed skillet (preferably nonstick); sautée $1/3$ cup chopped onion or shallot, $1/2$ clove garlic. Reduce heat to medium, stir in $1/2$ cup Arborio rice or short grain rice and $1/4$ cup white wine, cook 30 seconds. Add $1/2$ cup hot chicken broth, stir occasionally until absorbed. Gradually add another cup of broth, stirring in $1/3$ cup at a time until each addition is absorbed. This should take 20 to 25 minutes. Add 4 oz. frozen cooked shrimp, 4 oz. crabmeat or canned minced clams, and $1/2$ cup frozen peas with last $1/3$ cup of broth until rice is tender on the outside, a little crunchy on the inside. Sprinkle with 1 tsp. parmesan. 1 zucchini, steamed, sliced open lengthwise, with a spritz of fresh lemon juice and salt and pepper to taste.

3. Middle Eastern kabobs: Combine $3^1/2$ oz. ground sirloin with 1 tsp. each chopped parsley and minced green onions and a pinch of allspice. Shape into four balls and thread on a skewer. Grill meatballs for 8 minutes, until cooked all the way through, turning once.

   Minty chopped salad: Combine one chopped tomato, $1/2$ cup chopped cucumber, 1 to 2 tsp. fresh mint or $1/2$ tsp. dried, 1 tsp. olive oil, $1/2$ tsp. lemon juice, and $1/2$ cup frozen yogurt.

4. One-dish pasta dinner: To $1^1/3$ cups hot cooked ziti, macaroni or other short pasta add 3 oz. cooked skinless chicken breast or drained water packed, 1 cup fresh or frozen vegetables sautéed in $1^1/2$ tsp. olive oil (broccoli, cauliflower, rapini, work well). Add $1/2$ cup chopped fresh juicy tomatoes, 1 to 2 tsp. fresh chopped basil, or $1/2$ to 1 tsp. dried. 1 Tbsp. low-fat plain yogurt and salt and pepper to taste.

5. Shrimp fettucini: Heat $1/3$ cup marinara sauce, add 3 oz. cooked frozen shrimp, and simmer about two minutes. Combine with 1 cup cooked fettucini; top with 1 Tbsp. parmesan.

   Salad: 2 cups mixed greens and $1/2$ cup sliced cucumber.

   Tangerine.

6. Grilled grouper (or another fish of your choice) on gingered greens. Combine 1 Tbsp. fresh lemon juice, 2 tsp. reduced sodium soy sauce, $1/2$ tsp. sesame oil, and 2 Tbsp. fresh orange juice in a resealable plastic bag or shallow bowl. Add a 5 oz. raw grouper fillet (or another fish of your choice) and marinate 15 minutes. In a small nonstick skillet, heat canola oil over medium heat. Add 2 tsp. finely minced fresh ginger, stir for 30 seconds, add a thinly sliced carrot, sautée for 3 minutes, then add 1 cup roughly torn arugula or spinach leaves. Sautée until wilted, turn off heat, add two Tbsp. fresh orange juice. Meanwhile broil or grill the grouper until opaque all the way through (about 8 minutes total). Serve over greens.

   $1/2$ cup rice.

   $1/3$ cup frozen yogurt with 2 tsp. chocolate syrup.

7. Burger: Grill a 4-oz. raw ground sirloin patty until cooked through. Serve on a hamburger bun with mustard and/or catsup.

   Coleslaw for two (have half): Toss $1^1/2$ cups shredded cabbage and a shredded carrot, 3 Tbsp. light mayo, $1/2$ tsp. vinegar, $1/8$ tsp. sugar, and a few drops of Worcestershire sauce.

   Frozen juice bar (70 cal).

8. All-bean chili dinner (either use about 1 cup canned or make your own): Chili for three (have ¹/₃ of recipe): In 1 Tbsp. olive oil sautée 1 chopped onion with 1 chopped green pepper about 3 minutes, add 2 cloves minced garlic, sautée another 2 minutes. Add ¹/₂ tsp. ground cumin, 1 Tbsp. chili powder, and ¹/₂ tsp. dried oregano. Add 2 cups canned pinto or kidney beans, rinsed and drained, and ¹/₂ cup water and cook for about 15 minutes, adding water as needed. Garnish with chopped fresh cilantro.

³/₄ cup rice.

1 cup sliced strawberries.

9. Carry-out roasted chicken dinner: Chicken with skin removed—whole leg or whole breast.

2 cups steamed vegetables with a spritz of lemon.

1 slice garlic bread (four-in.-long slice of Italian bread brushed with 1 tsp. olive oil, sprinkled with garlic salt and pepper).

Tangerine.

10. Rosemary white beans and sausage: Beans (serves two, have half): In a tsp. of olive oil, sautée a small chopped onion, and a minced clove of garlic. Add 1¹/₂ cups of canned, rinsed white beans, rinsed and drained, scant tsp. fresh chopped rosemary or scant ¹/₂ tsp. dried, ¹/₂ tsp. dried thyme, and 2 Tbsp. white wine; simmer five minutes, adding water if necessary. Slice a 3 oz. link of turkey sausage, pan fry (no oil), and cook through, about eight minutes.

Slice of whole grain crusty bread.

Small green salad with 1 Tbsp. reduced-fat Italian dressing.

Ten high-calcium snacks averaging 110 calories, 235 mg calcium

1. $1/2$ cup nonfat or low-fat vanilla, lemon, or coffee yogurt.

2. Skim milk latté with 1 tsp. sugar.

3. Strawberry yogurt shake: In a blender combine: $1/4$ cup low-fat strawberry yogurt, $1/2$ cup skim milk, $1/4$ cup strawberries.

4. Low-fat nachos: 3 Tbsp. grated low-fat (no more than 5 g fat per oz.) cheddar, jack, or Jarslberg melted over seven baked tortilla chips garnished with salsa.

5. 4 rye crisp crackers (no fat) and 1 oz. reduced-fat (no more than 5 g per oz.) cheddar, Jarlsberg, or other cheese.

6. Parmesan popcorn (2 cups air-popped popcorn mixed with 2 Tbsp. grated parmesan cheese).

7. 1 to 2 cups vegetables dipped in $1/3$ cup yogurt dip. Dip: Put a cup of nonfat yogurt in a small strainer lined with a coffee filter. Let drip into a bowl in the fridge for at least an hour. Remove $1/3$ cup, add a dash of garlic salt, and 1 tsp. chopped parsley.

8. Skim milk hot chocolate: Add 2 tsp. chocolate syrup to 1 cup hot skim milk.

9. Orange creamsicle shake: Blend 2 ice cubes, $1/2$ cup calcium-enriched orange juice, $1/3$ cup 1% milk, 1 tsp. sugar, and $1/4$ tsp. vanilla extract.

10. Orange soda: 1 cup calcium-fortified orange juice with $3/4$ cup sparkling water.

Ten snacks averaging 150 calories

1. $^3/_4$ cup applesauce (125 cal).

2. Breakfast or snack bar (check label for no more than 150 cal and 3 g fat and at least 2 g fiber).

3. $1^1/_2$ oz. baked tortilla chips (about 30 chips), plain or with salsa.

4. 5 to 6 cups air-popped popcorn (check labels carefully of microwave popcorn for no more than 5 g fat per 5 cups (Pop Secret 94 Percent Fat Free Butter, 94 Percent Fat Free Natural, and Butter Flavor Light, or Orville Redenbacher's Smart Pop make the grade).

5. 1 to $1^1/_2$ oz. of pretzels.

6. $^3/_4$ cup cereal (check labels, should come to about 110 cal per cup, so this excludes most granolas) with $^3/_4$ cup milk.

7. 2 graham cracker rectangles, each spread with $^1/_2$ tsp. peanut butter and $^1/_2$ tsp. honey.

8. 2 to 4 whole grain crackers (check labels for no more than 3 g fat per oz.) with 1 oz. low-fat (no more than 5 g fat per oz.) cheese.

9. Any 2 fruits (here's an elegant option: Combine a sliced ripe mango with $^1/_2$ cup of raspberries).

10. $^1/_4$ of a six-in whole wheat pita dipped in $^1/_4$ cup hummos (hummos is a Middle Eastern spread make of garbanzo beans, tahini (sesame paste), fresh lemon juice, and garlic).

Fast-Food Fat and Calorie Counts

Here's a fat and calorie breakdown of the menus of some of the most familiar fast-food chains.

SUBWAY

Menu Item	Calorie Content	Fat Content (in grams)
6" Cold Subs (One standard sandwich includes: wheat bread, meat/poultry or seafood, onions, lettuce, tomatoes, pickles, green peppers, and olives.)		
Veggie Delite™	237	3
Turkey Breast	289	4
Turkey Breast and Ham	295	5
Ham	302	5
Roast Beef	303	5
Subway Club®	312	5
*Subway Seafood and Crab® (a processed seafood and crab blend)	347	10
B.L.T.	327	10
Cold Cut Trio	378	13
*Tuna	391	15
Subway Seafood and Crab® (a processed seafood and crab blend)	430	19

473

Menu Item	Calorie Content	Fat Content (in grams)
Classic Italian B.M.T.®	460	22
Tuna	542	32
6" Hot Subs		
Roasted Chicken Breast	348	6
Steak and Cheese	398	10
**Subway Melt®	382	12
Meatball	419	16
**Chicken Taco Sub	436	16
**Pizza Sub	464	22

Deli-Style Sandwiches (Standard deli-style sandwiches include: deli style roll, meat/poultry or seafood, onions, lettuce, tomatoes, pickles, green peppers, and olives.)

Turkey Breast	235	4
Ham	234	4
Roast Beef	245	4
*Tuna	279	9
Bologna	292	12
Tuna	354	18

Salads (Standard salad includes: meat/poultry or seafood, onions, lettuce, tomatoes, pickles, green peppers, and olives. Values do not include dressing.)

Veggie Delite™	51	1
Turkey Breast	102	2
Subway Club®	126	3
Roast Beef	117	3
Ham	116	3
Turkey Breast and Ham	109	3
Roasted Chicken Breast	162	4
*Subway Seafood and Crab®	161	8
**Steak and Cheese	212	8
B.L.T.	140	8
**Subway Melt™	195	10
Cold Cut Trio	191	11
*Tuna	205	13
**Chicken Taco	250	14
Meatball	233	14

Menu Item	Calorie Content	Fat Content (in grams)
Subway Seafood and Crab®	244	17
**Pizza	277	13
Tuna	356	30
Bread Bowl	330	4
Salad Dressings (Serving size = 1 Tbsp. One 2 oz. packet of dressing contains approximately four servings.)		
Creamy Italian	65	6
Fat-Free Italian	5	0
French	65	5
Fat-Free French	15	0
Thousand Island	65	6
Ranch	87	9
Fat Free Ranch	12	0
Condiments and Extras (Values given are for suggested serving size only.)		
Vinegar (1 tsp.)	1	0
Mustard (2 tsp.)	8	0
Light Mayonnaise (1 tsp.)	18	2
Bacon (2 slices)	45	4
Cheese (2 triangles)	41	3
Mayonnaise (1 tsp.)	37	4
Olive Oil Blend (1 tsp.)	45	5
Cookies (Serving size = 1 cookie.)		
Oatmeal Raisin	200	8
Chocolate Chunk	210	10
Chocolate Chip	210	10
Chocolate Chip M&M®	210	10
Peanut Butter	220	12
Sugar	230	12
White Chocolate Macadamia Nut	230	12
Double Chocolate Brazil Nut	130	12

* Made with light mayonnaise

** Indicates that value includes cheese or condiments.

Extra toppings are available on request, not included in the fat and calorie counts given above.

(Source: A Guide to Subway Nutrition, 1997)

BURGER KING

Menu Item	Calorie Content	Fat Content (in grams)
Burgers		
Whopper	640	39
Whopper w/Cheese	730	46
Double Whopper	870	56
Double Whopper w/Cheese	960	63
Whopper Jr.	420	24
Whopper Jr. w/Cheese	460	28
Big King	660	43
Hamburger	330	15
Cheeseburger	380	19
Double Cheeseburger	600	36
Double Cheeseburger w/Bacon	640	39
Sandwiches/Side Orders		
BK Big Fish	720	43
BK Broiler Chicken	530	26
Chicken Sandwich	710	43
Chicken Tenders (8 pieces)	350	22
*Broiled Chicken Salad	190	8
*Garden Salad	100	5
*Side Salad	60	3
French Fries (medium, salted)	400	21
Onion Rings	310	14
Dutch Apple Pie	300	15
Drinks		
Vanilla Shake (medium)	300	6
Chocolate Shake (medium)	320	7
Chocolate Shake (medium, syrup added)	440	7
Strawberry Shake (medium, syrup added)	420	6
Coca Cola® Classic (medium)	280	0
Diet Coke® (medium)	1	0
Sprite® (medium)	260	0
Tropicana® Orange Juice	311	0
Coffee	5	0
Milk (2% low fat)	130	5

Menu Item	Calorie Content	Fat Content (in grams)
Breakfast		
Croissan'wich w/Sausage, Egg, Cheese	550	42
Croissan'wich w/Sausage, Cheese	450	35
Biscuit	330	18
Biscuit w/Egg	420	24
Biscuit w/Sausage	530	36
Biscuit w/Bacon, Egg, Cheese	510	31
French Toast Sticks	500	27
Hash Browns (small)	240	15

* Without dressing

Calorie and fat totals do not include the value of additional condiments.

(Source: Burger King Nutritional Information, Burger King Corporation, 1996)

MCDONALDS

Menu Item	Calorie Content	Fat Content (in grams)
Sandwiches		
Hamburger	260	9
Cheeseburger	320	13
Quarter Pounder	420	21
Quarter Pounder w/Cheese	530	30
Big Mac	560	31
Arch Deluxe	550	31
Arch Deluxe with Bacon	590	34
Crispy Chicken Deluxe	500	25
Fish Filet Deluxe	560	28
Filet-o-Fish	450	25
Grilled Chicken Deluxe	440	20
Grilled Chicken Deluxe (plain, w/o mayo)	300	5
French Fries		
Small	210	10
Medium	450	22
Large	540	26

Menu Item	Calorie Content	Fat Content (in grams)
Chicken McNuggets/Sauces (Sauce serving size, 1 pkg.)		
4-piece	190	11
6-piece	290	17
9 piece	430	26
Hot Mustard	60	$3^1/_2$
Barbeque	45	0
Sweet 'N Sour	50	0
Honey	45	0
Honey Mustard	50	$4^1/_2$
Light Mayonnaise	40	5
Salads (w/o dressing.)		
Garden Salad	35	0
Grilled Chicken Salad Deluxe	120	$1^1/_2$
Salad Dressings/Toppings (Serving size, 1 pkg.)		
Croutons	50	$1^1/_2$
Caesar Dressing	160	14
Fat Free Herb Vinaigrette	50	0
Ranch	230	21
Red French Reduced Calorie	160	8
Breakfast		
Egg McMuffin	290	12
Sausage McMuffin	360	23
Sausage McMuffin w/Egg	440	28
English Muffin	140	2
Sausage Biscuit	470	31
Sausage Biscuit w/Egg	550	37
Bacon, Egg, and Cheese Biscuit	470	28
Biscuit	290	15
Sausage	170	16
Scrambled Eggs (2)	160	11
Hash Browns	130	8
Hotcakes (plain)	310	60
Hotcakes (two pats margarine and syrup)	570	16
Breakfast Burrito	320	20

Menu Item	Calorie Content	Fat Content (in grams)
Muffins/Danish		
Low-fat Apple Bran Muffin	300	30
Apple Danish	360	16
Cheese Danish	410	22
Cinnamon Roll	390	18
Desserts/Shakes		
Vanilla Reduced-Fat Ice-Cream Cone	150	$4^1/_2$
Strawberry Sundae	290	7
Hot Caramel Sundae	360	10
Hot Fudge Sundae	340	12
Nuts (for Sundaes)	40	$3^1/_2$
Baked Apple Pie	260	13
Chocolate Chip Cookie	170	10
McDonaldland Cookies (1 pkg.)	180	5
Shakes (small, all flavors)	80	9
Milk/Juices		
1% Low-fat Milk (8 fl. oz.)	100	$2^1/_2$
Orange Juice (6 fl. oz.)	80	0

BOSTON MARKET

Menu Item	Calorie Content	Fat Content (in grams)
Entrees		
$1/_4$ White Meat Chicken (w/o skin or wing)	160	$3^1/_2$
$1/_4$ White Meat Chicken (w/skin)	330	17
$1/_4$ Dark Meat Chicken (w/o skin)	210	10
$1/_4$ Dark Meat Chicken (w/skin)	330	22
$1/_2$ Chicken (w/skin)	630	37
Skinless Rotisserie Turkey Breast	170	1
Ham with Cinnamon Apples	350	13
Meat Loaf and Chunky Tomato Sauce	370	18
Meat Loaf and Brown Gravy	300	22
Original Chicken Pot Pie	750	34
Chunky Chicken Salad	370	27

Menu Item	Calorie Content	Fat Content (in grams)
Soup, Salad, and Sandwiches		
Caesar Salad Entree	520	43
Caesar Salad w/o Dressing	240	13
Chicken Caesar Salad	670	47
Chicken Soup	80	3
Chicken Tortilla Soup	220	11
Chicken Sandwich w/Cheese and Sauce	750	33
Chicken Sandwich w/oCheese or Sauce	430	$4^1/_2$
Chicken Salad Sandwich	680	30
Turkey Sandwich w/Cheese and Sauce	710	28
Turkey Sandwich w/o Cheese or Sauce	400	$3^1/_2$
Ham Sandwich w/Cheese and Sauce	760	35
Ham Sandwich w/o Cheese or Sauce	450	9
Meat Loaf Sandwich w/Cheese	860	33
Meat Loaf Sandwich w/o Cheese	690	21
Ham and Turkey Club Sandwich w/Cheese and Sauce	890	44
Ham and Turkey Club Sandwich w/o Cheese or Sauce	430	6
Hot Side Dishes		
Steamed Vegetables	35	$1/_2$
New Potatoes	130	$2^1/_2$
Whole Kernel Corn	180	4
Zucchini Marinara	80	4
Mashed Potatoes	180	8
Homestyle Mashed Potatoes and Gravy	200	9
Chicken Gravy	15	1
Rice Pilaf	180	5
Creamed Spinach	280	21
Stuffing	310	12
Butternut Squash	160	6
Macaroni and Cheese	280	10
BBQ Baked Beans	330	9
Hot Cinnamon Apples	250	$4^1/_2$
Green Bean Casserole	90	$4^1/_2$

Menu Item	Calorie Content	Fat Content (in grams)
Cold Side Dishes		
Fruit Salad	70	$1/2$
Mediterranean Pasta Salad	170	10
Cranberry Relish	370	5
Cole Slaw	280	16
Tortellini Salad	380	24
Caesar Side Salad	210	17
Baked Goods		
Corn Bread (1 loaf)	200	6
Oatmeal Raisin Cookie (1 cookie)	320	13
Chocolate Chip Cookie (1 cookie)	340	17
Brownie (1 cookie)	450	27
Honey Wheat Roll ($1/2$ roll)	150	$1 1/2$

Brand Name Calorie, Fat, and Fiber Counts

This table presents a selected list of brand-name foods found on the shelves of most major supermarkets and provides the fat, caloric, and fiber content of a serving of each. While this is not intended to be an exhaustive list, it will give you an idea of what's in those familiar brands you've been eating, and how similar foods compare with one another on the fat, calorie, and fiber fronts.

BRAND NAME	SERVING SIZE	CALORIES	FAT (G)	FIBER (G)
Breads and Rolls				
Sahara Regular White Pita Pockets	1 loaf	150	1	1
Sahara Regular Whole Wheat Pita Pockets	1 loaf	130	1	5
Pepperidge Farm 100% Whole Wheat	1 slice	60	1	1
Wonder 100% Stone-ground Whole Wheat	1 slice	80	$1^1/_2$	2

BRAND NAME	SERVING SIZE	CALORIES	FAT (G)	FIBER (G)
Candy				
Hershey's Hugs	8 pieces	210	12	0
Hershey's Chocolate Kisses	8 pieces	210	12	1
Hershey's Kisses w/Almonds	8 pieces	210	13	1
Hershey's Milk Chocolate Bar	1 bar	230	13	1
Hershey's Milk Chocolate w/Almonds	1 bar	230	14	1
Hershey's Sweet Escape Caramel and Peanut Butter	1 bar	150	5	<1
Milky Way, Dark	1 bar	220	8	1
Milky Way miniatures	5 pieces	190	7	0
Reese's Peanut Butter Cup	2 cups	240	14	1
Skittles Fruit Chews Original	1/4 cup	170	2	0
Starburst Fruit Chews Original	8 pieces	160	4	0
M&M's, Plain	1/4 cup	210	9	1
M&M's, Peanut	1/3 cup	220	11	1
Baby Ruth Bar	1 bar	280	12	2
Baby Ruth, King Size	1/3 bar	170	8	1
Butterfinger Bar	1 bar	280	11	1
Butterfinger, King Size	1/3 bar	170	7	0
Cookies and Crackers				
Animal Crackers	9 crackers	90	2	0
Archway Apple Filled	1 cookie	110	3	0
Archway Fat Free Granola	2 cookies	100	0	1
Archway Windmill Cookies	1 cookie	100	4	0
Frookie 50% Less Fat Chocolate Sandwich Cremes	3 cookies	130	4	0

BRAND NAME	SERVING SIZE	CALORIES	FAT (G)	FIBER (G)
Keebler E. L. Fudge Double Fudge	2 cookies	130	6	<1
Keebler Reduced Fat Fudge Stripe	3 cookies	130	4	0
Keebler Oatmeal Cookies	1 cookie	80	$3^1/_2$	<1
Keebler Club Crackers	5 crackers	80	4	0
Keebler 50% Reduced Sodium Club Crackers	4 crackers	70	3	<1
Pepperidge Farm Brussels	3 cookies	150	7	1
Pepperidge Farm Milano	3 cookies	180	10	<1
Pepperidge Farm Soft Baked Chocolate Chunk	1 cookie	130	6	2
Sunshine Ginger Snaps	7 cookies	130	4	<1
Sunshine Cheez-It Reduced Fat crackers	29 crackers	140	4	<1
Devonsheer Garlic Melba Rounds	5 rounds	60	$1^1/_2$	1
Devonsheer Plain Melba Rounds	5 rounds	50	0	1
Devonsheer Sesame Melba Rounds	5 rounds	60	$2^1/_2$	1
Wasa Fiber Rye	1 slice	30	1	2
Wasa Hearty Rye	1 slice	45	0	2
Wasa Lite Rye	1 slice	25	0	1
Wasa Sourdough Rye	1 slice	35	0	1
Rice, Wheat, Corn, and Rye Cakes				
Orville Redenbacher's Butter Mini Cakes	8 cakes	60	1	1
Quaker Apple Cinnamon Rice Cakes	1 cake	50	0	0
Quaker Butter Popped Corn Cakes	1 cake	35	0	0
Quaker White Cheddar Mini Rice Cakes	6 cakes	50	0	1

BRAND NAME	SERVING SIZE	CALORIES	FAT (G)	FIBER (G)
Butter				
Land O'Lakes Light Quarters	1 Tbsp.	50	6	0
Land O'Lakes Light Whipped	1 Tbsp.	35	4	0
Land O'Lakes Unsalted	1 Tbsp.	100	11	0
Margarine				
Country Morning Blend, Unsalted	1 Tbsp.	100	11	0
Country Morning Blend Light, Soft	1 Tbsp.	50	6	0
Promise Ultra Fat Free Soft	1 Tbsp.	5	0	0
Sour Cream				
Breakstone Sour Cream	2 Tbsp.	60	5	0
Breakstone Fat Free Sour Cream Substitute	2 Tbsp.	35	0	0
Cakes, Pastries, and Pies				
Pillsbury Thick 'n Fudgy Cheesecake Swirl Brownie	$1/16$ pkg.	170	9	<1
Pillsbury Thick 'n Fudgy Chocolate Brownie	$1/16$ pkg.	150	9	<1
Entenmann's Almond Topped Coffee Cake	$1/8$ cake	180	9	1
Entenmann's Reduced Fat Butter Loaf	$1/8$ loaf	140	4	0
Entenmann's Reduced Fat Chocolate Crumb Cake	$1/8$ cake	140	$2^1/2$	2
Sara Lee Reduced Fat Pound Cake	$1/4$ cake	280	11	<1
Cake Mixes				
Betty Crocker Sweet Rewards Devil's Food Reduced Fat (no cholesterol)	$1/12$ cake	210	6	1
Duncan Hines Angel Food Cake	$1/12$ cake	130	0	0

BRAND NAME	SERVING SIZE	CALORIES	FAT (G)	FIBER (G)
Duncan Hines Devil's Food (no cholesterol)	$1/12$ cake	280	15	1
Entenmann's Reduced Fat Cinnamon Buns	1 bun	190	4	1
Hostess Iced Honey Buns	1 bun	390	20	<1
Kellogg's Blueberry Pop Tarts	1 pastry	210	7	1
Kellogg's Low Fat Blueberry	1 pastry	190	3	1
Kellogg's Frosted Chocolate Fudge	1 pastry	200	5	1
Kellogg's Low Fat Frosted Chocolate Fudge	1 pastry	190	3	1
Cereals (Ready to Eat)				
Alpen Muesli	$1/3$ cup	200	3	4
Familia Muesli No Added Sugar	$1/2$ cup	200	3	5
Familia Regular Swiss Mixed	$1/2$ cup	210	3	5
General Mills Cheerios	1 cup	110	2	3
General Mills Cheerios Multigrain	1 cup	110	1	3
General Mills Fiber One	$1/2$ cup	60	1	13
General Mills Raisin Nut Bran	$3/4$ cup	210	4	5
General Mills Total Corn Flakes	$1 1/3$ cups	110	$1/2$	0
General Mills Total Raisin Bran	1 cup	180	1	5
Health Valley Organic Oat Bran Flakes	$3/4$ cup	100	0	4
Kashi Medley	$1/2$ cup	100	1	2
Kellogg's Bite Size Frosted Mini Wheats	1 cup	180	1	5
Kellogg's Cocoa Krispies	$3/4$ cup	120	1	0
Kellogg's Corn Flakes	1 cup	100	0	1

BRAND NAME	SERVING SIZE	CALORIES	FAT (G)	FIBER (G)
Kellogg's Cracklin' Oat Bran	$3/4$ cup	190	6	6
Kellogg's Frosted Mini Wheats	1 cup	180	1	5
Kellogg's Raisin Bran	1 cup	200	$1^1/_2$	5
Kelloggs Special K	1 cup	110	0	1
Kretschmer Wheat Germ	2 Tbsp.	50	1	2
Post 100% Bran	$1/2$ cup	80	1	2
Post Grape-Nuts	$1/2$ cup	200	1	5
Post Grape-Nuts Flakes	$3/4$ cup	100	1	3
Post Honeycomb	$1^1/_3$ cup	110	0	<1
Post Natural Bran Flakes	1 cup	90	$1/2$	6
Post Shredded Wheat'n Bran	$1^1/_4$ cups	200	1	8
Post Spoon Size Shredded Wheat	1 cup	170	$1/2$	5
Quaker 100% Natural Honey Raisin	$1/2$ cup	230	9	3
Quaker 100% Natural Low Fat w/Raisins	$2/3$ cup	210	3	3
Quaker Cap'N Crunch	$3/4$ cup	110	$1^1/_2$	1
Cheese, Cheese Products, and Cheese Substitutes				
Alpine Lace Fat Free Cheese Product	1 oz.	45	0	0
Cracker Barrel Sharp Light	1 oz.	80	5	0
Philadelphia Brand $1/3$ Less Fat Cream Cheese	2 Tbsp.	70	5	0
Laughing Cow Reduced Calorie Wedge	1 oz.	50	3	0
Cocoa Mixes				
Swiss Miss Fat Free	8 fl. oz.	50	0	<1
Swiss Miss Lite	8 fl. oz.	70	0	2
Swiss Miss Milk Chocolate	8 fl. oz.	140	3	<1

BRAND NAME	SERVING SIZE	CALORIES	FAT (G)	FIBER (G)
Ice Cream and Frozen Treats				
Betty Crocker Healthy Temptations Low Fat Ice Cream Sandwich	1 sandwich	80	$1^1/_2$	0
Good Humor Choco Taco	1 bar	310	17	1
Good Humor Chocolate Eclair	1 bar	170	9	1
Good Humor Fat Free Fudgsicle	1 bar	60	0	<1
Häagen-Dazs Raspberry Vanilla	1 bar	90	0	0
Klondike Original	1 bar	290	20	0
Klondike Reduced Fat No Sugar Added	1 bar	190	10	<1
Popsicle (Cherry, Orange, Grape)	1 pop	45	0	0
Popsicle Sugar Free (Cherry Orange, Grape)	1 pop	15	0	0
Edy's Fat Free Black Cherry Vanilla Swirl Frozen Yogurt	$1/_2$ cup	90	0	0
Edy's Fat Free Caramel Praline Crunch Frozen Yogurt	$1/_2$ cup	100	0	0
Edy's Fat Free Chocolate Frozen Yogurt	$1/_2$ cup	90	0	1
Häagen-Dazs Fat Free Chocolate Frozen Yogurt	$1/_2$ cup	140	0	<1
Häagen-Dazs Fat Free Vanilla Frozen Yogurt	$1/_2$ cup	140	0	0
Kemp's Fat Free Strawberry Frozen Yogurt	$1/_2$ cup	90	0	0
Kemp's Fat Free Vanilla Frozen Yogurt	$1/_2$ cup	100	0	0
Ben and Jerry's Cherry Garcia	$1/_2$ cup	240	16	0
Ben and Jery's Chunky Monkey	$1/_2$ cup	280	18	1

BRAND NAME	SERVING SIZE	CALORIES	FAT (G)	FIBER (G)
Edy's Fat Free Chocolate Fudge Ice Cream	1/2 cup	100	0	1
Edy's Fat Free Vanilla Ice Cream	1/2 cup	90	0	0
Edy's Grand Butter Pecan	1/2 cup	160	19	10
Edy's Grand French Vanilla	1/2 cup	160	10	0
Edy's Grand No Sugar Added Fat Free Vanilla Ice Cream	1/2 cup	80	0	0
Häagen-Dazs Butter Pecan Ice Cream	1/2 cup	320	24	<1
Häagen-Dazs Chocolate Ice Cream	1/2 cup	270	18	1
Häagen-Dazs Raspberry Sorbet and Vanilla	1/2 cup	190	9	<1
Häagen-Dazs Low Fat Chocolate Ice Cream	1/2 cup	170	2.5	<1
Häagen-Dazs Low Fat Vanilla Ice Cream	1/2 cup	170	2.5	0
Häagen-Dazs Orchard Peach Sorbet	1/2 cup	140	0	<1
Häagen-Dazs Raspberry Sorbet	1/2 cup	120	0	<1
Healthy Choice Cappuccino Chocolate Chunk Ice Cream	1/2 cup	120	2	1
Healthy Choice Vanilla	1/2 cup	100	2	1
Starbuck's Java Chip Ice Cream	1/2 cup	250	13	0
Starbuck's Low Fat Latte Ice Cream	1/2 cup	170	3	0
Gelatins				
Jello Regular (all flavors)	1/2 cup	80	0	0
Jello Sugar Free (all flavors)	1/2 cup	10	0	0

BRAND NAME	SERVING SIZE	CALORIES	FAT (G)	FIBER (G)
Puddings and Pie Fillings				
Hunt's Chocolate Light Snack Pack	1 container	100	0	0
Hunt's Vanilla Light Snack Pack	1 container	90	0	0
Hunt's Chocolate Snack Pack	1 container	150	6	0
Hunts Vanilla Snack Pack	1 container	160	6	0
Jello Chocolate Snack	1 container	160	5	0
Jello Free Chocolate Snack	1 container	100	0	0
Jello Free Vanilla Snack	1 container	100	0	0
Kozy Shack Chocolate	$1/2$ cup	130	3	1
Kozy Shack Rice Pudding	$1/2$ cup	130	$2^1/_2$	1
Toppings				
Hershey's Chocolate Flavored Syrup	2 Tbsp.	120	0	0
Smuckers Guilt Free Hot Fudge	2 Tbsp.	100	0	1
Salad Dressings and Mayonnaise				
Ken's Fat Free Honey Dijon	2 Tbsp.	40	0	1
Ken's Lite Honey Mustard	2 Tbsp.	70	4	0
Kraft Free Blue Cheese	2 Tbsp.	50	0	1
Kraft Free Caesar Italian	2 Tbsp.	25	0	
Walden Farms Fat Free Balsamic Vinaigrette	2 Tbsp.	15	0	0
Walden Farms Fat Free Blue Cheese	2 Tbsp.	25	0	0
Weight Watchers Caesar	2 Tbsp.	10	0	0
Weight Watchers Honey Dijon	2 Tbsp.	45	0	0
Hellmann's Light Mayonnaise	1 Tbsp.	50	5	0

BRAND NAME	SERVING SIZE	CALORIES	FAT (G)	FIBER (G)
Hellmann's Low Fat Cholesterol Free Mayonnaise	1 Tbsp.	25	1	0
Juices				
Martinelli Sparkling Cider	8 fl. oz.	140	0	0
Minute Maid Apple (from concentrate)	8 fl. oz.	100	0	0
Welch's Purple Grape (from Concentrate)	8 fl. oz.	170	0	0
Campbell's Regular Tomato	8 fl. oz.	50	0	1
Campbell's V-8	8 fl. oz.	50	0	1
Ocean Spray Cranapple	8 fl. oz.	160	0	0
Ocean Spray Lightstyle Cranapple	8 fl. oz.	40	0	0
Applesauce				
Musselman's Sweetened Cinnamon	$1/2$ cup	100	0	2
Musselman's Regular	$1/2$ cup	90	0	2
Musselman's Natural, Unsweetened	$1/2$ cup	50	0	2
Jellies, Preserves, and Spreads				
Musselman's Apple Butter	1 Tbsp.	30	0	<1
Polaner All Fruit Apricot	1 Tbsp.	40	0	0
Polaner Apricot Preserves	1 Tbsp.	60	0	0
Polaner Apricot Reduced Sugar	1 Tbsp.	25	0	0
Welch's Grape Jelly	1 Tbsp.	50	0	0
Peter Pan Smart Choice Creamy Peanut Butter	2 Tbsp.	180	11	2
Peter Pan Smart Choice Crunchy Peanut Butter	2 Tbsp.	200	12	2
Milk Substitutes				
Rice Dream Enriched Original	8 fl. oz.	120	2	0

BRAND NAME	SERVING SIZE	CALORIES	FAT (G)	FIBER (G)
Edensoy Original Extra	8 fl. oz.	130	5	0
Coffee Mate (liquid)	1 Tbsp.	20	1	0
Coffee Mate Fat Free (liquid)	1 Tbsp.	10	0	0
Coffee Mate Fat Free (powdered)	1 tsp	10	0	0
Coffee Mate Regular (powdered)	1 tsp	10	$1/2$	0
Pasta Products				
Dececco Whole Wheat Linguine	2 oz. dry	210	1	2
Mueller's Italian Style Penne Rigate	2 oz. dry	210	1	1
No Yolks Yolk Free Broad Egg Noodles	2 oz. dry	210	$1/2$	3
Pizza				
Celeste Cheese Pizza for One	1 pizza	470	21	4
Celeste Deluxe Pizza for One	1 pizza	540	29	6
Ellio's Cheese	1 slice	160	5	3
Lean Cuisine French Bread Cheese Pizza	1 pizza	350	8	4
Lean Cuisine French Bread Deluxe Pizza	1 pizza	330	6	5
Tombstone $1/2$ Less Fat Vegetable Pizza for One	1 pizza	360	10	5
Tombstone Light Vegetable Pizza	$1/2$ pizza	240	7	3
Pasta Sauce				
Classico Di Napoli	$1/2$ cup	50	1	2
Classico Sun Dried Tomato	$1/2$ cup	80	4	2
Contadina Fat Free Chunky Tomato	$1/2$ cup	45	0	2
Contadina Light Alfredo	$1/2$ cup	190	13	0
Healthy Choice Traditional	$1/2$ cup	4	$1/2$	3

BRAND NAME	SERVING SIZE	CALORIES	FAT (G)	FIBER (G)
Newman's Own Mushroom	1/2 cup	70	2	3
Prego Meat Flavored	1/2 cup	140	6	3
Prego Mushroom	1/2 cup	150	5	3
Prego Tomato and Basil	1/2 cup	110	3	3
Prego Traditional	1/2 cup	140	4	2
Progresso Red Clam	1/2 cup	80	3	1
Progresso White Clam	1/2 cup	120	9	0
Ragu Garden Style Garden Combo	1/2 cup	110	4	3
Ragu Garden Style Super Mushroom	1/2 cup	120	4	3
Ragu Light Chunky Mushroom	1/2 cup	50	0	2
Ragu Old World Style Traditional	1/2 cup	80	3	3
Weight Watchers Mushroom	1/2 cup	60	0	4

Snacks

BRAND NAME	SERVING SIZE	CALORIES	FAT (G)	FIBER (G)
Burns and Ricker Cinnamon Crisps	5 pieces	130	4	1
Burns and Ricker Garlic Crisps	5 pieces	130	4	1
Burns and Ricker Fat Free Bagel Crisp	5 pieces	100	0	1
Betty Crocker Sweet Rewards Fat Free Double Fudge Bar	1 bar	100	0	1
General Mills Fat Free Blueberry Snack Bars	1 bar	110	0	3
Health Valley Fat Free Blueberry Apple Bar	1 bar	140	0	3
Kellogg's Apple Cinnamon Nutri Grain Bars	1 bar	140	3	1
Kellogg's Blueberry Nutri Grain Bars	1 bar	140	3	1
Kudos Granola Chocolate Chip Bar	1 bar	120	5	1
Power Bar, Apple Cinnamon	1 bar	230	2 1/2	3

BRAND NAME	SERVING SIZE	CALORIES	FAT (G)	FIBER (G)
Power Bar, Banana	1 bar	230	2	3
Quaker Chocolate Chip Bar	1 bar	120	4	1
Quaker Low Fat Chocolate Chunk Bar	1 bar	110	2	1
Barbara's Blue Organic Corn Chips	15 chips	140	7	1
Dorito Nacho Cheese Chips	15 chips	140	7	1
Guiltless Gourmet Corn Chips	20 chips	110	1	2
Lays Original Baked Potato Chips	12 chips	110	$1^1/_2$	2
Louise's Fat Free Potato Chips	30 chips	110	0	2
Ruffles Reduced Fat Regular Potato Chips	16 chips	140	7	1
Smart Temptations Tortilla Chips	1 oz.	110	0	1
Tostito Original Baked Chips	9 chips	110	1	2
Utz Baked Potato Chips	12 chips	110	$1^1/_2$	2
Jolly Time Natural Light Microwave Popcorn	5 cups popped	120	5	7
Newman's Own Butter Flavor Microwave Popcorn	3/5 cups popped	170	11	3
Orville Redenbacher's Movie Theater Butter Microwave Popcorn	5 cups popped	180	13	4
Orville Redenbacher's Smart-Pop Movie Theater Microwave Popcorn	5 cups popped	90	2	5
Snyder's Fat Free Nibbler Pretzels	16 pretzels	120	0	<1
Snyder's Old Fashioned Sourdough Hard Salted Pretzels	1 pretzel	100	0	<1

BRAND NAME	SERVING SIZE	CALORIES	FAT (G)	FIBER (G)
Soups, Canned, or Condensed (prepared)				
Campbell's Beef Consomme	1 cup	25	0	0
Campbell's Chicken Noodle	1 cup	70	2	1
Campbell's Cream of Asparagus	1 cup	90	4	1
Campbell's Green Pea	1 cup	180	3	5
Campbell's Minestrone	1 cup	100	2	4
Campbell's Healthy Request Cream of Celery	1 cup	70	2	1
Healthy Choice Cream of Mushroom	1 cup	60	$1/2$	3
Progresso 99% Fat Free White Cheddar Potato	1 cup	140	$2^1/2$	2
Soups, Ready to Eat				
Campbell's Chunky Chicken Corn Chowder	1 cup	250	15	3
Campbell's Chunky Split Pea Ham	1 cup	240	4	4
Campbell's Healthy Request Hearty Minestrone	1 cup	120	2	3
Campbell's Home Cookin' Bean'N Ham	1 cup	180	$1^1/2$	9
Health Valley Fat Free 14 Garden Vegetable Soup	1 cup	80	0	4
Health Valley Fat Free 5 Bean Vegetable Soup	1 cup	140	0	13
Healthy Choice Bean and Ham Soup	1 cup	170	$1^1/2$	7
Healthy Choice Lentil Soup	1 cup	140	1	5
Progresso Hearty Black Bean Soup	1 cup	170	$1^1/2$	10
Progresso Lentil Soup	1 cup	140	2	7
Progresso Minestrone Soup	1 cup	120	2	5

BRAND NAME	SERVING SIZE	CALORIES	FAT (G)	FIBER (G)
Dry Mixes (prepared)				
Nile Spice Black Bean	1 pkg	170	$1^1/_2$	11
Nile Spice Lentil Curry Couscous	1 pkg	200	$1^1/_2$	4
Meat Substitutes				
Boca Burgers Chef Max's Favorite	1 burger	110	2	4
Green Giant Original Harvest Burger	1 burger	140	4	5
Morning Star Farms Garden Vegetable Patty	1 patty	100	$2^1/_2$	4
Wholesome and Hearty Foods Original Garden Burger	$2^1/_2$ oz.	140	$2^1/_2$	5
Teas				
Arizona Lemon Tea	8 fl. oz.	100	0	0
Lipton Diet Lemon Tea	8 fl. oz.	0	0	0
Lipton Sweetened Lemon Tea	8 fl. oz	90	0	0
Yogurt				
Yoplait Strawberry Custard Style	6 oz.	190	4	0
Yoplait Vanilla Custard Style	6 oz.	190	4	0
Breyer's Lowfat Strawberry	8 oz.	250	$2^1/_2$	0
Colombo Lowfat Vanilla	8 oz.	180	4	0
Colombo Lowfat Plain	8 oz.	130	4	0
Dannon Lowfat Vanilla	8 oz.	210	3	0
Dannon Lowfat Strawberry Fruit on the Bottom	8 oz.	240	3	1
La Yogurt Lowfat Strawberry	6 oz.	170	2	0
Colombo Strawberry Nonfat	8 oz.	200	0	0
Dannon Plain Nonfat	1 cup	120	0	0

BRAND NAME	SERVING SIZE	CALORIES	FAT (G)	FIBER (G)
Dannon Light Nonfat Strawberry	8 oz.	100	0	0
Yoplait Light Nonfat Strawberry	6 oz.	90	0	0
Yoplait Nonfat Strawberry	6 oz.	160	0	0

Blank Food Records
for You to Use

Here is the world's greatest tool for diagnosing your eating problems: the food record. Make at least 21 photocopies of the blank food records provided here. Chapter 10 describes how to fill it out; the main point is LEAVE OUT NOTHING. Every M&M, every packet of sugar or cream, and each glass of wine gets scribbled in.

To help you guesstimate your food group serving sizes, use the chart below; while not an exhaustive list, it gives you the idea. Then compare your daily tally for each food group with the Food Guide Pyramid in Chapter 4. You'll quickly see where you're overdoing it and which foods you may not be getting enough of.

Food Group	A Serving Size Is
Complex carbs	1 slice bread; $1/2$ cup cooked rice, pasta, or other grain; 1 oz. cold cereal; 1 medium baked potato
Vegetables	1 cup raw or 1 cup cooked (exclude potatoes and avocados)
Fruit	1 medium fruit, 1 cup chopped fruit, $3/4$ cup fruit juice

Food Group	A Serving Size Is
Dairy	1 cup milk or yogurt, 1 ounce cheese (See table in Chapter 4 for guidelines on reduced-fat versions of these foods. They're lumped under the Milk, Yogurt, Cheese group in the Food Guide Pyramid.)
High Protein	2 to 3 oz. lean meat, poultry, or fish. Vegetarian equivalent to an ounce of meat is $1/2$ cup beans (also knock off a complex carb serving), $1/3$ cup tofu, 2 Tbsp. peanut butter (also takes care of a fat serving). (Listed under Meat, Poultry, Fish, Dry Beans, Eggs and Nut group in the Food Guide Pyramid.)
Fat	1 tsp. oil, margarine, or butter, 1 Tbsp. mayo or salad dressing, a slice of bacon, 2 Tbsp. cream cheese or sour cream (Pyramid doesn't specify, but try to stay under 6 servings daily.)
Alcohol	12 oz. beer, 6 oz. wine, or 1 shot hard liquor (Again, no rules, but for weight loss, try to limit to 4 drinks a week.)
High Fat and/ or High Sugar	1 medium cookie, $1/2$ cup ice cream, small chocolate bar, a very thin slice of pie or cake, a handful of nuts, or $3/4$ oz. chips. (Try to limit to 3 servings per week.)

Food record for _____

Date _____

How Much of What Food	Food Group Guesstimate	Where/Time of Day	Hungry? (Not, a Little, Very)	Mood (Before/ After)

Day's tally

Dairy: _____	Carbs: _____	Fruit: _____	Alcohol: _____
Protein: _____	Fat: _____	Vegetables: _____	High Sugar/
			High Fat: _____

Food record for _____

Date _____

How Much of What Food	Food Group Guesstimate	Where/Time of Day	Hungry? (Not, a Little, Very)	Mood (Before/ After)

Day's tally

Dairy: _____   Carbs: _____   Fruit: _____   Alcohol: _____

Protein: _____   Fat: _____   Vegetables: _____   High Sugar/ High Fat: _____

Food record for _____

Date _____

How Much of What Food	Food Group Guesstimate	Where/Time of Day	Hungry? (Not, a Little, Very)	Mood (Before/ After)

Day's tally

Dairy: _____   Carbs: _____   Fruit: _____   Alcohol: _____

Protein: _____   Fat: _____   Vegetables: _____   High Sugar/ High Fat: _____

Food record for _____

Date _____

How Much of What Food	Food Group Guesstimate	Where/Time of Day	Hungry? (Not, a Little, Very)	Mood (Before/ After)

Day's tally

Dairy: _____ Carbs: _____ Fruit: _____ Alcohol: _____

Protein: _____ Fat: _____ Vegetables: _____ High Sugar/ High Fat: _____

Food record for _____

Date _____

How Much of What Food	Food Group Guesstimate	Where/Time of Day	Hungry? (Not, a Little, Very)	Mood (Before/ After)

Day's tally

Dairy: _____

Protein: _____

Carbs: _____

Fat: _____

Fruit: _____

Vegetables: _____

Alcohol: _____

High Sugar/ High Fat: _____

Food record for _____

Date _____

How Much of What Food	Food Group Guesstimate	Where/Time of Day	Hungry? (Not, a Little, Very)	Mood (Before/ After)

Day's tally

Dairy: _____ Carbs: _____ Fruit: _____ Alcohol: _____

Protein: _____ Fat: _____ Vegetables: _____ High Sugar/ High Fat: _____

Food record for _____

Date _____

How Much of What Food	Food Group Guesstimate	Where/Time of Day	Hungry? (Not, a Little, Very)	Mood (Before/ After)

Day's tally

Dairy: _____   Carbs: _____   Fruit: _____   Alcohol: _____

Protein: _____   Fat: _____   Vegetables: _____   High Sugar/ _____

High Fat: _____

Symbols

% daily value
    food labels, 94
    of supplements, 110

A

accepting weight, 17
addictions to food, 57
aerobic exercise, 416–432
    machines, 430–432
Afraid to Eat, 262
alcohol
    and calories, 65–66, 86
    obesity and, 81–82
Alzheimer's disease and exercise, 395
amphetamines, 203
ANAD (anorexia or bulimia sufferers), 58
anorexia nervosa, 27, 351–354
anticonvulsants, 117
antioxidants, 110
appetite suppressants
    drugs, 140–141, 208
    exercise, 320
apple-shaped bodies, 13–14
Asian diet, 180–181
Atkins' diet, 25
attitudes, 239–272
    about weight loss, 36–38
    during weight loss, 21
    toward obesity, 64
    young girls', 245
awareness of eating (grazing), 251–255

B

basal metabolic rate, *see* BMR
bee pollen, 115
beta-carotene, 103, 111
Beverly Hills Diet, The, 192–193
binge-eating disorders, 40–41, 57, 345–348
bingeing, 252, 344–345
birth control pills
    osteoporosis and, 352
    vitamin C and, 117
blood analysis, 234
BMI (body mass index), 5–9

BMR (basal metabolic rate), 67.
    See also metabolism
body appreciation, 246–248, 328
body fat
    measurement, 9–12
    models, 246
    normal, 246
body mass index, *see* BMI
body type
    alcohol burning and, 81
    diets based on, 190
bone strength, increasing, 20
botanical diets, 190–191
brain cells, and low-fat diets, 25
breakfast, 149, 250, 262
    menus, 464–466
breast cancer, and exercise, 387–388
breast-feeding and metabolism, 75
breathing problems, 18–19
bulimia nervosa, 27, 344, 348–351
burning calories, 66–68, 174

C

Cabbage Soup Diet, 189
caffeine and exercise, 380–381
calcium, 9
calories, 64–69, 299–303. *See also* low-calorie diets
    alcohol and, 65–66, 86
    brand name foods, 483–498
    burning, 66–68, 174
    carbohydrates and, 65–66, 85
    fast food, 473–481
    fat and, 65–66, 85
        food labels, 93
    food pyramid, 99–100
    restricting, 67
cancer and weight loss, 16
Carbohydrate Addicts LifeSpan Program, The, 185
carbohydrates, 86–88, 185
    and calories, 65–66, 85
    controlling, 287–288
    energy and, 87
    exercise and, 395–401
    fiber, 88
    food labels, 94

Index

cardiovascular disease, 10. *See also* coronary heart disease; heart disease
carotenoids, 103
cellulite, 228
cellulose-bile products, 219–220
changing lifestyle, 33
childhood obesity, 10
cholesterol
  exercise and, 387
  food labels, 95
  prescription medicine and vitamins, 118
Choose to Lose Weight Loss/Healthy Eating Program, 151–152
colon cancer, 27, 388
comfort food, 240
commercial weight loss chains, 52, 55, 134–155, 454
  appetite suppressant drugs, 140–141
  characteristics of, 136–137
  medically supervised, very low-calorie diets, 155–157
  prepackaged food, 140
complete proteins, 89
complex carbohydrates, 86
compulsive eating, 158. *See also* Overeaters Anonymous
control over eating, 39–40
cooking, 301-307
coronary heart disease, 15, 27, 385
counseling, 55, 129
cravings, 255–258
  bingeing and, 345
  maintenance and, 329

D

deaths and liquid protein diets, 27
dehydration, 289
depression
  and binge eating, 57
  bulimia and, 351
  eating disorders and, 396
  exercise and, 393
deprivation, 22–23, 328
detoxification, 175–176, 194
diabetes
  apple-shaped bodies, 13

exercise and, 388–389
obesity and, 27
weight loss and, 15–16
dieting and exercise, 379–380
diets
  all fruit, 27
  anorexia/bulimia, 27, 371
  Asian, 180–181
  Beverly Hills Diet, The, 192
  blood type as basis, 190
  body type as basis, 190
  botanical, 190–191
  bulimia, 27
  Cabbage Soup, 189
  deprivation, 22–23
  doctor-endorsed, 172
  fads, 25–28
  harmfulness, 20–22
  healthy, 176–179
  herbal, 190–191
  liquid meal replacement, 21, 181–183
  low-fat and obesity, 78–79
  Mayo Clinic Diet, 192
  myths, 22–25
  restrictive, 24
  risks, 25–28
  Rotation Diet, The, 193–194
  single foods, 189
  Weight Watchers, 21
  yo-yo cycle, 24
dinner menus, 467–471
diuretics, 118
doctors, background checks, 228
drugs (weight loss), 201–213. *See also* appetite suppressants, drugs
  amphetamines, 203
  appetite suppressant, 208
  eating disorders, 358–359
  fen/phen, 207
  hypertension and, 206
  illegal, 75
  leptin, 211–212
  Melanocortins, 212–213
  neuropeptide Y blocker, 212
  obesity, 202
  Orlistat (XENICAL), 209–211
  over-the-counter, 208–209
  precautions, 206–207
  risks, 203
Duke Diet and Fitness Center, 159–160

E

eating
  binge eating, 40–41, 57
  controlling, 39–40
  emotional eating, 41–42,
    50–51
  purging, 40–41
Eating Attitudes Test, 341–343
eating disorders, 339–374
  anorexia nervosa, 351–354
  binge-eating, 345–348
  bulimia nervosa, 348–351
  causes, 340– 343, 366–374
  depression and, 369
  exercise and, 379
  support, 454–456
  treatments, 354–366
eating habits goal, 50
emotional eating, 41–42, 50–51,
    240, 252, 258–260
energy levels, 19, 87
evaluating diets, 173–176
exercise, 79–80, 377–407
  aerobic exercise, 416–432
  Alzheimer's and, 395
  blood pressure and, 386
  breast cancer and, 388
  calorie burning, 67–68
  cautions, 135
  children and, 20
  cholesterol and, 387
  classes, 424–430
  colon cancer and, 388
  coronary heart disease and,
    385
  depression and, 393
  diabetes and, 388–389
  dieting and, 379–380
  eating disorders and, 379
  fat-burning, 402
  heart disease and, 385
  household chores, 75
  internal benefits, 385–393
  maintaining weight loss and,
    318–320
  mood and, 320, 393–395
  motivation, 413–416
  osteoarthritis and, 390
  osteoporosis and, 391–392
  Physical Activity Pyramid,
    414–415
  prostate cancer and, 388
  safety, 436–437
  self-esteem and, 394
  smoking and, 384
  stroke and, 385
  target heart rate, 418–419
  types, 409–444
  vitamin increases, 400–401
  workout partner, 416

F

fad diets, 25–28
failures as learning experiences,
    244, 328
fast food, 295–299
  fat/calorie counts, 473–481
  obesity and, 22
fasting, 194
fat, 89–92
  calories and, 65–66, 85
  food labels, 94
  food pyramid, 99
  monounsaturated, 90
  omega-3, 90–91
  omega-6, 91
  saturated, 91
fat genes. See genetics
fat-burning exercises, 402
fatty acids, brain cells and, 25
fen/phen, 207, 217-218
fiber, 86, 88, 221
  increasing intake, 287
  low-carbohydrate diets, 27
  pills, 218–219
  water and, 219
food
  addiction, 57
  as comfort, 240
  availability, 250
  habits, changing, 240–272
food diary, see food record
Food Guide Pyramid, 96–105
food labels, 92–96
food record, 275–280,
    499-507
fruits, 27
  as laxative, 193
  food pyramid, 98
  increasing intake, 284–286
  phytochemicals, 118–119

G

gaining weight, 63–83
gastric surgery, 56, 163
genetics, 69–74
gluttony , 24–25

goals, 36–38, 46–52
    changing eating habits, 50
    exercise, 49
    healthy-eating, 50
    realistic weight, 51–52
grains, increasing intake,
    286–287
grazing, 249–255
Green Mountain at Fox Chase,
    161–162

H

habits and goals, 50
hair analysis, 233
health benefits, 12–15, 19–20,
    385–393
health care costs for obese
    persons, 11
healthy diets, 176–181
healthy weight, 3, 12–20
heart disease. *See also* cardiovas-
    cular disease; coronary
    heart disease
    apple-shaped bodies, 13
    exercise and, 385
    *Program for Reversing Heart
        Disease, The*, 152–155
    vitamin B6 and, 117
    weight loss and, 15
height/weight charts, 5–6
herbs, 115, 220, 222
    herbal diets, 190–191
    herbal fen/phen, 217–218
high blood pressure
    exercise and, 386
    medication stoppage, 34
high potency vitamins, 110
high-fat foods, 295–299
high-protein/low-carbohydrate
    diets, 25
hip-to-waist ratio, 14
hospital-based programs, 55
hospitalization for anorexia, 365
household chores as exercise, 75
hypertension
    apple-shaped bodies, 13
    diet drugs, 206
    vitamin B6 and, 117

I–J–K

instructors (exercise), 438
insulin, 74, 183
insurance and eating disorder
    treatment, 358

internal health benefits of exer-
    cise, 385–393
iron, 111

Jenny Craig, 143–145
joint pain and weight loss, 17

keeping weight off, 4–5
ketones, 26

L

L.A. Weight Loss Centers,
    145–147
laxatives
    fruit as, 193
    vitamin absorption and,
        118
lean body mass, 68–69
LEARN Program, 148–149
liposuction, 168–169
liquid meal replacement diets,
    21, 55, 181–183
liquid protein diets and death,
    27
Living Without Dieting, 240
low resting metabolic rate, 72
low-calorie diets, 21
    exercise and, 27
    medically supervised, very
        low-calorie diets, 155–157
low-carbohydrate/high-protein
    diets, 185–188
low-fat diets
    brain cells and, 25
    cooking, 301–307
    foods, 274–275
    metabolism and, 75
    obesity and, 78–79
    snacks, 292
low-fat/high-carbohydrate diets,
    176–179
low-protein diets and heart
    problems, 27
lunch menus, 466–467

M

Ma Huang, 217
macrobiotic diet, 188–189
magnesium and diuretics, 118
Mayo Clinic Diet, 192
measurements
    body fat, 10-12
    bone density (body fat test),
        11–12

subcutaneous fat, caliper
measurement of, 10
waist-to-hip, 14
medically supervised, low-calorie
programs, 155–157
Medifast, 156
Mediterranean eating, 104–105,
179–180
mental health goal, 50–51
menus, 463–472
metabolism, 72, 75-76, 80–82, 383
Modern Methods diet, 187
monounsaturated fat, 90
mood and exercise, 320,
393–395
motivation, 325, 413–416
multivitamins, 113–118
muscle mass, 68–69
low-calorie diets, 27
myths regarding weight loss,
22–25

N

natural sources of vitamins, 114
niacin, 111
non-weight goals, 49–51
nurturing yourself, 25, 241–248
NutraSweet, 310–311
Nutri/System, 145–147
nutrition, 85–105
carbohydrates, 87
counseling, 45, 55
and exercise, 395–401
labels, 92–96, 95
nutritionists, 130–131

O

obesity
alcohol and, 81–82
breast cancer and, 27
breathing problems and,
18–19
colon cancer and, 27
compared to overweight, 5–7
coronary heart disease and,
15, 27
diabetes and, 27
drug treatment, 202
genes and, 69–74
insulin and, 74
ilow-fat diets and, 78–79
physiological factors in,
69–74
television and, 78

omega-3 fats, 90–91
omega-6 fats, 91
Optifast, 56, 156
Ornish, Dean, MD, 130, 178
osteoarthritis
exercise and, 390
weight loss and, 17–18
osteoporosis, 9
anorexia and, 354
birth control pills and,
352
exercise and, 391–392
Overcoming Binge Eating, 361
Overeaters Anonymous (OA),
55, 58, 158–159
overweight, 53, 63–83
analyzing reasons for, 47–48
causes, 196
compared to obesity, 5–7

P

pear-shaped bodies, 13–14
percent body fat, 9–12
Physical Activity Pyramid,
414–415
potassium and diuretics, 118
presecription medicines and
supplements, 117–118
*Program for Reversing Heart
Disease, The*, 152–155
prostate cancer and exercise,
388
protein, 88–89
calories and, 65–66, 85
exercise and, 395–401
food labels, 94
psychological support, 56–57
psychological trauma, 19
eating disorders, 339–374
purging, 40–41
Beverly Hills Diet and, 193
pyruvate, 222–223

Q–R

qualifications of nutritionists,
130–131

recipe makeovers, 305–307
recording food, 275–280
restaurant eating, 264–267
rewards for weight loss,
248–249
risks of dieting, 25–28
Rotation Diet, The, 193–194

S

saturated fat, 91, 94
scams, 226–228
sedentary lifestyles, 79–80
self-esteem, 248
    exercise and, 394
    weight loss and, 242
self-help groups, 55
self-nurturing, 241–248, 327
serving size (food labels), 93
set point of weight, 75–76
Shape Up America!, 7
single food diets, 189
sleep apnea, 18–19
sleep deprivation and weight, 264
Slim Fast, 181–183
slimming teas, 220
smoking
    exercise and, 384
    metabolism and, 80–82
    vitamin C and, 116–117
snacks, 252–253, 292, 471–472
social eating, 264–267
sodium, 114, 274
Solution, The, 150–151, 243
spiritual aspects of weight loss,
    172
splurges, 250
starch in vitamins, 114
storing calories, 65–66
stress
    and binge eating, 57
    bingeing and, 345
    maintenance and, 333–337
stretching, 436
stroke and exercise, 385
Strong Women Stay Slim, 385
Strong Women Stay Young, 385
sugar, 89, 114, 296
    food labels, 94
    substitutes, 307, 310–315
suicide and anorexia, 354
supplements, 107–125, 234. See
    also vitamins
    diet evaluation and, 174
    dosage level, 109
    minerals, chelated, 115
    multivitamin gimmicks,
        113–115
    natural sources, 114
    prescription medicine use
        and, 117–118
    smokers and C, 116–117
    weight loss claims, 213–226

support system, 268–271
    groups, 57–60, 157–159
    maintenance and, 331
    TOPS, 269
surgical options, 163–169
sweets, 293–295

T–U–V

target heart rate, 418–419
teas, 220
television and obesity, 78
therapists, interviewing, 45
thiamin, 111
Thin for Life, 240
TOPS, 55, 58, 158, 269
total fat (food labels), 94
trans fats, 91–92
treatment of eating disorders,
    354–366

UCP (uncoupling protein),
    213
uric acid (gout), 17

vegetable protein, 297
vegetables
    food pyramid, 98
    increasing intake, 282–284
vegetarians
    food pyramid, 101–104
    vitamin B12 and, 117
vitamins 111, 117–118, 235. See
    also supplements

W–X–Y–Z

waist-to-hip ratio, 14
walking, 402, 420–421
weight loss
    counselors, 45
    deciding to lose, 243
    exercise and, 400–401
    keeping it off, 4–5
    psychology of, 239–272
Weight Watchers, 21, 55,
    141–142
woman's multivitamins,
    113

yeast in vitamins, 114
yo-yo dieting myth, 24

zinc, 112, 118
Zone Diet, The, 183–185

The *Unofficial Guide*™ Reader Questionnaire

If you would like to express your opinion about dieting safely or this guide, please complete this questionnaire and mail it to:

The *Unofficial Guide*™ Reader Questionnaire
Macmillan Lifestyle Group
1633 Broadway, floor 7
New York, NY 10019-6785

Gender: ___ M   ___ F

Age: ___ Under 30   ___ 31–40   ___ 41–50
___ Over 50

Education: ___ High school   ___ College
___ Graduate/Professional

What is your occupation?

_____

How did you hear about this guide?
___ Friend or relative
___ Newspaper, magazine, or Internet
___ Radio or TV
___ Recommended at bookstore
___ Recommended by librarian
___ Picked it up on my own
___ Familiar with the *Unofficial Guide*™ travel series

Did you go to the bookstore specifically for a book on dieting safely?   Yes ___   No ___

Have you used any other *Unofficial Guides*™?
Yes ___   No ___

If Yes, which ones?

_____
_____
_____

What other book(s) on dieting safely have you purchased?

_____
_____
_____

Was this book:
___ more helpful than other(s)
___ less helpful than other(s)

Do you think this book was worth its price?
Yes ___ No ___

Did this book cover all topics related to dieting safely adequately? Yes ___ No ___

Please explain your answer:

_____
_____
_____

Were there any specific sections in this book that were of particular help to you? Yes ___ No ___

Please explain your answer:

_____
_____
_____

On a scale of 1 to 10, with 10 being the best rating, how would you rate this guide? ___

What other titles would you like to see published in the _Unofficial Guide_™ series?

_____
_____

Are _Unofficial Guides_™ readily available in your area? Yes ___ No ___

Other comments:

_____
_____
_____
_____

Get the inside scoop...with the *Unofficial Guides*™!

The Unofficial Guide to Alternative Medicine
ISBN: 0-02-862526-9   Price: $15.95

The Unofficial Guide to Buying a Home
ISBN: 0-02-862461-0   Price: $15.95

The Unofficial Guide to Buying or Leasing a Car
ISBN: 0-02-862524-2   Price: $15.95

The Unofficial Guide to Childcare
ISBN: 0-02-862457-2   Price: $15.95

The Unofficial Guide to Cosmetic Surgery
ISBN: 0-02-862522-6   Price: $15.95

The Unofficial Guide to Divorce
ISBN: 0-02-862455-6   Price: $15.95

The Unofficial Guide to Eldercare
ISBN: 0-02-862456-4   Price: $15.95

The Unofficial Guide to Hiring Contractors
ISBN: 0-02-862460-2   Price: $15.95

The Unofficial Guide to Investing
ISBN: 0-02-862458-0   Price: $15.95

The Unofficial Guide to Planning Your Wedding
ISBN: 0-02-862459-9   Price: $15.95

All books in the *Unofficial Guide*™ series are available at your local bookseller, or by calling 1-800-428-5331.

About the Author

Janis Jibrin can tell you everything you need to know about dieting safely. Janis is a registered dietitian with a Master of Science in Nutrition; she received her training counseling children and teens at Georgetown University Hospital. She counsels both adults and children on losing weight and a range of health and nutrition issues. Janis has written over 100 articles for publications such as *Parenting, Modern Maturity, Family Circle, Mademoiselle,* and *Prevention.* She co-authored *Dr. Health'nstein's Body Fun* (StarPress, 1994) a nutrition education CD-ROM for children which was developed by the Cancer Research Foundation of America. It won *Macworld's* "Ten Best CDs of the Year" award for 1995.